CONTENTS

Hazard analysis critical control point evaluations

PREFACE

Foodborne diseases cause considerable morbidity and mortality throughout the world, even though the principles for controlling most of these diseases are well established. Traditional approaches may therefore be considered to have failed to deal with the problem.

A relatively new approach to the prevention and control of foodborne diseases is the hazard analysis critical control point (HACCP) system. This system seeks to identify the hazards associated with any stage of food production, processing, or preparation, assess the related risks, and determine the operations where control procedures will be effective. Thus, control procedures are directed at specific operations that are crucial in ensuring the safety of foods.

This publication is intended for use by public health personnel who have been trained in food microbiology and technology and who are concerned with food safety and the prevention of foodborne disease. Drawing on principles used by a number of food-processing companies, it provides guidance on the assessment of risks that occur during the processing, preparation and storage of foods in homes, schools, food service establishments, cottage industries, and street markets. Emphasis is placed on assessing hazards and risks and identifying critical control points, rather than on control criteria and monitoring. This has been done because many of the places where HACCP evaluations will be made (e.g., homes, cottage industries and street stalls) do not readily lend themselves to sophisticated monitoring. Follow up of the hazard analyses should therefore focus on educating the people who prepare and store the foods.

This guide will assist in the planning of food safety and health education activities that focus on the hazards and technologies associated with the types of food commonly eaten and on foods that are processed and prepared by local inhabitants. Use of this approach should result in the best possible health protection at the lowest cost.

Many of the ideas presented here have been developed as a result of discussions with colleagues from the International Commission on Microbiological Specifications for Foods (ICMSF). The procedures for collecting clinical specimens and water samples have been taken from publications by the International Association of Milk, Food and Environmental Sanitarians (IAMFES).[a] The author is grateful to ICMSF and IAMFES for stimulation in this endeavour.

---

[a] Bryan, F.L. et al. *Procedures to investigate foodborne illness*, 4th ed. Ames, IA, International Association of Milk, Food and Environmental Sanitarians, 1987.

Thanks are also expressed to the following people, who reviewed early drafts of this guide:

Professor M. Abdussalam, formerly World Health Organization, Geneva; Dr R.H. Charles, Senior Medical Officer, Food and Hygiene, Department of Health, London, England; Dr L. Cox, Quality Assurance Department, Nestec, Vevey, Switzerland; Dr S. Michanie, Food Protection, Pan American Zoonoses Center, Buenos Aires, Argentina; Dr B.A. Munce, Microbiologist/Food Technologist, Qantas Airways Ltd, Qantas Jet Base, Mascot, New South Wales, Australia; Dr F. Quevedo, Head, Food Protection, Pan American Health Organization, Washington, DC, USA; Dr P. Teufel, Institute of Veterinary Medicine, Berlin, Germany; Dr M. van Schothorst, Head, Quality Assurance Department, Nestec, Vevey, Switzerland; Dr J.I. Waddington, WHO Regional Office for Europe, Copenhagen, Denmark.

Particular thanks are due to Dr T.A. Roberts, Head, Microbiology Department, AFRC Institute of Food Research, Reading, England, for detailed technical review.

INTRODUCTION

From the earliest religious edicts concerning food, innumerable ordinances, codes of practice, and laws concerning processing, handling and sale of foods have been promulgated by local, national and international bodies with the intention of protecting the public from adulterated food, fraud and foodborne illness. Several approaches have been used to implement these laws and to reduce the risks of foodborne diseases. These approaches can be classified into six categories (Bryan, 1986):

- surveillance of foodborne diseases;
- surveillance of foods;
- surveillance and training of people who handle foods;
- surveillance of facilities and equipment used for production or preparation of food;
- surveillance of food operations;
- education of the public.

Each of these approaches has its merits and its limitations. The degree of usefulness varies with time, place, and type of food operation (production, processing, preparation, storage, distribution, etc.).

Surveillance of foodborne diseases is essential to any rational control programme. Preventive and control measures must be based on the problems commonly found in the community, region or country. Surveillance data can indicate the prevalent foodborne diseases, common causative agents, places where mishandling occurs, and factors that contribute to outbreaks. In many developing countries, there are no such surveillance activities, and the information available may be scanty and unreliable. In that case, reliance must be put on data collected elsewhere for similar foods.

Surveillance of foods employs organoleptic evaluations, measurements of physical properties, chemical analyses, and microbiological testing. Microbiological testing, as a means of assessing whether a product is hazardous, is a relatively recent innovation (ICMSF, 1986a). It has been successfully used to evaluate the quality of drinking-water, but there are few examples of its successful application to food control. The primary limitations of this approach are:

(a) the difficulty of collecting and examining enough samples to obtain meaningful information;
(b) the time required to obtain results (usually several days); and
(c) the high cost.

A number of approaches have been used by health and food regulatory agencies to detect infected food workers and to prevent them from contaminating food. These have been based on medical history, physical examination, blood analysis, X-rays, and examination of faeces for parasites, shigellae, *Salmonella typhi* and other salmonellae. There are significant limitations to each of these examinations (WHO, 1989). People diagnosed as free from infection on the day of an examination may be in the incubatory phase of a disease, or may have mild, abortive, or atypical illness. Furthermore, infections may be acquired and terminated between examinations, which can never be scheduled at a frequency sufficient to prevent the spread of pathogens. Except for epidemiological purposes, such tests are unacceptably costly. Many microorganisms that are transmitted by foods are seldom, if ever, sought during routine examination of specimens from food handlers. Other conditions (e.g., tuberculosis and venereal diseases) that may be sought during examinations are not, in fact, transmitted by food.

An alternative to clinical examination of food handlers or the testing of specimens from them is training in safe food-handling practices. Understanding of such practices would give a far greater assurance of food safety than clinical examination. Managers of food-handling establishments have the primary responsibility for preventing conditions that can lead to outbreaks of foodborne disease stemming from their establishments. They have daily supervisory control of operations, whereas public health personnel may inspect each establishment only infrequently, and spend a relatively short period of time at each visit. Because of their policy-setting and supervisory responsibilities, managers can effect improvements in their establishments. They must, therefore, be aware of the kinds of operations that can lead to outbreaks of foodborne disease and insist that appropriate preventive measures be taken and monitored routinely. Food handlers must also be aware of hazards associated with faulty food-handling practices. They should understand the principles of food safety and the importance of specific food-handling practices associated with their job. Food hygiene professionals and specialists in food safety need to understand the epidemiology of foodborne diseases and the microbial ecology of foods and food-processing operations, so that measures to prevent diseases and spoilage can be devised or selected and given appropriate emphasis.

History has taught us that certain facilities — potable running water, adequate plumbing systems, toilet and hand-washing facilities, and functioning sewage disposal systems — are essential for preventing contamination and promoting personal hygiene in food-handling establishments. In many such establishments in developing countries, there is a need to improve the physical facilities; however, it is even more important to ensure the safety of food processing, preparation and storage operations, many of which can lead to proliferation of microorganisms, e.g., if food is prepared several hours before serving, or kept at room temperature.

Inspections for food safety should focus on the processes that the foods undergo, with particular attention to (*a*) possible sources of contamination to which foods are exposed, (*b*) modes of contamination, (*c*) effects of the process on the level of contamination, (*d*) probability of microorganisms surviving processing, and (*e*) chances that bacteria or moulds will multiply during processing or storage. Hence, food safety rests on controlling food operations from receipt of ingredients until the processed or prepared foods are distributed, sold, or eaten. Surveillance should emphasize operations rather than physical facilities.

Education of the public is essential to food safety. Teachers and students who are preparing to teach must be given information about food safety which they can introduce into their lessons at school. For immediate impact, however, adults must also be informed of hazardous practices associated with preparation and storage of the common foods in the area and appropriate measures to counter the hazards.

This guide describes a system for ensuring food safety — the hazard analysis critical control point (HACCP) system — which combines several of these approaches (in particular, surveillance of diseases, foods, and operations, and education) into an action-oriented programme to identify and reduce the foodborne disease problem. It concentrates mainly on the hazard analysis portion, since monitoring is often impracticable in the places for which this guide is intended (homes, street markets, etc.).

3

THE HACCP SYSTEM

The hazard analysis critical control point (HACCP) concept is a systematic approach to the identification, assessment and control of hazards. The system offers a rational approach to the control of microbiological hazards in foods, avoids the many weaknesses inherent in the inspectional approach and circumvents the shortcomings of reliance on microbiological testing. By focusing attention on the factors that directly affect the microbiological safety of a food, it eliminates wasteful use of resources on extraneous considerations, while ensuring that the desired levels of safety and quality are met and maintained.

Components of the system and definitions of terms

The HACCP system (Fig. 1) comprises the following sequential steps:

1. *Identification of hazards and assesssment of the severity of these hazards and their risks (hazard analysis), associated with growth, harvesting, processing, manufacture, distribution, marketing, preparation and/or use of a raw material or food product.*

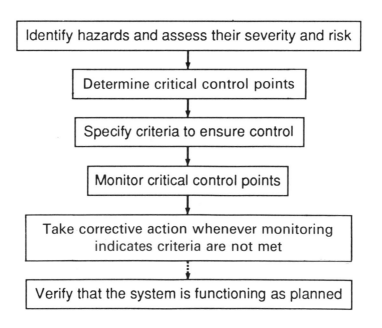

Fig. 1. Components of the HACCP system.

- **Hazard** means the unacceptable contamination, growth or survival in food of microorganisms that may affect food safety or lead to spoilage, and/or the unacceptable production or persistence in foods of products of microbial metabolism, e.g., toxins and enzymes.
- **Severity** is the magnitude of the hazard, or the seriousness of the possible consequences.
- **Risk** is an estimate of the probability of a hazard occurring.

Hazard analysis consists of an evaluation of all procedures concerned with the production, distribution and use of raw materials and food products to: (1) identify potentially hazardous raw materials and foods that may contain poisonous substances, pathogens, or large numbers of food spoilage microorganisms, and/or that can support microbial growth; (2) identify the potential sources and specific points of contamination; (3) determine the probability that microorganisms will survive or multiply during production, processing, distribution, storage and preparation for consumption; and (4) assess the risks and severity of the hazards identified.

2. *Determination of critical control points (CCPs) at which the identified hazards can be controlled.*

- **A CCP** is an operation (practice, procedure, location or process) at which control can be exercised over one or more factors to eliminate, prevent or minimize a hazard.

In some food processes, control of a single operation (CCP) can completely eliminate one or more microbial hazards, e.g., in pasteurization. It is also possible to identify control points at which a hazard can be minimized but not completely eliminated. Both types of CCP are important and must be controlled.

3. *Specification of criteria that indicate whether an operation is under control at a particular critical control point.*

- **Criteria** are limits of characteristics of a physical (e.g., time or temperature), chemical (e.g., concentration of salt or acetic acid), biological or sensorial nature.

It is important to select appropriate means to check that the hazard has been controlled at the CCP. Factors to be monitored may include: time and temperature for thermally processed foods; water activity (a_w) of certain foods; pH of fermented foods; chlorine level in can cooling water; humidity in storage areas for dry products; temperature during distribution of chilled foods; depth of product in trays to be chilled; instructions on labels of finished products describing recommended procedures for preparation and use by the consumer. All criteria selected should be documented or specified clearly and unambiguously, with tolerances where appropriate. Choice of control criteria will depend on usefulness, cost, and feasibility but they must provide high assurance of control.

5

4. *Establishment and implementation of procedures to monitor each critical control point to check that it is under control.*

   ● **Monitoring** involves the systematic observation, measurement and/or recording of the significant factors for control of the hazard. The monitoring procedures chosen must enable action to be taken to rectify an out-of-control situation, either before or during an operation.

   The monitoring must detect any deviation from the specification (loss of control) in time for corrective action to be taken before the product is sold or distributed. Five main types of monitoring are employed: observation, sensory evaluation, measurement of physical properties, chemical testing and microbiological examination.

5. *Implementation of appropriate corrective action when monitoring indicates that criteria specified for safety and quality at a particular critical control point are not met.*

6. *Verification, i.e. the use of supplementary information and tests to ensure that the HACCP system is functioning as planned.*

   Verification may be done by either quality control staff or health or regulatory agency personnel. It includes a review of the HACCP plan to determine whether all hazards have been detected, all critical control points identified, criteria are appropriate, and monitoring procedures are effective in evaluating operations. Records are reviewed and supplementary tests done to evaluate the effectiveness of the monitoring.

APPLICATION OF THE HACCP APPROACH

The HACCP approach can be applied to food safety in homes as well as in food processing and food service establishments (WHO/ICMSF, 1982). A Joint FAO/WHO Expert Committee on Food Safety recommended that studies using the HACCP approach be carried out in homes in developing countries, so that more information about the causes of food-associated hazards and preventive measures could be obtained (FAO/WHO, 1984). Such information could be used to focus health education and food safety programme activities on the factors of greatest importance in causing foodborne illness.

Unlike most traditional food-inspection activities, the HACCP approach is based on an understanding of the factors that contribute to outbreaks of foodborne disease and on applied research on the ecology, multiplication, and inactivation of foodborne pathogens. Even where data are not available, a hazard analysis can detect potential problems and identify the critical control points of an operation. Thus, food safety agencies can target their resources on the greatest public health risks in an establishment, rather than on general sanitation and superficial improvements. Although the initial hazard analysis will take longer than an inspection, valuable information about the food process will be obtained. Follow-up inspections to verify that the operators are monitoring the critical control points take less time. The benefits derived from greater assurance of food safety should offset the time spent on the initial hazard analysis and verification. Additional benefits will ensue from inspections of potentially hazardous operations to determine whether they are being monitored effectively, rather than from random inspections, when only a few high-risk operations may be in progress.

Experience has shown that the HACCP system provides a greater assurance of food safety than other approaches, such as traditional quality control by testing the end product. Furthermore, monitoring of critical control points is less costly and more effective than analysis of samples and inspection of processing plants.

In attempting to identify potential hazards, it is necessary to consider three areas:

- the raw materials used,
- processing procedures,
- the manner in which the product is used.

Food processing operations

In any particular processing plant, the hazards will depend upon:

- the source of ingredients,
- the formulation,
- the processing equipment,
- the duration of the process and storage, and
- the experience and/or attitudes of the personnel.

Hazard analyses should be carried out on all existing products and processing lines, and on any new products that a processor intends to manufacture. Changes in the source of raw materials, product formulation, processing procedures, packaging, distribution, or use of a product indicate the need for re-evaluation, because any of these changes might adversely affect safety or shelf-life.

The HACCP approach can be applied to foods processed in cottage industries as well as to those processed in complex, technically advanced manufacturing plants. In the former, it may be necessary to use simple monitoring procedures, but they must be sufficiently accurate and reproducible to provide unambiguous and quantifiable results.

Food service operations

A wide variety of foods are prepared in food service establishments. The main food service systems can be classified as cook/serve, cook/hold hot, cook/chill, cook/freeze or assemble/serve. The HACCP system is applicable to food prepared by any of these systems. Critical control points are similar in any one system, but more than one system may be in operation in an establishment.

Raw foods of animal origin, freshly caught fish, shellfish, raw products of vegetable origin, cereals, fruits, dairy products, ices, juices and iced drinks are sold on streets and in markets in many countries. Some of these foods are cooked on the street, or are processed, prepared and cooked in cottage industries, food service establishments or homes long before they are sold or eaten. Risks will vary depending on:

- the food source;
- the methods used to freshen, preserve, process and prepare the foods;
- the duration and conditions of holding and display; and
- the interval between heating and consumption.

The HACCP approach can be used to identify hazards and evaluate risks associated with the preparation and holding of foods sold on the street (Bryan et al., 1988). Preventive measures can then be applied at the most hazardous stages of preparation, storage or display and wherever control is feasible.

Homes

One might expect considerable variation in food preparation practices in individual homes, but the types of food, fuel and energy sources, cooking facilities, economic resources and cultural influences often result in considerable uniformity within subgroups of a society. Therefore, the HACCP approach can be used to obtain information about hazards associated with preparation and storage of foods in homes, to assess risks, and to identify critical control points. The data generated from such analyses can be used in health education courses and campaigns, and in school curricula to disseminate information on foods and practices that entail a high risk.

Other

The HACCP approach can also be applied to the production and harvesting of crops, raising of livestock and poultry, fishing, harvesting of shellfish and the transportation, storage and marketing of foods (ICMSF, 1988).

Data accumulated during hazard analyses and experience in monitoring critical control points can be used to train professional staff and food workers and to educate the public. Training and educational programmes must become an integral part of food safety activities and should be given high priority.

WHERE TO CONDUCT A HACCP EVALUATION

It is not practicable to try to conduct a hazard analysis in every home and every commercial food establishment. Priorities must be established depending on the incidence of disease, recognized food-associated problems, the qualifications of quality control personnel in industry and of food safety officers in regulatory agencies, and the targets and goals of the food safety agency. The selection of places to perform the analyses should be based on a classification of the population or establishments (e.g. by region, ethnic and/or socioeconomic group, presence of infants or young children in the family, type of food service establishment, class of food). Whenever possible, epidemiological data should be used in making the selection.

The selection of places to be studied can be based on four factors (Bryan, 1982): food property, food operation, volume of food prepared (measured as average daily patronage), and susceptibility of consumer.

The "food property" factor primarily concerns the epidemiological history of foods prepared and served in an establishment and is determined from local, national or international data. It takes into account the characteristics of the food (e.g. pH, water activity) and gauges its potential for supporting rapid growth of infectious or toxigenic microorganisms.

The "food operations" factor assesses the procedures that the foods usually undergo that expose them to contamination, that might fail to destroy contaminants, or during which the contamination increases, e.g., improper holding of foods. It takes into account the cultural patterns of food preparation, equipment and facilities available, and the food service system used.

The "volume of food prepared" or average daily patronage is another risk factor. Often, when the same dish is served to many people, a large amount of the food is prepared hours, or even days, in advance to ensure quick service. If, during the interval between preparation and serving, these foods are not held under conditions that prevent bacterial growth, a hazard is created. The risks increase with the time of holding.

The susceptibility of the consumer is another risk factor. People who are more susceptible to disease than the general population (e.g. hospital patients, infants or the elderly) are examples of high-risk populations.

If hazard analyses are to be performed in homes, to gather information and focus attention for education of the public, they should be conducted in the regions with the highest incidence of diarrhoeal disease. Families with children being treated for diarrhoea should be studied first. In areas with high infant mortality, households with children of weaning age should also be selected for analysis. Matched control families, with no recent history of diarrhoea, may also be investigated. Alternatively, households may be selected where there has been a recent episode of typhoid fever, non-typhi salmonellosis, hepatitis A, cholera, or other foodborne disease. If outbreaks of foodborne disease or reported cases of illness are attributed to food processed in homes or cottage industries, hazard analyses should also be performed in those places if feasible.

In selecting commercial establishments in which to conduct HACCP analyses, priority should be given to: those associated with outbreaks of foodborne disease; those that prepare foods known to be common vehicles of etiological agents of foodborne disease; and places where hazardous foods are prepared in advance of serving, where they are likely to be stored in a way that allows microbial growth, and where reheating may not be sufficient to inactivate the pathogens or toxins. Where diarrhoea is common among visitors to the area, programmes should include places frequented by tourists.

Where there is no national or local surveillance of foodborne disease, epidemiological or research data from other countries where the same foods are prepared in a similar way may indicate probable vehicles of foodborne pathogens or toxins. For example, Chinese-style boiled and fried rice dishes prepared in restaurants in Australia, Europe, Japan, and the United States of America have been reported to be vehicles of *Bacillus cereus*; such dishes prepared in restaurants and homes in other countries may thus be expected to pose similar risks. Processed food that has been identified as a health hazard, e.g. one that has been frequently rejected by importing countries or that is highly likely by its nature to cause disease, is also a logical candidate for a HACCP investigation.

ANALYSING HAZARDS AND ASSESSING THEIR SEVERITY AND RISKS

A hazard may be an unacceptable level of foodborne disease-causing agents or of products of microbial metabolism. An "unacceptable" level may be only one cell of salmonella or shigella or 100 000 or more *Bacilllus cereus* or *Clostridium perfringens* per ml or gram. A hazard can also mean contamination of food by organisms that cause spoilage, so that spoilage occurs within the expected shelf-life of the product. Hazards also relate to survival of undesirable microorganisms or persistence of toxins after heating, and to multiplication of microorganisms when food is held: (*a*) at room temperature or warm outside temperature for several hours; (*b*) warm — but not hot — in ovens or other hot-holding devices; (*c*) in cold storage facilities, in large quantities or at an insufficiently low temperature. Hazards may also be caused by chemical substances that reach food inadvertently through various agricultural practices, or during food processing, preparation or storage. Hazards may also result from chemicals that are added to foods in excess of functional or culinary needs; that leach into highly acidic foods from containers, pipes or their toxic coatings; or that reach foods accidentally.

The first step in the HACCP system is hazard analysis. Technical expertise is required to assess hazards and their severity, and to predict risks. Incorrect predictions will not provide the security desired and will increase costs.

Review of epidemiological data

Data on factors that are known to have contributed to outbreaks of foodborne disease, or practices or situations that have led to outbreaks can help to identify potential hazards. Contributory factors have been found to be remarkably similar in Australia (Davey, 1985), Canada (Todd, 1983), the United Kingdom (Roberts, 1982), and the United States of America (Bryan, 1978, 1988), and can be classified according to whether the outbreak was the result of contamination, microbial survival, or microbial growth. Listed below are the most common contributory factors in outbreaks of foodborne disease in the above-mentioned countries.

Factors related to contamination

- Raw foods (e.g., raw meat and poultry) are often contaminated at source with salmonellae, *Campylobacter jejuni*, *Clostridium perfringens*, *Yersinia enterocolitica*, *Listeria monocytogenes*, or

Staphylococcus aureus. In some regions, raw fish are often contaminated with *Vibrio parahaemolyticus* and non-01 *Vibrio cholerae.* Rice and other grains often harbour *Bacillus cereus*, and herbs and spices may be contaminated with *C. perfringens.*

- Infected persons (e.g. nasal carriers of *S. aureus*, persons in the incubation period of hepatitis A, persons infected with Norwalk agent, or carriers of *Shigella*) touched foods that were not subsequently adequately heat processed.
- Contaminants were spread by workers' hands, cleaning cloths, or equipment, from raw foods of animal origin to cooked foods or to foods that were not subjected to further heating (cross-contamination).
- Equipment (e.g. slicers, grinders, cutting boards, knives, storage vats, containers, pipelines) was not properly cleaned.
- Foods were obtained from unsafe sources (e.g. shellfish, raw milk, raw-egg products, home-canned low-acid foods, mushrooms).
- High-acid foods were stored in containers, or conveyed through pipelines, that contained toxic metals, such as antimony, copper, cadmium, lead, or zinc, causing leaching or migration of the toxic substance into the food.
- Contaminated food or ingredients were eaten raw or not sufficiently heat processed.
- Substances were added to foods in excess of culinary needs (e.g., monosodium glutamate) or processing needs (e.g., sodium nitrite).
- Poisonous substances, such as pesticides, reached foods as a result of carelessness, accidents, improper storage, or because they had been mistaken for food ingredients.
- Food became contaminated during storage, e.g. through exposure to leaking or overflowing sewage, or to sewage backflow.
- Contaminants penetrated cans or packages through seam defects or breaks.
- Food was contaminated by sewage during growth or production.

Factors related to survival of microorganisms

- Food was cooked or heat-processed for an insufficient time or at an inadequate temperature.
- Previously cooked food was reheated for an insufficient time or at an inadequate temperature.
- Food was inadequately acidified.

Factors related to microbial growth

- Cooked food was left at room temperature.
- Food was improperly cooled (e.g., stored in large pots or other large containers in a refrigerator).

- Hot food was stored at a temperature that permitted multiplication of bacteria.
- Food was prepared half a day or more before serving (and then stored improperly).
- Fermentation (and thus acid formation) was inadequate or slow.
- Inadequate concentrations of curing salts were added or curing time was too short.
- Low- and intermediate-moisture foods had elevated water activity (a_w), or there was condensation on these foods.
- The environment selectively permitted certain pathogens to multiply either by providing favourable conditions, e.g. vacuum packaging, or by inhibiting competitive microorganisms.

During hazard analysis of an operation, each phase should be evaluated to determine whether any of the above situations have occurred, are occurring, or are likely to occur.

Reviewing operations

Preparation for analysis

Visit several establishments of the type in which hazard analyses are planned. Observe the situation and talk to the people in charge, such as the manager of a food establishment, shopkeeper, street vendor, or homemaker to obtain information about the type of foods usually prepared, the ways in which they are prepared, and when they are prepared. Explain the purpose of the study and its expected duration. Try to determine the degree of cooperation that can be expected and whether any special equipment will be needed. Choose the place where the analyses will be performed, make arrangements for the visit, and coordinate date and time of arrival. Emphasize that you are performing a scientific investigation, not an inspection, and that the data will not be used to condemn or embarrass anyone. Tell the people involved that their tolerance and cooperation will greatly assist the Ministry of Health (or other agencies involved in the study) to understand patterns of food preparation and processing within the country or cultural group, and that the results of the study will be used as a basis for a health education campaign. Ask them to prepare or process foods in their usual way, telling them that you will be watching, taking certain measurements, and possibly collecting samples.

Interviewing responsible persons

Ask the managers and the people who prepare foods about each step of the operation. Take as complete a history of the processing or preparation of the foods under investigation as possible. This history should include the sources of foods and ingredients, the people who handled the items, the procedures and equipment used, all potential sources of contamination during handling, and the time and temperature conditions to which the foods were exposed. Talk to the people responsible for each operation. Obtain recipes or product formulae or composition, if possible. Note the sequence of operations, from arrival of the ingredients until their distribution, sale, or consumption; note all temperature settings and the duration of each step. At processing establishments, for example, the investigation may cover the conditions under which animals are held prior to slaughter, the slaughter itself, dehairing, defeathering, washing, eviscerating, heat-processing, cooling, freezing, drying, fermentation, acidification, smoking, packaging and storage. At food service operations and in homes, the investigations will probably study receipt of food, storage, preparation, cooking, handling after cooking, hot-holding, cooling, reheating, and serving of foods. Study also the operations in establishments where the ingredients were previously stored or processed, and the storage methods and preparation practices used after the products left those establishments. For more information see Bryan et al. (1987).

Observing operations

During a hazard analysis, specific evaluations of products and operations are necessary. Concerns about products include formulation, processing, and conditions of intended distribution and use. Answers to the following questions should be obtained:

Regarding formulation or recipe

1. What raw materials or ingredients are used?
2. Are microorganisms of concern likely to be present on or in these materials, and if so what are they?
3. Do any of the ingredients have toxic properties or contain toxic substances?
4. If preservatives are used, are they at concentrations able to prevent the growth of microbes of concern?
5. Are any of the ingredients used in quantities too high or too low for culinary needs?
6. Will the pH of the product prevent microbial growth or inactivate particular pathogens?
7. Will the a_w of the product prevent microbial growth?

Regarding food processing and preparation

1. Can a contaminant reach the product during preparation, processing, or storage?
2. Will microorganisms or toxic substances of concern be inactivated during cooking, reheating, or other processes?
3. Could any microorganism or toxin of concern contaminate the food after it has been heated?

15

4. Could any microorganism of concern multiply during preparation or storage?
5. How does the package or container affect survival and/or growth of microorganisms?
6. What is the time taken for each step of processing, preparation, storage and display?

Regarding the expected use of prepared foods

1. Is the food expected to be held hot, chilled, frozen or at ambient temperature after it leaves the plant or store?
2. Will the time–temperature exposure during reheating inactivate microorganisms and toxins of concern?
3. If the food is held after reheating, will it be held hot or at ambient temperature?
4. Will the food be handled or otherwise exposed to potential contamination?

Answers to these questions may indicate possible hazards and provide information on severity and risks. It may sometimes be necessary to inoculate a product with particular foodborne pathogens and to subject it to the conditions that exist during distribution, storage, use and handling, to determine whether those conditions permit multiplication of the microorganisms. The protocol and interpretation of the test results should be supervised by a food microbiologist. If appropriate, samples of foods should be collected and tested for microorganisms such as *S. aureus*, *Escherichia coli*, or salmonellae, to confirm observations or to detect problems that may have occurred during periods when observations were not made. Testing of samples can never take the place of observation, but results can provide supportive data and perhaps confirm hypotheses. Small numbers of microbes may not be detected, however, and the reliability of counts is limited if only a few samples are tested.

Evaluate the effectiveness of cleaning of utensils and equipment by:

● observing the cleaning procedures;
● measuring the temperature and/or concentration of detergent and disinfectant solutions, and the contact time;
● examining the appearance of equipment after cleaning; and, under some circumstances,
● swabbing or taking contact samples from surfaces.

Measuring temperature of food

Measure the temperature of foods with thermocouples or thermometers, to evaluate whether they will support microbial growth (see pp. 31–34). Use bayonet-type thermocouples long enough to reach the point in the

16

internal regions of the food (often the geometric centre) at which temperature is to be measured. If practicable, insert most of the shaft of the probe into the product being examined.

If a bayonet-type thermometer is used, insert the tip of the thermometer beyond the geometric centre. Raise or lower the thermometer to locate the highest temperature of a food being cooled, or the lowest temperature of a food being heated.

To measure the temperature on the surface of a product press or attach a thermocouple with a button end on the surface, insert an open-ended thermocouple just under the surface, or point a reflecting potentiometer at the surface. Plug the thermocouple leads into a potentiometer and take readings at appropriate time intervals or record the data automatically. Measure time with a watch, or a chart moving at a known speed.

Measure the temperature of foods during or after certain operations (e.g., during or on completion of cooking or reheating, and during the period immediately following, when the temperature continues to rise). For food cooked in a retort or pressure cooker, evaluate the functioning of the retort, the pressure and time of processing, the venting procedure, the adequacy of the container seals, and whether the cooling is done hygienically.

Measure the temperatures and holding time of foods being held hot or cold, to determine whether they could permit multiplication of bacteria; if so, evaluate whether bacteria are likely to multiply rapidly or slowly. Note the rate at which foods cool during storage at room temperature and in refrigerators or other cooling devices. Estimate probable cooling rates and the potential for microbial growth from the dimensions of the containers and the depth of the food in them. See whether lids are used (they impede cooling but may prevent further contamination and transfer of moisture and odour), whether containers are stacked on top of or against each other (which impedes cooling), and the location of containers in refrigerators (which may affect cooling and likelihood of cross-contamination). (For further information, see Bryan, 1981; Bryan & Bartleson, 1985.)

If you suspect that any step in the processing or preparation of the food may have permitted survival or growth of microorganisms, collect samples of foods at appropriate stages and test for total numbers of aerobic mesophiles or for pathogens of concern (see pp. 19–23). Use caution in interpreting the results of the laboratory analysis as the counts follow a probability distribution and individual measurements may be distributed over a considerable range.

Clean and disinfect thermocouples and thermometers between each use. Heat-treat thermocouples by inserting the sensors into a pan of boiling water, or dipping them into 95% ethanol (ethyl alcohol) and immediately flaming them. Repeat the flaming three times. Make sure that the flame is extinguished before the sensor is returned to the ethanol. If the ethanol in the container catches fire, immediately replace the lid on the container to cut off the supply of oxygen. Disinfect thermometers by inserting the bayonet or bulb into boiling water for a few seconds, or into a tube containing a 100 mg/l (100 ppm) solution of sodium hypochlorite for 30 seconds. In certain situations, it may be feasible to keep a pot of water boiling to disinfect thermometers and thermocouples.

Measuring pH of food

Several types of electrode can be used to measure the pH of foods. Some electrodes are encased in bayonet shafts that can be inserted into food. Others commonly used for testing the pH of laboratory media have a flat end that can be placed on the surface of the food being tested. If a conventional laboratory probe made to test the pH of liquids is used, the food to be tested must either be in liquid form, or be ground, or blended with distilled water that has recently been boiled and cooled (pH 7). The electrode is attached to a pH meter which must be calibrated, as recommended by the manufacturer, with at least two standard buffers (usually pH 4.0, 7.0 or 10.0). Compensate for temperature before each series of tests. Clean the electrode and rinse three times with boiled distilled water or buffer of pH 7 between each measurement. A squirt-type water bottle is useful for this purpose.

Measuring water activity of food

To measure the water activity (a_w) of a food, put a sample in a vapour-tight holder; the holder should be large enough for a representative sample, but small enough to permit equilibration of the sample within a reasonable time. Since temperature influences a_w, the holder should be placed in a constant-temperature cabinet, in which the temperature does not fluctuate more than 0.3 °C. A fan within the cabinet will help maintain a uniform temperature. Temperature fluctuations in the sample will be minimized if the holder with attached sensor is kept in a polystyrene box. With some instruments, the holder assembly is kept in a water-bath or is automatically cooled or heated to maintain a constant temperature. (See Troller et al., 1984, for more information.)

Use a standard salt (e.g., $MgCl_2$, NaCl, KCl, KNO_3, K_2SO_4) or sulfuric acid solution to calibrate the hygrometer to specific a_w values, according to the manufacturer's instructions. The equilibrium relative humidity values for certain salts at 30 °C are: $MgCl_2$, 32.44±0.14; NaCl, 75.09±0.11; KCl, 83.62±0.25; KNO_3, 92.31±0.60; K_2SO_4, 97.00±0.40 (Greenspan, 1977). Select standard salts or H_2SO_4 solutions with a_w values close to those of the samples to be tested. Calibrate the instrument frequently to ensure a high degree of accuracy (e.g., whenever the drift exceeds 2–3%). This may require monthly recalibration.

Place the sample in a small plastic dish and put the dish in the holder with the sensor attached. Allow the sample to equilibrate; this may take from 20 minutes to 24 hours, depending on the size of the holder, the equipment used, and the type of sample. The water activity is determined from the digital readout, recorder plot or calibration curve. Whenever possible, test duplicate samples and take the average of the results. Equilibrium is usually considered to be achieved when two consecutive hourly readings differ by less than 0.01 units (for direct readout equipment), or when a plateau is reached (on recording equipment) (Troller et al., 1984).

Collecting food samples

If laboratory facilities are available to support the study, take samples of foods at different stages during, before or after an operation, to determine the impact of all previous operations on contamination and survival and multiplication of microorganisms. Collect samples of food aseptically using sterile or disinfected utensils, and place them in sterile jars or sterile plastic bags.

The sample of food should be large enough for all the analyses to be performed; a sample of approximately 200 g or 200 ml is usually enough. If only one test is to be done, a smaller portion may be sufficient. Check the amounts needed with the laboratory. In situations where it is impractical to collect the amount of food needed (e.g., from homes or street stalls), collect smaller portions and request the laboratory to adapt its procedures accordingly.

Before collecting the samples, record the temperature of the room, refrigerator, or hot-holding unit in which the food is stored. Then either (*a*) measure and record the temperature of the food remaining after the sample has been collected, or (*b*) if plastic bags are used to hold the samples, remove the excess air from the bag, wrap the filled bag around the sensing portion of the thermometer, and hold it in place until the temperature stabilizes.

Label all containers with a code that identifies the establishment, together with a sample number. If the sample is hot, immerse it in running water, or in a bowl of water or container of ice, until it is cold to the touch. Rapidly chill samples of perishable foods that are not frozen at the time of collection to below 4.4 °C, and keep them below this temperature until they can be examined. Do not freeze food samples because certain foodborne bacteria (such as Gram-negative bacteria and vegetative forms of *C. perfringens*) die off rapidly during frozen storage. Pack samples with a refrigerant that will maintain the desired temperature during transit, and transport them to the laboratory in an insulated container as quickly as possible.

Send to the laboratory a copy of a log with code number, date, time of sampling, type of sample, and type of test required, together with the sample. Keep a copy of the log.

The equipment needed for collecting, holding, and transporting samples includes the following (Bryan et al., 1987):

Sterile sample containers: disposable plastic bags (e.g. 'stomacher'-type); wide-mouth jars (capacity 150–1000 ml) with screw caps; bottles for water samples (bottles for chlorinated water should contain enough sodium thiosulfate to provide a concentration of 100 mg per ml of sample); foil or heavy wrapping paper; metal cans with tight-fitting lids.

Sterile and wrapped implements for sample collection: spoons, scoops, tongue-depressor blades, butcher's knife, forceps, tongs, spatula, drill bits, metal tubes (1–2.5 cm in diameter, 30–70 cm in length), pipettes, scissors, swabs, sponges, Moore swabs (compact pads of gauze made from 120 × 15 cm strips, tied in the centre with long, strong twine or wire).

Sterilizing agents: 95% ethanol, propane torch.

Refrigerants: commercial refrigerant in plastic bags; liquid in cans; rubber or heavy-duty plastic bags or bottles that can be filled with water and frozen; heavy-duty plastic bags for ice; canned ice.

General equipment: fine-point felt-tip marking pen; roll of adhesive or masking tape; cotton; electric drill (if frozen foods are to be sampled); matches; 0.1% peptone water or buffered distilled water (5 ml in screw-capped tubes); test-tube rack; insulated chest or polystyrene box; reporting forms.

Clothing (optional): laboratory coat, hat, disposable plastic gloves and boots.

Collecting environmental samples and clinical specimens

Depending on the circumstances and the hazards, it may be useful to collect other types of samples and specimens. Collection of water samples, for instance, while not usually part of a HACCP evaluation, may be needed if the source of the water is subject to pollution, since water is an ingredient in many foods, and is used for washing hands, utensils and food containers, and in certain operations that may be critical control points.

In certain regions, water may be thought to be the main vehicle for enteric pathogens that cause diarrhoeal diseases, while, in reality, food may be a more important vehicle. Testing is required to confirm or refute the various hypotheses. A HACCP evaluation might also be done in conjunction with an environmental survey, to evaluate risks associated with the environment and with food. Instructions for collecting water samples are given in Annex 1.

The collection of specimens from people is not usually part of a hazard analysis. However, when the analysis is part of an investigation of a disease outbreak or a follow-up of people being treated for diarrhoeal disease, it may be appropriate to collect specimens in order to find additional cases, to trace sources of contamination, or to compare cases with matched controls. It may also be useful to collect appropriate specimens if the street vendor or people in the household, cottage industry, or food service establishment being investigated complain of, or are reported to have, symptoms of diarrhoeal disease, or if signs of other gastrointestinal disease are observed. In particular, wherever possible, faecal specimens should be obtained from infants with diarrhoea.

The equipment needed for collecting specimens includes: cartons with lids for stool specimens; bottles containing preservative solution for transport of specimens; protective canisters or cartons; sterile swabs; sterile sponges; rectal swab sets; sterile gauze pads, 10×10 cm; and tubes of transport media. Procedures for collecting specimens are described in Annex 2.

Testing samples for microorganisms

A description of the procedures for testing food samples is beyond the scope of this manual (see ICMSF, 1978; Speck, 1984). The tests to be performed will depend on what information is needed to support the hazard analysis, the type of food concerned, and the types of microorganisms expected in the samples or specimens.

Plate counts for samples of foods obtained immediately after cooking, and again after holding, provide information on the microbial growth occurring during the holding period. Information on microbial inactivation can be obtained from counts on raw materials, on samples taken immediately after cooking, and on samples of the cooked foods after storage, before and after reheating. When only a few samples are taken, considerable variation in counts may occur. Nevertheless, these tests have been found to be useful and can be performed in most laboratories.

E. coli, coliforms, faecal coliforms, and Enterobacteriaceae are useful indicators of contamination of heat-processed foods. *Staphylococcus aureus* can be used as an indicator that cooked food has been handled by human beings, as well as an indicator of time–temperature abuse of food carrying a risk of foodborne disease. Salmonellae have been used as indicators of the inadequacy of heat processing (e.g., in egg pasteurization) or of contamination of heat-processed foods of animal origin.

Epidemiological information may indicate that certain foods should be tested for particular pathogens or indicator organisms (Table 1). For

Table 1. Tests that may be considered for specific foods

Food	Appropriate tests
Acidified food	pH
Beans, pinto, red, black or navy	*C. perfringens, B. cereus*
Canned food (primarily home-canned)	pH
Cereals and food containing cornstarch	*B. cereus*
Cheese	*S. aureus, Brucella* spp, pathogenic *E. coli, L. monocytogenes*
Confectionery products	salmonellae, a_w
Cream-filled baked goods, custards	*S. aureus*, salmonellae, *B. cereus*; pH, a_w
Eggs and egg products	salmonellae, β-haemolytic streptococci
Fish	*V. parahaemolyticus, V. cholerae*
Fruits and vegetables, raw	parasites, *Shigella* spp, pathogenic *E. coli, L. monocytogenes*
Ham	*S. aureus*
Mayonnaise	pH (*S. aureus*, salmonellae if pH > 4.5)
Meat, meat products, and foods containing meat	salmonellae, *C. perfringens, S. aureus, C. jejuni, L. monocytogenes, Y. enterocolitica*, pathogenic *E. coli*
Meat, fermented	*S. aureus*; pH, a_w
Meat, ground or shredded	*C. perfringens, B. cereus, Shigella* spp, salmonellae, *S. aureus*
Milk, dried, and milk formula	salmonellae, *S. aureus, B. cereus*
Milk, raw	salmonellae, *S. aureus, C. jejuni, L. monocytogenes, Y. enterocolitica*, β-haemolytic streptococci
Potatoes and tubers	*B. cereus* (*S. aureus* if cooked items handled)
Poultry, poultry products, and foods containing poultry	salmonellae, *C. perfringens, S. aureus, C. jejuni, L. monocytogenes, Y. enterocolitica*
Rice	*B. cereus*
Salads containing cooked and cut ingredients (e.g., ham, tuna, potato, egg)	*S. aureus*
Salads of mixed vegetables, meat, poultry or fish	*S. aureus, L. monocytogenes*, salmonellae, β-haemolytic streptococci, *Shigella* spp, pathogenic *E. coli*; pH
Shellfish	*V. parahaemolyticus, V. cholerae*, possibly other vibrios
Smoked or dried meat, poultry, fish products	salmonellae, *S. aureus, L. monocytogenes*, a_w
Soft drinks, fruit juices and concentrates held in metallic containers or vending machines	Metals such as copper, zinc, cadmium, lead, antimony, tin; pH
Soups, stews, gumbos, chowders, gravies	*B. cereus, C. perfringens*
Vegetables, cooked	*B. cereus*

example, rice, cereal products, beans, milk and potato products could be tested for *B. cereus*, fish and shellfish for *V. parahaemolyticus*, cooked meat and poultry products, gravies, and beans for *C. perfringens*. If laboratory resources are limited, enrichment procedures may be used with both raw foods (to determine the source of contamination) and recently cooked foods (to determine whether microorganisms have survived cooking), and counts made on cooked foods that have been held for long periods after cooking (to determine whether microorganisms have multiplied).

Close collaboration between field and laboratory personnel is essential. The field investigator should tell the laboratory why the sample was collected and what tests are required. Information on the use of routine microbiological tests for foods and their limitations is given in Annex 3. The significance of specific microorganisms in foods is considered in the above-mentioned texts (ICMSF, 1978; Speck, 1984) and in the report of the Subcommittee on Microbiological Criteria for Foods (1985).

Analysis of specific operations

Homes

When conducting a hazard analysis in a household, ·describe the characteristics of the family and the environment as well as any techniques used that could affect food safety. The information recorded should include the following:

- family name and address or location;
- number of persons living in the household, the number of children and their ages;
- occurrence of diarrhoea in the last month;
- number of rooms or bedrooms (this gives an indication of crowding and may relate to person-to-person spread of disease);
- types of foods usually eaten and those prepared on the day of the visit, including recipe and source of ingredients;
- types of foods fed to infants alone or in combination (e.g., breast milk, raw milk, pasteurized milk, dried milk, canned milk, milk formula, family foods, special foods);
- facilities for preparing, preserving and storing foods, including type of fuel and availability of a refrigerator;
- foods epidemiologically associated with illness, if applicable;
- source of water, method of treatment (if any), and method of storage;
- method of sewage disposal;
- season of year, and date.

A simple form, relevant to the local situation, should be devised to record appropriate aspects of this information. The information should be considered in relation to possible sources and modes of contamination, and the likelihood that pathogens will survive cooking or processing and multiply during storage. The following factors are of particular importance.

- *Ingredients and recipe.* Whenever possible, obtain the recipe for the food being investigated; at least, list the ingredients and relative proportions. Note the use of meat, poultry, fish, eggs, milk, and other foods of animal origin, spices, cereals and foods grown in soil or water. Ascertain whether pathogens are likely to be associated with these foods.
- *Preparation and processing.* Determine each step of the preparation and processing. Consider any operation that has an effect on microorganisms, e.g., heat, acidification, drying, modification of atmosphere. Determine the type of equipment used and the fuel source. Observe actual or potential modes of contamination, including contamination from persons handling the foods and cross-contamination. Measure temperatures and times of each step of the procedure. Collect samples for measurement of pH and a_w, for testing to determine the presence of microorganisms, or for time–temperature simulations or other studies, as applicable.
- *Storage.* Measure the length of time that foods are stored and, if possible, the temperature of the foods during storage. Pay particular attention to any period during which they are within the temperature range that permits rapid microbial growth (21–49 °C, 70–120 °F). Observe the type and size of container in which the foods are stored, whether they are covered, and where they are kept.

Annex 4 gives more detailed information on potential hazards and appropriate control action for a number of specific foods that might be prepared in homes.

Food processing in cottage industries

The hazards associated with food processing operations in cottage industries will vary with the type of food and the process used; however, some general principles can be described.

- Certain ingredients, especially those of animal origin, are likely to contain pathogens; for example, raw meat, poultry, and fish frequently harbour a variety of enteric pathogens; spices, sugar, and starch may contain bacterial spores; water may be contaminated by enteric pathogens or microorganisms that cause spoilage; mycotoxins may form in cereals and nuts. If the process does not inactivate the microorganisms or toxic substances, the ingredients become of considerable concern, particularly for people who are more susceptible than healthy adults, such as infants, the elderly, and those who are sick or malnourished.
- Processes that fail can create hazards. For example, pasteurization,

retorting, and sometimes preheating are intended to kill particular groups of microorganisms, but inadequate heating times or too-low temperatures can permit their survival. Certain chemicals (e.g., salt, nitrites, acids) inhibit microbial growth, but if concentrations are too low or the mixture is not properly blended, the process can fail. During fermentation, the fermenting flora inhibit growth of undesirable microbes, and their metabolic products kill pathogens. If fermentation is delayed, however, microbial growth may occur, with the formation of toxins which will survive subsequent fermentation. Slow or incomplete drying, or defective packaging of dried products, may also permit growth of microorganisms. Improper refrigeration or prolonged storage of perishable foods in refrigerators can result in either spoilage or growth of certain foodborne pathogens.

● Another concern to food processors is the possibility of mishandling of the product by food handlers or preparers of food in homes; when assessing product stability, the potential consequences of such abuse should be borne in mind. Factors to be considered include the extent of the heat process, the pH and water activity of the product, the presence of preservatives that inhibit growth of certain microbes or germination of bacterial spores, and temperature during distribution and storage. Any change in packaging should be evaluated for its effect on the growth of microbes that survive processing. Particular attention should be paid to products that can support the growth of foodborne pathogens. Information should be gathered about the ways in which the product is likely to be handled by the public. The processor may need to build additional safeguards into the process, place a warning on the label, or alert purchasers in other ways.

Annex 5 gives more detailed information on critical control points and monitoring procedures for a number of specific foods that might be processed in cottage industries.

Food service establishments, food stalls, and other retail outlets

In establishments where foods are prepared, displayed, served, or sold, the source of the foods, and the likelihood of their being contaminated on arrival at the establishment or during handling, should be evaluated. Recipes of formulated (composite) foods should be assessed for the types and amounts of ingredients that are likely to contain pathogens, as well as for other substances (e.g., acid, salt, sugar, garlic) that act as stabilizers. Cooking and reheating practices should be evaluated to determine whether they are sufficient to inactivate pathogens and denature any toxins. The conditions after heating should be assessed to determine whether spores that survive heat treatment are likely to germinate, whether the resulting vegetative cells will be able to multiply, and whether microorganisms that reach the food after heating will be able to multiply. For this purpose, some or all of the following actions will be necessary at the various steps of the operation.

- *Receiving*. Assess incoming foods for appearance, quality, temperature, pH, a_w, and type of packaging. Note any damage to packaging and estimate the possible types and quantities of contaminants. Note the source of the food and, if possible, the processing history. It may be appropriate to obtain information on the manufacturer's quality assurance or HACCP programme.
- *Storage*. Appraise methods of storing raw, frozen, chilled and dry foods, to identify any situations that could permit contamination or promote microbial growth.
- *Handling of raw products*. Assess the handling of raw products, reconstitution of dehydrated foods, thawing of frozen foods, and preparation of foods to be served without subsequent heating, to identify operations during which contamination could occur.
- *Formulation*. Review the formulation of foods and, if appropriate, measure pH and a_w.
- *Cooking*. Measure the highest temperature attained at the geometric centre of foods after cooking, or record the time–temperature exposure of foods during cooking, to determine whether pathogens of concern could survive the cooking.
- *Handling of cooked foods*. Appraise the handling of cooked foods to identify potential modes of contamination.
- *Hot holding of cooked foods*. Measure the time for which foods are held hot and their temperature to determine whether pathogens could survive and multiply.
- *Holding of cooked foods at room temperature*. Observe whether cooked foods are kept at room temperature and, if so, measure the temperature and the duration to determine whether pathogenic bacteria could multiply or generate toxins.
- *Cooling*. Measure the depth of food being cooled, or the temperature of food at intervals during cooling, to determine whether pathogenic bacteria could multiply.
- *Reheating*. Measure the highest temperature attained at the geometric centre of foods after reheating, or record the time–temperature exposure of foods during reheating to determine whether pathogens could survive reheating.
- *Cleaning of equipment and utensils*. Determine whether cleaning and disinfection procedures are adequate to remove pathogens from equipment and utensils or to inactivate them.
- *Storage of final product*. Determine the characteristics of prepared food (pH, a_w, and microbiological quality, as applicable) to assess the type of storage needed.
- *Personnel*. Assess the knowledge of personnel regarding the safe handling of foods.

Annex 6 gives more detailed information on potential hazards and appropriate control action for a number of specific food service operations.

Food-flow diagrams

From the information obtained during the interviews and from observations, draw a food-flow diagram. (Use pencil so that changes can be made later, if necessary.) Draw a separate flow chart for every food that was investigated. Represent each operation by a rectangle and use arrows to indicate direction of flow. Notes or symbols can be used to indicate hazards, including: (a) the probable type of contamination, (b) the possibility of survival of microorganisms or toxic substances during heating or other potentially lethal processes, and (c) the possibility of multiplication of pathogenic bacteria or toxigenic moulds. Examples of symbols are given in Table 2. Indicate on the chart critical control points and, if space permits, criteria for control and parameters to be monitored. For each operation, note the temperature and duration of the process, the size of any containers used, the depth of food in the containers, and any other relevant information.

Examples of food-flow diagrams are given in Fig. 2–4. Potential sources of contamination and operations that might allow survival or multiplication of contaminants are illustrated by the symbols given in Table 2. Fig. 2 represents preparation of rice in households in a rice-growing village. Rice may be associated with foodborne illness caused by *B. cereus*, the spores of which are frequently found in raw rice. Cooking does not control the problem because the spores survive. The critical control point is the holding of the cooked rice between preparation and serving; the time of holding should therefore be monitored. Significant

Table 2. Symbols used in food-flow diagrams

Symbol	Interpretation
⚠	Possibility that food or water initially contaminated with foodborne pathogens
△	Possibility of contamination with foodborne pathogens from surfaces or equipment in contact with foods
▽	Possibility of contamination with foodborne pathogens from person who handled food
□	Process step
⌋⌊	Possible process step, but not always carried out
↓	Direction of flow
CCP	Critical control point: monitoring procedure
⊗	Destruction of vegetative bacteria if boiled or cooked to near boiling temperatures, but spores survive
○	Possibility of survival of microorganisms
⊕	Possibility of multiplication of bacteria
⊖	Bacterial growth unlikely
S	Spores

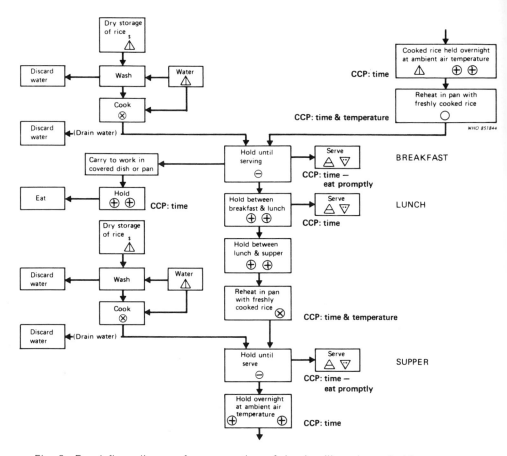

Fig. 2. Food-flow diagram for preparation of rice in village households.

microbial growth can occur in rice that has been held at room or warm-outside temperatures for 4 hours or more. Covering the rice may increase the hazard by trapping moisture.

Fig. 3 represents the preparation of acidified shrimp paste. Acidification is the critical control point. The type and amount of acid ingredients and the pH should be monitored; this is obviously not practical in village households, so monitoring is done by taste to ensure that the product is sufficiently sour. (This method is not completely reliable but may be the only practical option.)

Fig. 4 shows the steps in the preparation of a milk–water–sugar formula for feeding an infant. The critical control points are the boiling of the water used to dilute the concentrated milk, the cleaning and disinfection of the bottle, and the holding of the opened container of milk and the prepared formula. Temperature is "measured" by observing the boiling of the water used in the formula and to disinfect the bottles. The holding

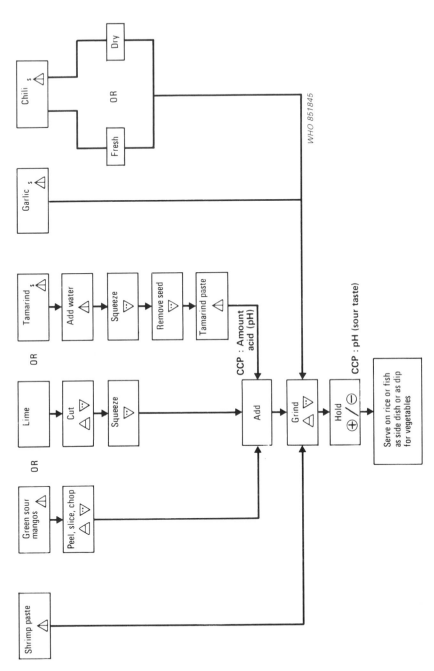

Fig. 3. Food-flow diagram for preparation of nam prik (acidified shrimp paste).

WHO 851845

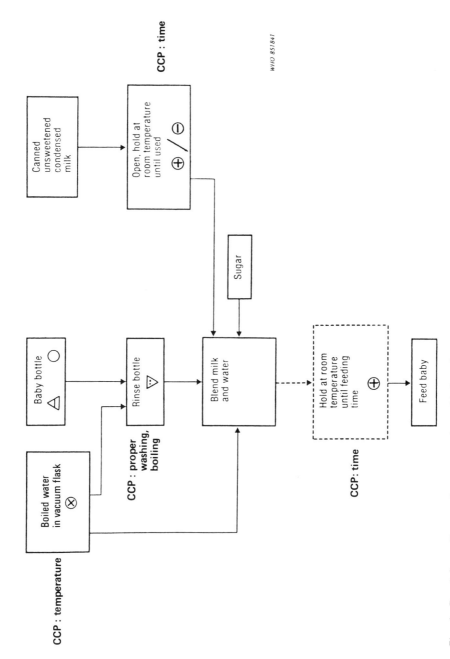

Fig. 4. Food-flow diagram for preparation of infant formula from milk, water and sugar.

of the formula is a critical control point, and the time of holding is monitored.

Analysing measurements

Plot temperature measurements against time on graph paper. Compare the temperatures recorded with the optimum temperatures for growth and multiplication of microorganisms of concern (see Table 3). For example, in interpreting heating curves, note the highest temperature reached and the combined time–temperature exposure, to determine whether the pathogens of concern could have survived the heating process. In interpreting cooling curves, note the time during which the temperature of the food is within a range that permits multiplication of the bacteria of concern (see Table 3).

Compare the temperatures attained during heat processing, cooking, and reheating to certain reference temperatures (e.g., 74 °C), or time–temperature values (e.g., 55 °C (130 °F) for 2 hours, 60 °C (140 °F) for 12 minutes) that are lethal for the microorganisms of concern. Mathematical techniques are available for calculating the probability of survival or destruction of the microorganisms expected to be present in the food being investigated. For examples of the use of these techniques, see Genigeorgis & Riemann, 1979, and Stumbo, 1973.

Compare the temperature, pH and a_w values measured with the ranges within which pathogens multiply or are killed. Where relevant and practicable, compare any conclusions with the results of microbial analyses.

Table 3. Limiting conditions for multiplication of some common foodborne pathogenic bacteria

Organism	Temperature (°C)			pH Minimum	a_w Minimum
	Minimum	Maximum	Optimum		
Bacillus cereus	5	49	30	4.4–4.9	0.91–0.95
Campylobacter jejuni	30	45	42–43	4.9	—
Clostridium botulinum[a]					
Group I, A, B, F	10	48	—	4.6	0.94
Group II, B, E, F	3.3	45	—	5.0	0.97
C. perfringens	15	50	43–45	5.0	0.96–0.97
Escherichia coli	15	—	37–45	5.0	—
Listeria monocytogenes	0	45	—	4.0	—
Salmonella spp	5.2	45.6	43	4.1–4.5	0.94–0.95
Shigella spp	—	—	37	—	—
Staphylococcus aureus	6.7	45	35–37	3.8–4.5	0.83–0.85
Vibrio cholerae	10–15	43	37	5.0	0.97
V. parahaemolyticus	5	43	37	5.0	—
Yersinia enterocolitica	0	—	32–34	6.8	—

[a] Group I = proteolytic; group II = saccharolytic ("non-proteolytic").

31

Examples

Fig. 5 shows the time–temperature curves for various foods prepared in a village household. It can be seen that the temperatures reached by the moist foods were high enough (>74 °C (165 °F)) to kill vegetative pathogenic bacteria. Subsequently, the leftovers were held for approximately 12 hours within a temperature range (21–49 °C) that permits germination of bacterial spores and rapid multiplication of pathogenic bacteria. During reheating, temperatures sufficient to inactivate vegetative forms of bacteria (but not to destroy heat-stable toxins) were attained in all foods except the left-over rice. The left-overs were then kept at ambient temperature until lunchtime and were eaten without reheating. Left-over food from lunch remained at ambient temperature until suppertime. In these conditions, bacterial growth might be expected to occur.

Fig. 6 shows the time–temperature curve for foods during preparation and holding in an urban household. High temperatures were reached during cooking, but the food was then held for several hours at room temperature, during which time spores could germinate and the emerging vegetative forms multiply. Only one food was subsequently reheated. Left-overs remained at room temperature (near the optimum for growth of *B. cereus*, which is likely to be found in rice) for up to 12 hours. (For further information on interpreting time-temperature curves, see Bryan et al., 1981; Bryan & Bartleson, 1985.)

Use graphs and tables such as those shown in discussions with managers and supervisors of operations to emphasize hazards and point out the locations of critical control points. Such material can also be used in training sessions for professional staff or managers of food operations, and in public education programmes.

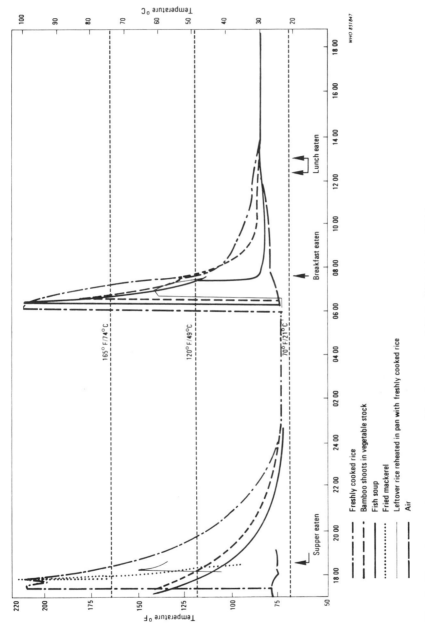

Fig. 5. Time–temperature exposure of foods prepared in a village household.

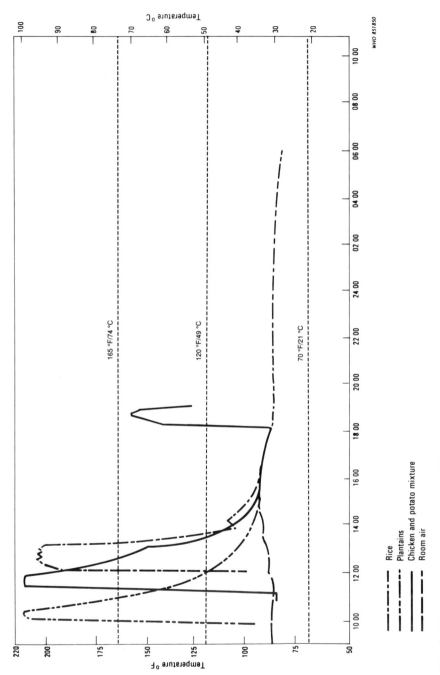

Fig. 6. Time–temperature exposure of foods prepared in an urban household.

IMPLEMENTATION OF A HACCP SYSTEM

Selecting critical control points

A critical control point, as defined on page 5, is a point in an operation
at which control can be exercised to eliminate, prevent or minimize
a hazard. Not every hazard requires a specific control measure:
sometimes a control measure taken at one critical control point reduces
the need for control measures at preceding points in the chain (e.g.,
irradiation of packaged poultry). At other times, a combination of
control measures must be used at successive critical control points. In
other operations (e.g., processing of raw meat and raw poultry), the
hazard of contamination with salmonellae cannot be eliminated except
by irradiation and other critical control points at best only reduce the risk
of contamination. If a hazard cannot be eliminated, or if a critical control
point cannot be monitored, particular attention must be given to other
critical control points, before or after the operation, that can be
effectively controlled and monitored.

Selection of critical control points depends on:

(a) the likely hazards, their estimated severity and risk in relation to what
    constitutes unacceptable contamination of food, or survival or
    growth of microorganisms;
(b) the operations to which the product is subjected during processing
    and preparation; and
(c) subsequent use of the product.

Because incoming foods may contain pathogens, their purchase and
receipt may be considered to be critical control points. One or more steps
in the preparation (e.g., cooking) may eliminate or greatly reduce the
hazard. If this is not the case, the food should be obtained from a safe
source (e.g., shellfish from certified or non-polluted waters) or tested
for contamination (e.g., dried eggs should be tested for salmonellae).

Formulation may also be a critical control point, particularly if the
ingredients affect the pH or a_w of the formulated food, or if they are likely
to contain pathogens. Thorough mixing is essential to ensure uniform
distribution of ingredients that lower pH or a_w.

Certain aspects of processing may be critical control points. For example,
heat processing inactivates many pathogenic microorganisms and others
that cause spoilage. Cooling may be a critical control point for heat-
processed foods and for cold-stored products. Drying in itself does not
kill pathogens, but the low a_w of the finished product may inhibit growth
of microorganisms. Acidification may be a critical control point if the

final pH is sufficiently low. In cured products, the concentration of salt and nitrites and the resulting a_w must be specified and monitored to ensure safety. Specific conditions of temperature and humidity select and promote multiplication of particular microorganisms during fermentation. Control of these conditions and/or the use of starter cultures, or cultures from a previous batch, are essential for the safe production of fermented products. The resulting pH should be monitored, as should the a_w if the products are dried. In other products, such as mayonnaise, the nature and concentration of acid should be controlled and monitored.

The environment is sometimes considered to be a critical control point, particularly when potentially hazardous foods are dried, blended, and packaged. The source and treatment of water used as an ingredient, or for cooling or cleaning, may be critical to the safety of a product. The cleaning of equipment used in the processing of foods, particularly equipment used for heated foods or for ready-to-eat meat products, is a critical control point. The handling of foods can also be considered to be a critical control point; training and education of food-handling personnel are thus essential preventive measures. If foods are to be packaged, the atmosphere in the package and thus the type of packaging material may be critical control points.

In food service operations and in homes, cooking is often a critical control point, although bacterial spores may survive. It should be noted, however, that the beneficial effects of cooking may be nullified by contamination of the cooked food. Critical control points for cooked foods include: handling, hot-holding, cooling, and reheating (see examples in Fig. 2–4).

Critical control points will depend on the food being prepared, the equipment available, and the cultural habits of the preparer. Nevertheless, critical control points for a particular system are usually the same wherever used (see Table 4). Further specific critical control points for various operations are listed in Annexes 4–6.

Specifying criteria

Once the critical control points have been identified, applicable control measures should be implemented. These measures must be practicable and economically feasible, and must ensure food safety. For each point, criteria must be specified that will ensure the safety of the product. Examples of criteria are: end-point temperatures attained after heat processing; time–temperature exposure adequate to inactivate microorganisms of concern; the pH or a_w of the final product; temperatures during cooling or hot-holding; the concentration of chlorine in water used to cool cans. Each criterion must be expressed in a clear and unambiguous statement, with specification of acceptable tolerances.

Table 4. Common critical control points in food service systems

System	Receipt	Formulation	Handling of raw ingredients	Cooking	Hot-holding	Cooling	Handling of cooked products	Reheating
Cook/serve				X				
Prepare/serve cold	X	X[a]						
Cook/hold hot			X	X	X		X	
Cook/chill				X		X	X	X
Cook/freeze				X		X	X	X
Assemble/serve	X						X	X

[a] Sometimes a critical control point.

Monitoring critical control points

Monitoring of critical control points is essential to ensure that the specified criteria are being met. Foods can be monitored in many ways depending on the type of control point and the instruments and equipment available.

Monitoring should aim to detect any deviation from the established criteria. It usually depends on observations, or physical or chemical measurements (e.g., temperature, pH, concentration of salt). Results should be obtainable immediately so that the process can be quickly adjusted if necessary. Microbiological tests are therefore of limited usefulness, since they may not be available for several days. Some of these procedures can be applied in food service establishments and cottage industries; monitoring may also be done in homes but, in that case, simpler approaches are often chosen.

If the receipt of raw materials constitutes a critical control point, the quality of these materials should be monitored, using a statistically sound sampling plan, to determine whether they are within acceptable microbiological limits (ICMSF, 1986b). Spices, sugar, and starches, for example, may need to be tested for numbers of thermophilic spores before use in certain operations (e.g., in low-acid canned foods), since such spores survive retorting and can germinate under conditions of high-temperature storage. However, monitoring of spices and sugars is not necessary when they are to be used in carbonated beverages, because the pH of the product will prevent the germination of any bacterial spores present. The small amounts of spices and sugars used in family meals do not greatly affect the quality or safety of the foods, so monitoring in the home is unnecessary (WHO/ICMSF, 1982). Nuts should be examined for signs of mould or aflatoxin, and fish for honeycomb decomposition; any affected products should be immediately rejected. Dried, frozen, or liquid eggs may need to be monitored for salmonellae before use in formulated foods.

When formulation of acidified products is a critical control point, monitoring may be by measurement of pH. For example, the safety of salads that contain mayonnaise should be monitored by checking that the pH is below 4.6. Such monitoring is feasible in a processing plant, but not in a home. If monitoring of pH is not practicable, or if the pH exceeds 4.6, product safety can be evaluated by monitoring the time that the food is kept before being eaten or, if a refrigerator is available, the temperature of the ingredients before formulation, the temperature of the finished product, and the rate of temperature reduction during cooling.

Heating processes may be monitored in a number of ways. In food processing plants, heat treatment of foods is often monitored with indicating and recording thermometers. Flow-diversion valves may be used to ensure that fluids that are not at a sufficiently high temperature are recycled. In canning operations, temperature, pressure, and duration of heating should be monitored to ensure that the temperature–time exposure is sufficient to inactivate the spores of pathogens of concern. If the cooking process in a food service establishment is designated as a critical control point, the internal temperature of cooked foods should be monitored when they are removed from the cooking device, and after the post-cooking temperature rise. If a microwave heating unit is used, temperatures should be monitored at or near the surface of the food, as well as inside the food, immediately after it has been removed from the unit.

In homes in industrialized countries, the temperature of foods such as turkeys, casseroles or large cuts of meat should be monitored during cooking using bayonet-type meat thermometers. Simple but less precise monitoring procedures include: observation of changes in the texture or colour of foods (e.g. uncured pork turns white on cooking); observation of the flow and colour of juices; cooking at a prescribed oven temperature for a specific time per pound of product. In homes in developing countries, monitoring is often limited to observing whether a mixture that contains fluid boils and whether it is thoroughly mixed during the boiling process. It should be understood, however, that even though a fluid may bubble, the solid food in the mixture may not be thoroughly heated. No additional monitoring is required when foods are eaten promptly after thorough cooking.

If cooked foods are to be held hot for more than one hour, the temperature should be monitored at regular intervals (e.g. every 2 hours) to ensure that it does not fall to within the range in which pathogenic bacteria can multiply, or that it does so only for a short time. In food service establishments, the internal temperature of foods should be monitored; if food is held in a container without a lid or in a unit (e.g., steam table, bain-Marie) where heat comes from the bottom or the sides, then temperatures at or near the surface should be monitored, and observations made of the frequency and efficiency of stirring.

Cooked foods should be monitored to ascertain for how long they are left at room temperature. In homes and street markets, the only practical control measure is to ensure that foods are not held for more than 5 hours (preferably less) after cooking, unless they can be refrigerated, held hot, or reheated.

Handling of foods after cooking can be monitored in a number of ways. Observations can be made to determine whether cross-contamination could occur:

- from raw food to workers' hands to cooked food;
- from raw food to equipment to cooked food processed on or in the same equipment;

- from cloths used to wipe areas where raw and then cooked foods are handled; or
- as a result of dripping from raw foods that are stored above cooked foods.

By observation, one can determine whether cooked foods have been touched or whether improperly cleaned equipment has been used to handle or hold the cooked foods. Monitoring of the handling of cooked foods is not always practical in homes, but an understanding of hazards and personal and food hygiene, and supervision of family members by the homemaker can serve as a safeguard.

For some foods, cooling may be a critical control point, and monitoring of the cooling procedures is essential. This can be done either by measuring the volume (particularly the depth) of the food being cooled or by measuring temperature before cooling and at intervals during cooling. A single measurement of the temperature of a food being cooled provides information for only one moment and is thus of limited value. Additional monitoring may include observing whether lids or covers are used and ensuring that there is an air space above, below, and between items. Measurement of air temperature in the refrigerator is of limited value in measuring the cooling rates of cooked foods. In developing countries where refrigerators are not easily affordable, monitoring is often limited to time of holding at room or outside ambient temperature.

Reheating of cooked foods must be monitored in the same way as the initial cooking. Monitoring of foods at this stage is particularly important because poor storage practices may have allowed the proliferation of large numbers of microorganisms in the cooked food. In homes in developing countries, the only way of monitoring liquid foods may be to ensure that they are thoroughly mixed and that they are reheated at least to boiling point.

An alternative form of monitoring may be to collect and test samples of finished products for microorganisms of concern. This is acceptable only if the product remains with the processor until the results of testing are available. For example, infant formulae, dried milk and dried eggs are often tested for salmonellae, and only distributed if the results of the tests are acceptable. Whenever samples are collected, a statistically sound sampling plan is essential (ICMSF, 1986a). The sampling plan should be based on an assessment of the severity and risk of hazards and on the expected use and storage of the food after sampling. Record-keeping is essential in large processing plants and should be considered in certain other operations, but is not practical in homes.

Taking corrective action

If monitoring indicates that a process is out of control, or that established criteria are not being met, immediate action must be taken. The specific action will depend on the process being monitored and may include reheating or reprocessing, increasing temperature, decreasing a_w, decreasing pH, extending the processing time, adjusting the concentration of certain ingredients, adjusting the processing at a later stage, rejecting incoming lots, diverting the product to use as animal feed, or discarding the product. The decision will be based on the hazards, their severity, and the risks involved and on the expected use of the product.

One of the positive features of the HACCP approach is that unacceptable contamination, process failure, or the existence of conditions that would permit multiplication of undesirable microorganisms can be detected as it occurs or shortly afterwards, so that immediate corrective action can be taken.

VERIFICATION

Food-processing establishments

Upon completion of the initial study, a HACCP system should be drawn up for the establishment, by either health personnel, quality control personnel, or outside consultants. This should then be carefully reviewed by technically qualified supervisors from the establishment and officials of the food safety programme, and if necessary, in consultation with specialists familiar with the processing and preparation of the foods concerned. The plan should include:

- a flow diagram of the various processes;
- a list of significant potential hazards;
- an indication of the critical control points;
- specification of the criteria for control;
- details of the monitoring procedures to be applied at each critical control point; and
- action to be taken when the operation is out of control.

Once the plan has been approved by all concerned, it should be returned to the manager of the establishment. A copy should be kept for review by quality-control and regulatory personnel before follow-up visits are made.

Routine monitoring of the critical control points of a food operation is the responsibility of the manager of the establishment, but food safety programme supervisors will need to verify the appropriateness of control criteria and critical control points, and inspectors will need to verify the extent and effectiveness of the monitoring. Verification may include:

- checking records of time–temperature readings;
- observing operations at critical control points;
- making measurements to confirm the accuracy of the monitoring;
- collecting samples;
- conducting special studies, e.g. inoculated pack or challenge test, with regard to the safety of products; and
- interviewing staff about the way they monitor critical control points.

Furthermore, the composition of food products and operational procedures should be reviewed to determine whether any changes have been made since the HACCP system was established. If so, it may be necessary to select different critical control points or modify the monitoring procedures.

USING HACCP DATA TO IMPROVE FOOD SAFETY

People who conduct HACCP evaluations can make a significant contribution to improved health and welfare and to economic development, by providing leadership to the food industry and the public. They are also ideally placed to guide the development of educational programmes so that the food industry and the public are informed of significant risks associated with food processing and food preparation practices, and of practical and economical ways to prevent or eliminate hazards.

Guiding health strategies

Information obtained during HACCP evaluations should be used for planning and setting priorities for health programmes. Control measures will have to be chosen or devised to deal with the hazards identified. These should be pointed out during routine inspections of food establishments, and should be the basis for regulations adopted to cope with existing or potential problems in food safety. Cumulative data generated during hazard analyses and experience in monitoring critical control points should be used to train staff of the health department.

Health education

Once the major risks associated with the processing and preparation of foods have been identified, and the relevant cultural patterns and social structures understood, educational materials should be developed, and training and educational efforts implemented, to increase awareness of the risks and how they can be avoided. Appropriate measures may include:

- modification of curricula at universities;
- training of public health personnel;
- training of managers and other staff in the food industry;
- health education of the public during home visits by public health workers;
- provision of relevant information to mothers and low-income families when food is distributed;
- discussions with interested community groups, such as mothers' clubs and consumer groups;
- preparation of educational films, leaflets, posters, and announcements for radio and television;
- teaching of food safety in schools.

REFERENCES

BRYAN, F.L. (1978) Factors that contribute to outbreaks of foodborne disease. *Journal of food protection,* **41:** 816–827.

BRYAN, F.L. (1981) Hazard analysis of foodservice operations. *Food technology,* **35**(2): 78–87.

BRYAN, F.L. (1982) Foodborne disease risk assessment of foodservice establishments in a community. *Journal of food protection,* **45:** 93–100.

BRYAN, F.L. (1986) New approaches for the control of foodborne diseases. In: *Proceedings of the Second World Congress on Foodborne Infections and Intoxications. Vol. 1.* Berlin, Institute of Veterinary Medicine, pp. 70–81.

BRYAN, F.L. (1988) Risks of practices, procedures and processes that lead to outbreaks of foodborne diseases. *Journal of food protection,* **51:** 663–673.

BRYAN, F.L. & BARTLESON, C.A. (1985) Mexican-style foodservice operations; hazard analyses, critical control points and monitoring. *Journal of food protection,* **48:** 509–524.

BRYAN, F.L. ET AL. (1981) Hazard analysis, in reference to *Bacillus cereus,* of boiled and fried rice in Cantonese-style restaurants, *Journal of food protection,* **44:** 500–512.

BRYAN, F.L. ET AL. (1987) *Procedures to investigate foodborne illness,* 4th ed. Ames, IA, International Association of Milk, Food, and Environmental Sanitarians.

BRYAN, F.L. ET AL. (1988) Critical control points of street-vended foods. *Journal of food protection,* **51:** 373–384.

DAVEY, G.R. (1985) Food poisoning in New South Wales: 1977–84. *Food technology, Australia,* **37:** 453–456.

FAO/WHO (1984) *The role of food safety in health and development*: report of a Joint FAO/WHO Expert Committee on Food Safety. Geneva, World Health Organization (WHO Technical Report Series, No. 705).

GENIGEORGIS, C. & RIEMANN, H. (1979) Food processing and hygiene. In: Riemann, H. & Bryan, F.L., ed., *Foodborne infections and intoxications,* 2nd ed. New York, Academic Press, pp. 613–713.

GREENSPAN, L. (1977) Humidity fixed points of binary saturated aqueous solutions. *Journal of research of the National Bureau of Standards — A. Physics and chemistry,* **81A:** 89–96.

ICMSF (1978) *Microorganisms in foods. 1. Their significance and methods of enumeration,* 2nd ed. Toronto, University of Toronto Press.

ICMSF (1986a) *Microorganisms in foods. 2. Sampling for microbiological analysis: principles and specific applications*, 2nd ed. Toronto, University of Toronto Press.

ICMSF (1986b) *Prevention and control of foodborne salmonellosis through application of the hazard analysis critical control point system.* Unpublished WHO document WHO/CDS/VPH/86.65. Available on request from Veterinary Public Health, World Health Organization, 1211 Geneva 27, Switzerland.

ICMSF (1988) *Microorganisms in foods. 4. Application of the hazard analysis critical control point (HACCP) system to ensure microbiological safety and quality.* Oxford, Blackwell Scientific Publications.

ROBERTS, D. (1982) Factors contributing to outbreaks of food poisoning in England and Wales 1970–1979. *Journal of hygiene*, **89:** 491–498.

SPECK, M.L., ed. (1984) *Compendium of methods for the microbiological examination of foods*, 2nd ed. Washington, DC, American Public Health Association.

STUMBO, C.R. (1973) *Thermobacteriology in food processing*, 2nd ed. New York, Academic Press.

Subcommittee on Microbiological Criteria for Foods, Committee on Food Protection, Food and Nutrition Board, National Research Council (1985) *An evaluation of the role of microbiological criteria for foods and food ingredients.* Washington, DC, National Academy Press.

TODD, E.C.D. (1983) Factors that contribute to foodborne disease in Canada, 1973–1977. *Journal of food protection*, **46:** 737–747.

TROLLER, J.A. ET AL. (1984) Measurement of water activity. In: Speck, M.L., ed., *Compendium of methods for the microbiological examination of foods*, 2nd ed. Washington, DC, American Public Health Association, pp. 124–134.

WHO (1989) *Health surveillance and management procedures for food-handling personnel:* report of a WHO Consultation. Geneva, World Health Organization (WHO Technical Report Series, No. 785).

WHO/ICMSF (1982) *Report of WHO/ICMSF meeting on hazard analysis critical control point system in food hygiene.* Unpublished WHO document, VPH/82.27. Available on request from Veterinary Public Health, World Health Organization, 1211 Geneva 27, Switzerland.

SELECTED FURTHER READING

Food microbiology and foodborne diseases

AYRES, J.C. ET AL. *Microbiology of foods*. San Francisco, Freeman, 1980.

BANWART, G.J. *Basic food microbiology*, 2nd ed. New York, Van Nostrand Reinhold (AVI), 1989.

DOYLE, M. *Foodborne bacterial pathogens*. New York, Dekker, 1989.

FRAZIER, W.C. & WESTHOFF, D.C. *Food microbiology*, 4th ed. New York, McGraw-Hill, 1988.

HOBBS, B.C. & ROBERTS, D. *Food poisoning and food hygiene*, 5th ed. Baltimore, Edward Arnold, 1987.

International Commission on Microbiological Specifications for Foods. *Microbial ecology of foods. Vol. 1. Factors affecting life and death of microorganisms*. New York, Academic Press, 1980.

International Commission on Microbiological Specifications for Foods. *Microbial ecology of foods. Vol. 2. Food commodities*. New York, Academic Press, 1980.

JAY, J.M. *Modern food microbiology*, 3rd ed. New York, Van Nostrand Reinhold, 1986.

RIEMANN, R. & BRYAN, F.L. *Foodborne infections and intoxications*, 2nd ed. New York, Academic Press, 1979.

The HACCP system

BRYAN F.L. Hazard analysis critical control point. What the system is and what it is not. *Journal of environmental health*, **50:** 400–401 (1988).

Committee on the Microbiological Safety of Foods. *The microbiological safety of foods, Part 1*. London, Her Majesty's Stationery Office, 1990.

SIMONSEN, B. ET AL. Report from the International Commission on Microbiological Specifications for Foods (ICMSF). Prevention and control of foodborne salmonellosis through application of hazard analysis critical control point (HACCP). *International journal of food microbiology*, **4:** 227–247 (1987).

TOMPKIN, R.B. The use of HACCP in the production of meat and poultry products. *Journal of food protection*, **53:** 795–803 (1990).

Application of HACCP system to food-processing operations

BAUMAN, H.E. The HACCP concept and microbiological hazard categories. *Food technology*, **28:** 30, 32, 34, 78 (1974).

BAUMAN, H.E. The hazard analysis critical control point concept. In: Felix, C.W., ed., *Food protection technology*, Chelsea, MI, Lewis Publishers, 1987, pp. 175–179.

HABERSTROH, C. ET AL. HACCP: making the system work. *Food engineering*, Aug: 70–80 (1988).

ITO, K. Microbiological criteria critical control points in canned foods. *Food technology*, **28:** 16–48 (1974).

PETERSON, A.C. & GUNNERSON, R.K. Microbiological critical control points in frozen foods. *Food technology*, **28:** 37–44 (1974).

SILLIKER, J.H. Principles and application of the HACCP approach for the food processing industry, In: Felix, C.W., ed., *Food protection technology*. Chelsea, MI, Lewis Publishers, 1980, pp. 81–89.

Application of HACCP system to food service operations

BOBENG, B.J. & DAVID, B.D. HACCP models for quality control of entree production in hospital food service. 1. Development of hazard analysis critical control point models. *Journal of the American Dietetic Association*, **7:** 534–539 (1978).

BRYAN, F.L. Hazard analysis critical control point approach: epidemiologic rationale and application to foodservice operations. *Journal of environmental health*, **44:** 7–14 (1981).

BRYAN, F.L. Application of HACCP to ready-to-eat chilled foods. *Food technology*, **44**(7): 70–77 (1990).

BRYAN, F.L. & McKINLEY, T.W. Hazard analysis and control of roast beef preparation in foodservice establishments. *Journal of food protection*, **42:** 4–18 (1979).

BRYAN, F.L. ET AL. Time–temperature survey of a restaurant that specializes in barbecued food. *Journal of food protection*, **43:** 595–600 (1980).

BRYAN, F.L. ET AL. Time–temperature conditions of *gyros. Journal of food protection*, **43:** 346–353 (1980).

BRYAN, F.L. ET AL. Hazard analyses of fried, boiled, and steamed Cantonese-styled foods. *Journal of food protection*, **45:** 410–421 (1982).

CREMER, M.L. & CHIPLEY, J.R. Microbiological problems in the foodservice industry. *Food technology*, **34:** 59, 68, 84 (1980).

DAHL, C.A. ET AL. Cook/chill foodservice systems with a microwave oven: aerobic plate counts from beef loaf, potatoes, and frozen green beans. *Journal of microwave power*, **15:** 95–105 (1980).

GUZEWICH, J.J. Practical procedures for using the HACCP approach in food service establishments by industry and regulatory agencies. In: Felix, C.W., ed., *Food protection technology*, Chelsea, MI, Lewis, 1987, pp. 91–100.

MATTHEWS, M.E. Monitoring the critical points in food service operations. In: *Microbial safety of foods in feeding systems*. Washington, DC, National Academy Press, 1982, pp. 158–168.

MUNCE, B. Hazard analysis critical control points and the food service industry. *Food technology in Australia*, **36:** 214–217, 222 (1984).

SNYDER, O.P. JR. Applying the hazard analysis and critical control points system in food service. Foodborne illness prevention. In: *Proceedings of the Second World Congress on Foodborne Infections and Intoxications, Vol. II*. Berlin, Institute for Veterinary Medicine, 1986, pp. 1018–1024.

SNYDER, O.P. Microbiological quality assurance in foodservice operations. *Food technology*, July: 122–130 (1986).

Application of HACCP system in homes

BRYAN, F.L. Safety of ethnic foods through the application of the hazard analysis critical control point approach. *Dairy and food sanitation*, **8:** 654–660 (1988).

ZOTTOLA, E. & WOLF, I. Recipe hazard analysis — RHAS — A systematic approach to analyzing potential hazards in a recipe for food preparation/preservation. *Journal of food protection*, **44:** 560–564 (1981).

Application of HACCP approach by health agencies

BRYAN, F.L. Procedures for local health agencies to institute a hazard analysis critical control point program for food safety assurance in foodservice operations. *Journal of environmental health*, **47:** 241–245 (1985).

GUZEWICH, J.J. Statewide implementation of a HACCP food service regulatory program. *Journal of environmental health*, **49:** 148–152 (1986).

A_w and its measurement

BEUCHAT, L.R. Influence of water activity on growth, metabolic activities and survival of yeasts and molds. *Journal of food protection*, **46:** 135–141 (1983).

LABUZA, T.P. ET AL. Water activity determination: a collaborative study of different methods. *Journal of food science*, **41:** 910–917 (1976).

RODEL, W. ET AL. Measurement of water activity (a_w) value of meat and meat products. *Fleischwirtschaft*, **59:** 849–851 (1979).

SPERBER, W.H. Influence of water activity on foodborne bacteria — a review. *Journal of food protection*, **46:** 142–150 (1983).

TROLLER, J.A. Water relations of foodborne bacterial pathogens — an updated review. *Journal of food protection*, **49:** 656–670 (1986).

TROLLER, J.A. & CHRISTIAN, J.H.B. *Water activity and food.* New York, Academic Press, 1978.

Sampling and testing foods

BRYAN, F.L. Procedures to use during outbreaks of foodborne illness. In: Lennette, E.H. et al., ed., *Manual of clinical microbiology*, 4th ed. Washington, DC, American Society for Microbiology, 1985.

CORRY, J.E.L. ET AL. *Isolation and identification methods for food poisoning organisms.* London, Academic Press, 1982.

GABIS, D.A. ET AL. Sampling plans, sample collection, shipment and preparation for analysis. In: Speck, M.L., ed., *Compendium of methods for microbiological examination of foods*, 2nd ed. Washington, DC, American Public Health Association, 1984.

SANDERS, A.C. ET AL. Foodborne illness — suggested approaches for the analysis of foods and specimens obtained in outbreaks. In: Speck, M.L., ed., *Compendium of methods for the microbiological examination of foods*, 2nd ed. Washington, DC, American Public Health Association, 1984.

SCHMIDT-LORENZ, W. *Sammlung von Vorschriften zur mikrobiologischen Untersuchung von Lebensmitteln.* [*Collection of methods for the microbiological examination of foods.*] Weinheim, Verlag Chemie, 1983.

COLLECTION OF WATER SAMPLES

Water samples can be collected in a number of ways, depending on the source.

From a tap or pump

Before taking a water sample from a tap, allow the water to run to waste (for 5–10 seconds for line samples and up to 5 minutes for source samples). Adjust the flow of water so that any sodium thiosulfate present in the sample bottle (to neutralize chlorine) will not be flushed out. Keep the sample container closed until just before collection. Hold the bottle near the base, fill without rinsing, and immediately replace the stopper or cap, and secure the hood, if attached. Leave an air gap of 2.5 cm to facilitate mixing.

If a plastic sample bag is used instead of a bottle, tear off the top, and open it by pulling the side tabs apart. Grasp the end wires and place the bag under the flowing water. Remove the bag before it is completely filled and squeeze out most of the air; fold over the top of the bag several times, and secure it by twisting the end wires.

From a dug well

Attach a stone or metal weight to a sampling bottle. Tie a clean piece of string to the bottle and lower the weighted bottle into the well. Immerse the bottle completely in the water and allow to fill. Once the bottle is full, pull it out of the well, discard the first 2–3 cm of water to provide an air space, and place a tight-fitting stopper or cap on the bottle.

From a container

Collect samples from buckets, jars, pans and other vessels either by pouring a portion into a sample container or by dipping a suitable sterile vessel into the water. Use a forward and upward motion, so that the hand remains behind the bottle. Then pour the water into the sample bottle or bag.

From water bodies

To collect samples from rivers, lakes, reservoirs, springs, shallow wells, step wells, and toilet tanks, hold the sample bottle or bag at the bottom and plunge it neck down to a depth of 15 cm below the surface. Turn the bottle the right way up and allow it to fill. Use a sweeping continuous, arc-shaped motion, against the flow of the stream. If possible, when taking samples from bodies of water avoid wading, because it often stirs up the bottom. Piers or other similar structures, or the front end of a drifting or slow-moving boat, are good sampling stations. If wading is unavoidable, wade upstream and keep moving forward until sample collection is completed.

Concentration methods

Concentration of microorganisms using swabs, filtration, or absorption is particularly important when waterborne pathogens are sought. Suspend Moore swabs or sponges, secured by strings or wires, overnight or for as long as possible (up to 5 days) in a water vessel, drum, stream, lake, sewer, latrine pit or drain. Bacteria can also be concentrated by filtering water through membrane filters, diatomaceous earth, or other filter media. For membrane filters, pass several litres of water through a sterile filter. Using aseptic techniques, transfer the filter to the surface of a selective enrichment medium held in an agar substrate in a saturated sterile absorbent pad, or suspend in a solution of enrichment broth, as used in the method of isolation.

More information on methods of sampling water can be found in Bryan et al.[a] and Greenberg et al.[b]

---

[a] BRYAN, F.L. ET AL. *Procedures to investigate waterborne illness.* Ames, IA, Association of Milk, Food and Environmental Sanitarians, 1979.

[b] GREENBERG, A.E. ET AL. *Standard methods for the examination of water and wastewater*, 15th ed. Washington, DC, American Public Health Association, 1981.

COLLECTION OF CLINICAL SPECIMENS

If collecting a specimen from a person who is vomiting, instruct the person to vomit directly into a clean receptacle or lavatory. Transfer a spoonful of the vomit to a sterile specimen container or a small glass jar that has been thoroughly cleaned and boiled in water for approximately 15 minutes. Take the specimen directly to the laboratory, if practicable; if not, refrigerate it or add transport medium (see p. 53), but do not freeze it.

If the person has diarrhoea or has had diarrhoea in the previous month, obtain either a stool specimen or a rectal swab. Rectal swabs should only be taken by a trained medical practitioner, nurse, technician, or microbiologist. If this is not practicable, provide the person with a stool specimen container and either a disposable plastic or wooden spoon or tongue depressor. A clean container (such as a jar or milk carton that can be sealed and later disinfected, burned, or otherwise disposed of in a sanitary manner), and a clean spoon or short stick can be used if laboratory supplies are not available.

If there are flush toilets, tell the person to collect the stool specimen by one of the following methods:

1. Put two sheets of newspaper under the toilet seat and push them down slightly in the centre, without letting them touch the water in the bowl. Defecate on to the newspaper; using a clean spoon or other utensil transfer a spoon-size portion of faeces into a specimen container, or a clean glass or plastic container.
2. Float a paper towel on the surface of the water in the toilet bowl. Defecate on to the towel; using a spoon, tongue depressor, or stick, collect a spoon-size specimen of the faeces from above the water line and transfer it to the specimen container.

If there are no flush toilets; use one of the following methods:

1. Tell the person to defecate directly into a specimen container or other dry container.
2. Give the person a swab and a tube containing transport medium. Tell the person to press the cotton-wrapped end of the swab into the top of the faeces, or on to faecally soiled toilet paper; a twisting motion should be used to pick up some excrement. The excrement-coated swab should then be broken off into the sample tube.
3. If faecal specimens cannot be easily obtained otherwise, give the person a pad of paper tissues and a sterile specimen bottle containing liquid transport medium. Tell him or her to use the tissues or toilet paper to wipe the anus after defecation and then to put them into the specimen container.

To collect specimens from an infant, rub a sterile cotton or alginate tipped swab or sponge over the anal region after the infant has defecated. Use a disposable plastic glove or a piece of sterile paper to handle the sponge so as not to introduce contaminants. Alternatively, rub the sponge or a moistened sterile swab over the soiled portion of the infant's napkin (diaper). Put the sponge into a sterile jar; break the tip of the swab into a tube of enrichment broth or transport medium.

Collect samples from latrines, sewers, sewage-contaminated water courses, and overflow from toilets by inserting Moore swabs into the faecal matter or stream, secured with a string or wire. Transport the samples to the laboratory in plastic bags. These specimens will provide information about pathogens likely to infect people in a particular household or neighbourhood. The data can indicate which microorganisms should be tested for in food samples.

If you cannot deliver faecal specimens to the laboratory immediately, do one of the following:

1. Transfer a spoon-size portion of stool from the container to a specimen bottle containing transport medium.
2. Push a swab into the faecal matter and transfer it to a tube containing transport medium.
3. Refrigerate the specimen at or below 4.4 °C. Transport media (e.g., Cary-Blair, Amies', or Stuart's transport medium, or buffered glycerol saline) preserve pathogens and prevent them from being overgrown by normal faecal flora.

If it appears that animals or their faeces may be sources of food contamination, collect specimens of droppings. If the droppings have a loose and liquid consistency insert a swab into one or more of them. If the dropping is dry, pick it up using a spoon, tong, tongue depressor or disposable plastic glove. Put the swabs directly into a tube of enrichment broth or transport medium. Put the dried faeces into a sterile jar or plastic bag.

For additional information on specimen collection, see Bryan et al. (1979, 1987).[a]

---

[a] BRYAN, F.L. ET AL. *Procedures to investigate waterborne illness.* Ames, IA, Association of Milk, Food and Environmental Sanitarians, 1979; BRYAN, F.L. ET AL. *Procedures to investigate foodborne illness.* Ames, IA, International Association of Milk, Food and Environmental Sanitarians, 1987.

TESTS THAT MIGHT BE USED DURING HAZARD ANALYSIS, MONITORING OR VERIFICATION[a]

Test	Purpose	Limitations
Aerobic plate (colony) count	Indicates (a) compliance with microbial criteria for certain foods (e.g., milk, shellfish); (b) compliance with purchase specifications; (c) adherence to good manufacturing practices High counts indicate that food supports microbial growth, particularly in samples taken sequentially	Measures only the microbial flora that is able to produce colonies in the medium used and under the conditions of incubation Rigid adherence to standard test conditions required High counts eventually develop in all perishable foods, even if initial counts are low and food is stored under acceptable temperature conditions Usefulness depends on point at which sample was taken Measures only living cells Counts decrease during storage in frozen or dried form and in acidic products Of little value for retorted and fermented foods Of little value in assessing quality Does not differentiate between types of bacteria No direct relationship to presence of pathogens, and therefore to the safety of the food
a_w	Indicates whether certain microorganisms can grow in foods; provides information on shelf stability	Equipment not available in many field laboratories Instruments need periodic calibration
Bacillus cereus	Indicates presence and number of *B. cereus* per g or ml (cause of both vomiting and diarrhoea) High counts indicate that growth has occurred	Competitive organisms often overgrow *B. cereus* in certain foods *B. cereus* commonly found in low numbers in many foods (spores can withstand usual heat treatments) Several tests are required for confirmation

[a] Other tests that might be considered during investigations of outbreaks of foodborne disease and the monitoring of critical control points have been reviewed by the Subcommittee on Microbiological Criteria for Foods of the National Research Council (*An evaluation of the role of microbiological criteria for foods and food ingredients*, Washington, DC, National Academy Press, 1985).

Test	Purpose	Limitations
Campylobacter jejuni	Indicates presence or number of *C. jejuni* per g or ml (cause of enterocolitis)	Tests require selective enrichment/plating and filtration
		Elevated optimal growth temperature
		Test requires atmosphere with reduced oxygen
		Test not yet performed in many food laboratories; methods under development but not yet standardized
Clostridium botulinum	Indicates presence and number of *C. botulinum* and possibly its neurotoxins (cause of neurotoxic disease; fatalities are not uncommon)	Expertise needed in testing and in interpreting results
		Tests require: anaerobic atmosphere; identification of toxin in laboratory animals
		Toxins and antitoxins needed
Clostridium perfringens	Indicates presence and number of *C. perfringens* per g or ml (cause of enteritis)	Small numbers likely to be present in foods
		Spores survive usual heat treatments
	High counts indicate that growth has occurred	Vegetative cells significantly decrease in refrigerated and frozen foods
		Test requires anaerobic atmosphere
Coliforms	Indicates contamination after processing (heating, irradiation, chlorination). Used as indicator of post-process contamination of water and milk	No value for monitoring raw foods
		Coliforms are sublethally stressed by freezing
	High counts indicate that growth has occurred	Use requires thorough understanding of production, processing, and preparation practices
		Coliforms may become established on equipment and grow in environment
		Does not indicate faecal contamination *per se*
Enterobacteriaceae	Indicates contamination after processing	Does not indicate faecal contamination *per se*
		Use requires thorough understanding of production, processing and preparation practices
		Enterobacteriaceae may grow in environment
		No value for monitoring raw foods
Enterococci	Indicates presence or number of enterococci (faecal streptococci)	Enterococci may survive pasteurization
		Can live on the surface of green plants
	Has been used as an indicator of poor sanitation	May become established on equipment and persist in environment for long periods
		Small numbers normally present on many foods

Hazard analysis critical control point evaluations

Test	Purpose	Limitations
Enterococci (cont.)		Fermented foods may contain large numbers
		Not a reliable indicator of faecal contamination
		Thorough understanding of role and significance of enterococci, and hence normal population levels in a food, required for appropriate interpretation of test result
		Little useful significance because of many limitations
Escherichia coli (indicator)	Best available indicator of possible faecal contamination, hence risk of presence of enteric pathogens and potential health hazard Indicates contamination after processing or process failure Large numbers may indicate that growth has occurred	Does not provide proof of presence or absence of enteric pathogens Often present on raw products of animal origin Large numbers in foods may be due to growth in product during processing (e.g., cheese) or on equipment Confirmation by indole, methyl red, Voges-Proskauer, citrate tests required Most probable number (MPN) method time-consuming, costly, imprecise; injured cells are inhibited
Escherichia coli (pathogenic)	Indicates presence of invasive, toxigenic or haemorrhagic strains of _E. coli_ (cause of diarrhoea, sometimes bloody)	Identification of pathogenic strains through animal and tissue-culture testing which is expensive and requires trained personnel Test result not always clear cut
Faecal coliforms	Indicates probable faecal contamination (more indicative than coliforms, but less so than _E. coli_) Indicates sanitary quality of water in which shellfish grow	Proportion of _E. coli_ from faecal sources not established; ratio of _E. coli_ to other organisms giving positive reaction needs to be established for each food Faecal coliforms may become established on equipment and grow in environment Faecal coliforms are sublethally stressed by freezing
Listeria monocytogenes	Indicates presence of _L. monocytogenes_ (cause of meningitis, encephalitis, stillbirths, abortions, and neonatal infections)	Cold enrichment often required Serotyping provides little information about source; need to have isolates phagetyped, which can be done in only a few typing centres
pH	Indicates whether certain microorganisms can grow in foods	Instruments need calibration

Test	Purpose	Limitations
	May indicate ability of food to destroy microorganisms	
	Low values indicate shelf stability	
Pseudomonas aeruginosa	Indicates human (skin) contamination	Can multiply in water and other substances of low nutrient level
	Indicator of hazards of bottled water for infants	
	P. aeruginosa may cause diarrhoea in infants	
Salmonellae	Indicates presence of salmonellae (cause of gastroenteritis and enteric fever)	Routine procedures require series of tests which take several days
	On heat-processed foods, indicates survival or contamination after processing (often cross-contamination)	Serotyping for epidemiological purposes, and for associating strains isolated from foods, people and environment, often needs to be done in reference laboratories (sometimes outside the country)
	Used as indicator of hazards in dried eggs, dried milk, and infant formulae	
	MPN procedures can give estimate of numbers	MPN procedure cumbersome and expensive and probably not very accurate
Shigella	Indicates presence of shigellae (cause of dysentery)	Routine procedures require series of tests which take several days
		Procedures for isolation from foods based on clinical procedures and not well developed
		Serotyping often necessary for confirmation and identification of source
Staphylococci (as indicator)	Indicates contamination after processing by persons who handled food	Small numbers not unusual in foods handled by or exposed to people
	High counts indicate that growth has occurred and possible presence of enterotoxins; thus can indicate a potential health hazard	
Staphylococcus aureus	Indicates presence or number of *S. aureus* per g or ml and possible presence of enterotoxins (cause of gastroenteritis)	Confirmation by coagulase testing required
	Indicates possible handling by workers	Presence and even large numbers of *S. aureus* do not necessarily indicate toxigenic strain or presence of enterotoxin

Hazard analysis critical control point evaluations

Test	Purpose	Limitations
Staphylococcus aureus (cont.)	High counts indicate that growth has occurred, and potential health hazard	Specific tests for enterotoxins require expertise, special procedures, and toxins and antitoxins, which are not available in most laboratories
Streptococcus pyogenes	*Indicates presence of S. pyogenes* (cause of septic sore throat and scarlet fever)	Routine method not available for food; clinical procedures used
		Test requires microaerophilic environment
Time–temperature	Indicates whether certain microorganisms would be killed or survive a process	Gives information only for portion of food in which sensor of thermometer or thermocouple located
	Indicates whether certain microorganisms could multiply and how fast	Measurement of both time and temperature needed for rational interpretation
Vibrio cholerae	Indicates presence of *V. cholerae* (cause of diarrhoea and sometimes extreme dehydration and electrolyte imbalance)	Test requires alkaline enrichment to inhibit competitive organisms
		Serotyping and biochemical tests required for confirmation
Vibrio parahaemolyticus	Indicates presence and estimate of numbers of *V. parahaemolyticus* per g (cause of gastroenteritis)	Method of enumeration time-consuming and inaccurate
		Method for identifying pathogenic strains complicated
Yersinia enterocolitica	Indicates presence of *Y. enterocolitica* (cause of gastroenteritis and ileitis)	Suitable method for isolation from foods not available; modified enrichment procedures for clinical isolations
		Confirmation and differentiation from closely related species time-consuming
		Isolates must be tested for pathogenicity

HAZARDS, CRITICAL CONTROL POINTS AND MONITORING PROCEDURES FOR FOODS THAT MIGHT BE PREPARED IN HOMES, IN SMALL FOOD SHOPS AND BY STREET VENDORS

The table overleaf gives examples of hazards associated with the preparation of some common foods in homes and small food service establishments, together with appropriate control actions and monitoring procedures. The information is based on studies by Bryan et al. (1986, 1988a,b) and Michanie et al. (1987, 1988a,b). (CCP) indicates a control point at which a hazard can be reduced, but not eliminated.

References

BRYAN, F.L. ET AL. (1986) *Phase II: Food handling. Hazard analysis critical control point evaluations of foods prepared in households in a rice-farming village in Thailand.* Rome, Food and Agriculture Organization of the United Nations.

BRYAN, F.L. ET AL. (1988a) Hazard analyses of foods prepared by inhabitants near Lake Titicaca in the Peruvian Sierra. *Journal of food protection*, **51**: 412–418.

BRYAN, F.L. ET AL. (1988b) Hazard analyses of foods prepared by migrants living in a new settlement at the outskirts in Lima, Peru. *Journal of food protection*, **51**: 314–323.

MICHANIE, S. ET AL. (1987) Critical control points for foods prepared in households in which babies had salmonellosis. *International journal of food microbiology*, **5**: 337–354.

MICHANIE, S. ET AL. (1988a) Hazard analyses of foods prepared by inhabitants along the Amazon River. *Journal of food protection*, **51**: 293–302.

MICHANIE, S. ET AL. (1988b) Critical control points for foods prepared in households whose members had either alleged typhoid fever or diarrhea. *International journal of food microbiology*, **7**: 123–134.

Food	Operation	Hazards	CCP	Control actions	Monitoring procedures
Rice, lentils, beans, pulses, chickpeas	Receiving	Bacterial spores present (*B. cereus, C. perfringens*)			
	Washing	Enteric pathogens in water		Enteric pathogens killed	
	Cooking (boiling, steaming)	Spores survive			
	Holding	Spores germinate and resulting cells multiply if food held for several hours	CCP	Serve/eat promptly after preparation; hold hot (>55°C)	Measure time of holding; measure temperature at intervals; stir
	Cooling	Bacterial multiplication continues until product cold	CCP	Cool rapidly in shallow pans	Measure depth of food in pans
	Reheating, frying	Heat-stable toxins survive reheating; pathogens survive inadequate reheating	(CCP)	Reheat thoroughly	Measure temperature at centre
Potatoes	Receiving	Bacterial spores present (*B.cereus, C. perfringens*)			
	Washing	Enteric pathogens in water		Enteric pathogens killed	
	Cooking (boiling)	Spores survive			
	Cutting or handling	Contamination by handler (*S. aureus*, shigellae, hepatitis A virus, Norwalk virus)	(CCP)	Avoid touching cooked foods	Observe practices
	Holding	Spores germinate and resulting cells multiply if food held for several hours	CCP	Serve/eat promptly after preparation; hold hot (>55°C)	Measure time of holding; measure temperature at intervals; stir
	Cooling	Bacterial multiplication continues until product cold	CCP	Cool rapidly in shallow pans	Measure depth of food in pans
	Reheating	Heat-stable toxins survive reheating; pathogens survive inadequate reheating	(CCP)	Reheat thoroughly	Measure temperature at centre
Vegetables	Receiving	Bacterial spores present (*B. cereus, C. botulinum*)			
	Washing	Enteric pathogens in water			

Trimming, cutting, handling	Contamination by handler (*S. aureus*, shigellae, hepatitis A virus, Norwalk virus)			
Cooking	Spores survive	(CCP)	Enteric pathogens killed	
Holding	Spores germinate and resulting cells multiply if food held for several hours	CCP	Serve/eat promptly after preparation; hold hot (>55°C) for several hours	Measure time of holding; measure temperature at intervals; stir
Cooling	Bacterial multiplication continues until product cold	CCP	Cool rapidly in shallow pans	Measure depth of food in pans
Reheating	Heat-stable toxins survive reheating; pathogens survive inadequate reheating	(CCP)	Reheat thoroughly	Measure temperature at centre
Chicken, meat dishes — Receiving	Pathogens present (salmonellae, campylobacters, yersiniae, *C. perfringens*, *S. aureus*); handling transfers microbes from meat surfaces to hands, equipment and utensil surfaces; cloths pick up microbes from surfaces			
Addition of bread or spice. Cutting, puncturing	Bacterial spores present (*C. perfringens*, *B. cereus*). Internal contamination from surfaces or implements			
Cooking	Pathogens survive inadequate cooking; spores survive	CCP	Enteric pathogens killed	Measure end-point temperature; measure time–temperature exposure

Food	Operation	Hazards	CCP	Control actions	Monitoring procedures
Chicken, meat dishes (cont.)	Cutting or handling	Contamination by handler (S. aureus, shigellae, hepatitis A virus, Norwalk virus); cross-contamination from raw products via hands, equipment, utensils, surfaces and cleaning cloths	(CCP)	Avoid touching cooked foods: use clean equipment and utensils; avoid contact with anything that has been used in raw food areas	Observe practices; measure concentration of disinfectant solution and contact time
	Holding	Spores germinate and resulting cells multiply if food held for several hours	CCP	Serve/eat promptly after preparation; hold hot (>55 °C)	Measure time of holding; measure temperature at intervals; stir
	Cooling	Bacterial multiplication continues until product cold	CCP	Cool rapidly in shallow pans	Measure depth of food in pans; observe whether lid used and pans stacked; measure temperature of cooling unit
	Reheating	Heat-stable toxins survive reheating; pathogens survive inadequate reheating	(CCP)	Reheat thoroughly	Measure temperature at centre
Egg dishes	Receiving	Pathogens present (salmonellae); handling transfers microbes from shells to hands			
	Cooking	Pathogens survive inadequate cooking	CCP	Enteric pathogens killed	Measure time of boiling; observe coagulation
	Peeling, cutting or handling	Contamination by handler (S. aureus, shigellae, hepatitis A virus); cross-contamination from shells via hands	(CCP)	Avoid touching cooked foods: use clean equipment and utensils; avoid contact with anything that has been used in raw food area	Observe practices; measure concentration of disinfectant solution and contact time
	Holding	Spores germinate and resulting cells multiply if food held for several hours	CCP	Serve/eat promptly after preparation; hold hot (>55 °C)	Measure time of holding; measure temperature at intervals; stir
	Cooling	Bacterial multiplication continues until product cold	CCP	Cool rapidly in shallow pans	Measure depth of food in pans; observe whether lids used and pans stacked; measure temperature of cooling unit

Step	Hazard		Control	Monitoring
Reheating	Heat-stable toxins survive reheating; pathogens survive inadequate reheating	(CCP)	Reheat thoroughly	Measure temperature at centre
Fish dishes				
Receipt	Pathogens present (*V. cholerae*, *V. parahaemolyticus*); handling transfers microbes from fish surfaces to hands, equipment, utensils, surfaces; cloths pick up microbes from surfaces			
Addition of bread or spice; Cutting, puncturing	Bacterial spores present (*C. perfringens*, *B. cereus*) Internal contamination from surfaces or implements			
Cooking	Pathogens survive inadequate cooking; spores survive	CCP	Enteric pathogens killed	Measure end-point temperature; measure time–temperature exposure
Cutting or handling	Contamination by handler (*S. aureus*, shigellae, hepatitis A virus, Norwalk virus); cross-contamination from raw products via hands, equipment, utensils, surfaces, and cleaning cloths	(CCP)	Avoid touching cooked food; use clean equipment and utensils; avoid contact with anything that has been used in raw food areas	Observe practices: measure concentration of disinfectant solution and contact time
Holding	Spores germinate and resulting cells multiply if food held for several hours	CCP	Serve/eat promptly after preparation; hold hot (>55 °C)	Measure time of holding; measure temperature at intervals; stir
Cooling	Bacterial multiplication continues until product cold	CCP	Cool rapidly in shallow pans	Measure depth of food in pans; observe whether lids used and pans stacked; measure temperature of cooling unit
Reheating	Heat-stable toxins survive reheating; pathogens survive inadequate reheating	(CCP)	Reheat thoroughly	Measure temperature at centre

Food	Operation	Hazards	CCP	Control actions	Monitoring procedures
Milk	Receiving	Pathogens present (salmonellae, campylobacters, yersiniae, brucellae, streptococci, *S. aureus*); microbes transferred from hands to udder and milk during milking; microbial contamination from improperly cleaned equipment; microbial growth during storage and delivery			
	Heating	Spores survive heating; vegetative pathogens survive inadequate heating	CCP	Pasteurize or boil	Ensure that the milk boils
	Holding	Spores germinate and resulting cells multiply if milk held for several hours	CCP	Serve/drink promptly after preparation	Measure time of holding
	Cooling	Bacterial multiplication continues until product cold	CCP	Cool rapidly in small containers	Measure depth of milk in containers
	Reheating	Heat-stable toxins survive reheating; pathogens survive inadequate reheating	(CCP)	Reheat thoroughly	Measure temperature at centre
Milk-based concentrate (*khoa*)	Receiving	Pathogens present (salmonellae, campylobacters, yersiniae, brucellae, streptococci, *S. aureus*); microbes transferred from hands to udder and milk during milking; microbial contamination from improperly cleaned equipment; microbial growth during storage and delivery			
	Boiling to concentrate		CCP		Ensure that milk boils for sufficient time

Process step	Hazard		Control measure	Monitoring
Handling of concentrate	Contamination by handler (S. aureus, shigellae, hepatitis A virus); contamination from equipment, utensils, surfaces and cleaning cloths	(CCP)	Avoid touching cooked foods; use clean equipment and utensils; avoid contact with anything that has been used in raw food area	Observe practices; measure concentration of disinfectant solution and contact time
Storage, delivery	Microbial growth	CCP	Store cold	Measure depth of product to ensure rapid cooling; measure temperature of cooling unit
Khoa-based confectionery				
Mixing with other ingredients, forming into balls	Contamination by handler (S. aureus, shigellae, hepatitis A virus); contamination from equipment, utensils, surfaces and cleaning cloths	(CCP)	Avoid touching cooked foods; use clean equipment and utensils	Observe practices
Heating	Spores survive heating; vegetative pathogens survive inadequate heating	CCP	Pasteurize or boil	Measure temperature; ensure that temperature >75 °C is attained
Cooling	Bacterial contamination from cooling water	CCP	Use safe water	
Cutting, filling, topping	Contamination by handler (S. aureus, shigellae, hepatitis A virus); contamination from equipment, utensils, surfaces and cleaning cloths	(CCP)	Avoid touching cooked foods; use clean equipment and utensils	Observe practices
Storage	Microbial growth	CCP	Store cold	Measure temperature of cooling and holding units

COMMON CRITICAL CONTROL POINTS AND EXAMPLES OF MONITORING PROCEDURES FOR FOOD-PROCESSING OPERATIONS

Process	Food	Critical control point	Monitoring procedures
Receipt of raw product	Fruit and vegetables	Fertilization	Observe sewage disposal practices and whether faeces are used as fertilizer
		Irrigation	Observe practices to determine whether sewage reaches irrigation water
		Washing and freshening	Conduct sanitary survey of water source
	Meat, poultry, eggs	Receipt	Observe/smell for signs of spoilage
		Cleaning of equipment	Observe for possibility of cross-contamination; observe effectiveness of cleaning procedures
		Chilling and cold storage	Measure size of batch, time of cooling, temperature of chilled product, time of storage
		Packaging	Observe whether vacuum is effective; observe type of wrap/package
	Fish	Receipt	Observe/smell for signs of spoilage
		Chilling and cold storage	Measure temperature of product and time of storage
		Cleaning of equipment	Observe for possibilities of cross-contamination; observe effectiveness of cleaning procedures
	Shellfish	Harvesting from water free from pollution and with low levels of indicator organisms	Sample water and test for faecal indicator organisms; survey for sewage outflows
Freezing	Fruits, vegetables	Blanching	Measure temperature and time
		Freezing	Measure time–temperature exposure during freezing; observe whether product is frozen
		Storage of thawed product	Measure temperature of product and time held after thawing
	Meat, poultry	Freezing	Measure time–temperature exposure during freezing; observe whether product is frozen

Process	Food	Critical control point	Monitoring procedures
	Fish and shellfish	Storage of thawed product	Measure temperature of product and time held after thawing
		Freezing	Measure time–temperature exposure during freezing and observe whether product is frozen
		Storage of thawed product	Measure temperature of product and time held after thawing
Pasteurization	Milk	Pasteurization	Measure time–temperature exposure; observe indicator thermometer and recording charts; evaluate function of flow diversion valve, check pump speed, and time flow through holding tubes; check plates for leaks (high-temperature, short-time pasteurization), collect samples and test for phosphatase
		Cooling, holding, filling	Inspect cleanliness of equipment, take swabs from contact surfaces; inspect valves; collect samples and test for coliforms
		Cold storage	Measure temperature of product and time of storage
	Roast beef, turkey	Pasteurization	Measure time–temperature exposure
		Slicing, packaging	Observe for possibility of cross-contamination from raw to cooked product via personnel, equipment, cleaning cloths; observe handling of cooked product
		Air-chilling	Measure size of product and time–temperature exposure
		Water-chilling	Measure residual and free chlorine levels and pH of water
Canning/retorting	Vegetables, meat, fish	Retorting	Observe operation of retorts; measure temperature after exhausting, observe filling of cans, determine whether size of can and type of product appropriate for process, record time–temperature distribution and pressure; measure product pH; observe can-handling equipment
		Cooling	Measure residual and free chlorine levels and pH of water

Hazard analysis critical control point evaluations

Process	Food	Critical control point	Monitoring procedures
Canning/retorting (cont.)	Fruits (high-acid)	Heat-processing	Observe operation of retorts; record time–temperature exposure and pressure; measure product temperature after exhausting; observe filling practices; observe can-handling equipment
		Cooling	Measure residual and free chlorine levels and pH of water
Canning/retorting of products containing added salt and nitrite	Luncheon meats	Heat-processing	Observe operation of retorts, water baths or ovens; measure time–temperature exposure and pressure
		Formulation	Check pH, a_w, concentration of NaCl or $NaNO_2$ (as appropriate)
		Cooling	Measure residual and free chlorine levels and pH of water; observe cans for damage during cooling and drying
Drying	Milk/eggs	Pre-heating and pasteurization	Measure time–temperature exposure; observe indicator thermometer and recording charts; evaluate function of flow diversion valves; collect samples and test for phosphatase
		Environment	Collect samples from air filters, sweepings, dust collectors, tailings and test for salmonellae
		Packaging	Check integrity of package
		Holding of final product	Collect samples and test for salmonellae, measure a_w
	Coconut	Pasteurization	Measure time–temperature exposure; observe indicator thermometer and recording chart
		Grating and shredding	Observe operations for possibility of contamination
		Packing	Check integrity of package
		Holding of final product	Collect samples and test for salmonellae, measure a_w
	Chocolate	Raw product	Collect samples and test for salmonellae
		Roasting of beans	Measure time–temperature exposure
		Environment	Collect environmental samples and test for salmonellae; observe moisture control
		Holding of final product	Collect samples of product and test for salmonellae

Process	Food	Critical control point	Monitoring procedures
	Dry-blended infant formula	Ingredients	Collect samples and test for salmonellae
		Environment of blending and packaging areas	Collect environmental samples and test for salmonellae
		Holding of final product	Collect samples and test for salmonellae, measure a_w
	Meat and fish	Formulation	Check concentration of NaCl
		Drying	Measure time of drying; measure a_w; measure temperature of dryer
	Nuts	Drying	Evaluate rapidity of drying process. Measure humidity of storage facilities
Fermentation	Meat products	Fermentation	Check temperature and humidity of fermentation chamber or room; observe whether starter culture is used; check frequency of transfer of culture; test speed of fall in pH
		Formulation	Check concentration of NaCl, NO_2, NO_3, sugar
		Heating	Measure product temperature: observe indicator thermometer and recording chart
		Drying	Measure time of drying
		Final product	Measure pH, a_w; check appearance of product
		Fermentation	Measure temperature and humidity of fermentation chamber or room
	Vegetables, fish	Formulation	Check concentration of NaCl
		Final product	Measure pH, a_w; check appearance of product
	Milk, cheese, yoghurt	Pre-heating or pasteurization	Measure time–temperature exposure; observe indicator thermometer and recording chart
		Fermentation	Measure product temperature; check type, amount and purity of starter culture
		Aging	Measure duration of aging
		Packaging	Observe integrity of package
Acidification	Fish	Formulation	Check concentration and type of acid
		Blending	Observe thoroughness of blending
		Marinating	Measure duration of marinating, check effectiveness of mixing, measure pH

Hazard analysis critical control point evaluations

Process	Food	Critical control point	Monitoring procedures
Acidification (cont.)	Mayonnaise	Formulation	Check type and amount of organic acid used
		Blending	Observe thoroughness of blending
		Final product	Measure percentage of organic acid and pH

HAZARDS, CRITICAL CONTROL POINTS AND MONITORING PROCEDURES FOR COMMON FOOD SERVICE OPERATIONS

The table below gives examples of hazards associated with some common food service operations, together with appropriate control actions and monitoring procedures. The information is adapted from Bryan, F.L., Microbiological hazards of feeding systems. In: *Microbiological safety of foods in feeding systems*, Washington, DC, National Academy Press, 1982 (ABMPS Report No. 125), pp. 64–80.

Operation/ critical control point	Hazards	Control measures	Monitoring procedures
Purchase/receipt	Pathogens on raw foods; foods obtained from unsafe sources	Obtain foods from safe source	Set purchase specifications and check for compliance on receipt
Frozen storage	Microbial growth in thawed goods	Maintain frozen until use	Observe whether foods are frozen; measure temperature of freezer
Refrigerated storage	Microbial growth if temperatures too high or duration of storage too long; cross-contamination	Maintain cold temperature; rotate stock	Observe condition of food; measure food and unit temperature, observe storage practices; measure duration of storage; look for potential routes of contamination
Dry storage	Break in package; high moisture; poisons stored near foods; sewage backflow or drippage from pipes; vectors	Maintain low temperature and humidity; store poisons elsewhere; protect foods from contamination	Observe storage practices
Thawing	Bacterial growth; contamination of area by thaw water; incomplete thawing	Thaw at temperatures and within times that do not permit multiplication of common pathogenic bacteria	Observe thawing practice; feel whether product completely thawed
Reconstitution (rehydration)	Contamination during rehydration; bacterial growth	Use safe water and clean utensils and containers; use food promptly or refrigerate in small volumes	Observe practices

Hazard analysis critical control point evaluations

Operation/ critical control point	Hazards	Control measures	Monitoring procedures
Preparation	Cross-contamination from raw products; contamination from food handlers and dirty equipment and utensils	Avoid handling raw foods and then cooked foods; avoid touching foods that are not to be heated subsequently	Observe practices
Cooking	Pathogens survive inadequate time–temperature exposure; spores survive	Adequate time–temperature exposure	Measure temperature at geometric centre of food
Handling of foods that are not subsequently heated	Cross-contamination from raw products; contamination from hands, equipment, or utensils	Avoid handling raw foods and then cooked foods; avoid touching foods that are not to be heated subsequently; exclude ill persons from working with food; ensure personal hygiene of food service workers	Observe practices; observe personnel for signs of illness; receive reports of illness or significant symptoms
Holding at room or warm outside temperatures	Bacterial growth	Limit time of such holding; hold hot or cool	Observe practices; measure time of holding
Hot-holding	Bacterial growth	Hold foods at temperatures at which pathogenic bacteria do not multiply	Measure temperature of foods at intervals
Cooling	Pathogenic bacteria multiply	Cool foods rapidly in shallow containers or use other method of rapid cooling; store as close to freezing as feasible	Measure depth of food; measure temperature of food after cooling; observe storage practices
Reheating	Microbial pathogens may survive; heat-stable toxins will survive	Adequate time–temperature exposure	Measure temperature at completion of reheating
Cleaning of equipment and utensils	Failure to remove pathogens from surfaces	Wash, rinse, disinfect	Observe practices; measure concentration of disinfectant solution and contact time

INSIDERS' GUIDE®

FUN WITH THE FAMILY™ SERIES

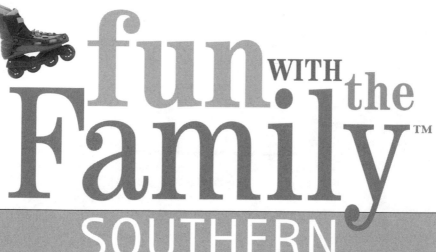

fun WITH the Family™

SOUTHERN CALIFORNIA

HUNDREDS OF IDEAS FOR DAY TRIPS WITH THE KIDS

LAURA KATH AND PAMELA PRICE

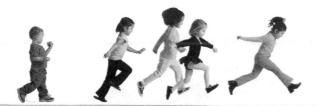

FIFTH EDITION

INSIDERS' GUIDE®

GUILFORD, CONNECTICUT
AN IMPRINT OF THE GLOBE PEQUOT PRESS

To buy books in quantity for corporate use or incentives, call **(800) 962–0973, ext. 4551,** or e-mail **premiums@GlobePequot.com.**

INSIDERS' GUIDE®

Copyright © 1996, 1998, 2000, 2003, 2005 by The Globe Pequot Press

Text design by Nancy Freeborn and Linda Loiewski
Maps created by Rusty Nelson © The Globe Pequot Press
Spot photography throughout © Photodisc and RubberBall Productions

ISSN 1541-8952
ISBN 0-7627-3442-6

Manufactured in the United States of America
Fifth Edition/Second Printing

To Anna Kath, my indomitable mom!
—Laura Kath

To Leona Effress, my dynamic, delightful mother!
—Pamela Price

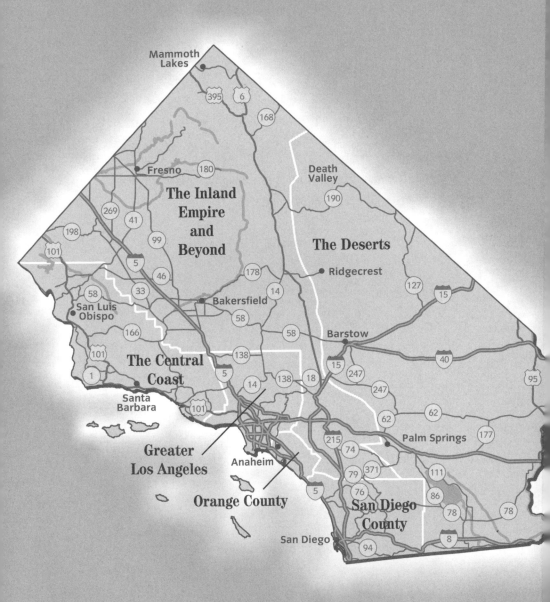

Contents

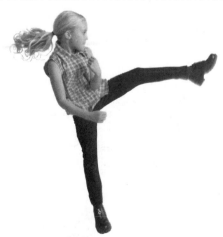

Acknowledgments

Researching the best family fun throughout Southern California could not have been accomplished without the invaluable assistance of so many generous individuals, organizations, and attractions. From the tips of our fingers to our achy feet, we gratefully acknowledge just a few of the many (and hereby apologize if we've neglected to mention anyone).

Anaheim/Orange County Visitor and Convention Bureau; Barnstorming Adventures; California Office of Tourism (Leona Reed); Catherine Boire PR; Disneyland Resort; Bob Gourley and family; Janet Newcomb Public Relations; Janis Flippen Public Relations; Vern Lanegrasse, the Hollywood Chef; Los Angeles Convention and Visitors Bureau; Long Beach Area Visitors and Convention Bureau; Maris Somerville Associates Public Relations; Omni Hotel San Diego; Oxnard Convention and Visitors Bureau; Palm Springs Bureau of Tourism; Palm Springs Desert Resorts Convention and Visitors Bureau; Riverside Convention and Visitors Bureau; San Diego Convention and Visitors Bureau (Robert Arends); San Diego North County Visitors and Convention Bureau; San Luis Obispo Chamber of Commerce; Santa Barbara Conference and Visitors Bureau; SeaWorld; Solvang Visitors Bureau; Steve Valentine PR; Susan Bejeckian Public Relations; Universal Studios; Ventura Visitors and Convention Bureau.

Pamela would like to thank Bernard Bubman, who introduced her to his favorite family-friendly places around Los Angeles. Pamela thanks her son Tony for his outspoken opinions on what families will find festive in Southern California and her son Artie for his enthusiasm in exploring dozens of attractions on and off the road map. Pamela values broadcasting "wonder woman" Jackie Olden for her incredible support. Pamela also thanks her mother, Leona Effress, for showcasing this book in her Palm Springs gift shop.

Laura especially appreciates her supportive family members and friends who are always eager to explore the wonders of SoCal attractions with her. Many thanks to travel partner Brian Scally for companionship and camaraderie, especially during our many research trips! Laura gratefully acknowledges the long-standing "author encouragement" provided by Amrit Joy, Fred Klein, Rev. Sandra Cook, Dr. Vida Makowski, Peggy Wentz, and Lee Wilkerson. Ultimately, Laura will always treasure "the Kath Party" for providing her very first "fun with the family" car trips!

Last but never least, we acknowledge the supportive staff at The Globe Pequot Press for giving us the opportunity to write about all this Southern California fun starting back in 1994!

Introduction

Southern California is a kaleidoscope—no matter which way you turn, something amazing appears! There is just no way we can include every fun-worthy thing and place for your family in a volume this size. However, we do believe that this guide will give you and your family a very practical, yet comprehensive way to experience the Golden State, starting from the Central Coast and heading south all the way to the Mexican border.

Both of us, along with our families, have traveled thousands of miles by trains, planes, automobiles, horses, mules, and aching feet to discover the best in Southern California family fun. We are very proud of our adopted home state—Pamela originally hails from Minnesota and Laura from Michigan—and have spent more than fifty combined years as journalists researching and describing life on the "left coast" of the United States. We are thrilled to share the adventure with you!

We believe the most important element to family fun in Southern California is time. Be sure you allow yourself and the kids plenty of it. Concentrated in this golden nugget of real estate are enough activities, sights, sounds, and sensations to fill a dozen or more visits. Be sure to carefully select the elements that satisfy your family's unique tastes. Don't "kid" yourself, Southern California is not as "laid-back" as you might think. Just ask any parent who has been done in by a day at an amusement park or managed to hit one of our famous freeway rush hours near dinnertime. Distance between activities can be deceptive. Five miles does not necessarily mean five minutes away. Be sure you plan "kick back" time—to relax on a beach or park bench and to soak up some of Southern California's 300-plus days of sunshine. Don't worry, we will be sure to save more for your next visit—promise!

If you and your family seek natural beauty, Southern California offers you the Pacific Ocean and its awesome beaches—some favorites include Moonstone Beach near Cambria, East Beach in Santa Barbara, Venice Beach near Santa Monica, and the pristine sands of Coronado. The mountain ranges, inland valleys, rivers, and freshwater lakes such as Nacimiento, Casitas, Big Bear, and Arrowhead are wonderful total recreation zones. Deserts such as Anza-Borrego, Palm Springs, Mojave, and Death Valley provide amazing contrasts to the palm-lined shores.

How about recreation? Participant or spectator, you can experience it all here. Teams such as basketball's Los Angeles Lakers, hockey's Mighty Ducks of Anaheim, baseball's L.A. Dodgers and Anaheim Angels, and football's San Diego Chargers offer the thrill of professional action. Needless to say, waterfront activity should rate high on your list when visiting Southern California—boating, fishing, sailing, sunbathing, surfing, and swimming are what "California dreams" are made of. If you visit between December and April, whale-watching along the Pacific is an absolute must-see thrill. You and the kids can get into the swing of golf and tennis at hundreds of public facilities. Of course, biking and hiking trails abound to explore, yet they preserve all the area's natural beauty. Don't forget to pack a picnic basket and take time to smell the perennially blooming flowers.

You can visit natural parks full of wildlife and sea life or human-made amusement parks stocked with thrills. Southern California museums are filled with hands-on displays of fun things from archives to outer space. Be certain to include the magnificent J. Paul Getty Museum as well as the California Science Center in Los Angeles. California's history, rich with Native American, Spanish, and Mexican influences, provides your family with plenty of cultural diversity education, not to mention the thrill of deciphering foreign names—like San Luis Obispo, Port Hueneme, Ojai, and Temecula!

We have also included some of our preferred accommodations, family-friendly dining, and shopping places to make your stay more enjoyable. We hope you will take the time to try some one-of-a-kind places to eat and stay that are not part of national chains. But let's be honest here—your kids would never forgive you if you didn't make a stop at a Planet Hollywood, Hard Rock Cafe, Nike Town, or Tower Records, all headquartered here.

Southern California is blessed with hundreds of annual special events—starting with January's immensely popular Rose Parade in Pasadena, right through holiday lighted boat parades all along the coast. There is always Carpinteria's Avocado Festival or the Historic Route 66 Jamboree. Since festivals have varying dates from year to year, we have included phone numbers you can call for specifics.

Southern California is like an endless summer vacation. Where else can you travel from the desert to a futuristic metropolis to some mountain snow skiing and, finally, take in the sunset at the beach—all in one day, all year-round? Would you expect anything less from the birthplace of Hollywood and Disneyland?

In this edition we have provided special sections under many area listings entitled "Where to Stay" and "Where to Eat"—describing just a few of the many outstanding establishments available for your family's enjoyment. Dollar signs provide a very general sense of the price range for each property. For meals, the prices are per individual dinner entrees, without tax or gratuity. For lodging, the rates are for a double-occupancy room, European plan (no meals unless indicated), exclusive of hotel "bed tax" or service charges.

Please keep in mind that meal prices generally stay the same throughout the year, but lodging rates fluctuate seasonally and by day of the week. Higher rates generally prevail in the summer season and holidays (when more fami-lies are on the go). Always be sure to inquire about special packages and promotional discounts.

Rates for Lodging

$	up to $50
$$	$51 to $75
$$$	$76 to $99
$$$$	$100 and up

Rates for Restaurants

$	most entrees under $10
$$	most entrees $10 to $15
$$$	most entrees $16 to $20
$$$$	most entrees more than $20

Admission prices for attractions are in dollar signs, which indicate the following price ranges:

Rates for Attractions

$	up to $5 per person
$$	$5 to $10 per person
$$$	$11 to $20 per person
$$$$	more than $20 per person

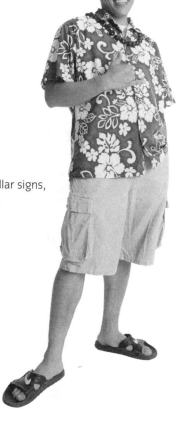

Please let us know what you like about our *Fun with the Family Southern California* guidebook. What other activities or attractions do we need to include in future editions? We really value your impressions. Write us today in care of The Globe Pequot Press, P.O. Box 480, Guilford, CT 06437.

Imagination, recreation, relaxation, nature, geography, cultural diversity, and history—complemented by a warm, sunny year-round climate—are waiting here for you. We know this guidebook will map out memorable family fun you will treasure and want to repeat, because Southern California makes every visitor feel young at heart. Enjoy!

Attractions Key

The following is a key to the icons found throughout the text.

SWIMMING		**FOOD**	
BOATING / BOAT TOUR		**LODGING**	
HISTORIC SITE		**CAMPING**	
HIKING / WALKING		**MUSEUMS**	
FISHING		**PERFORMING ARTS**	
BIKING		**SPORTS/ATHLETICS**	
AMUSEMENT PARK		**PICNICKING**	
HORSEBACK RIDING		**PLAYGROUND**	
SKIING/WINTER SPORTS		**SHOPPING**	
PARK		**PLANTS /GARDENS /NATURE TRAILS**	
ANIMAL VIEWING		**FARMS**	

the Central Coast

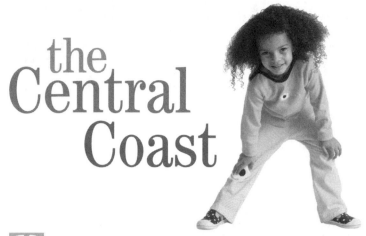

The Central Coast has always been considered the northern edge of Southern California. However, there is really a midwestern feeling of friendliness and hospitality in the three geographically close yet economically diverse counties of San Luis Obispo, Santa Barbara, and Ventura. You have all the quintessential Southern California trademarks here—great year-round weather, fun-filled recreation, and attractions; and, of course, sandy beaches woven between wide-open fields planted with veggies and fruit, soaring foothills, mountains, streams, and the glittering Pacific—all presented by locals with warm graciousness. With fewer people than the megalopolises to the south, the Central Coast is much more laid-back and casual.

So much about the Central Coast says "welcome" to your family. Hearst Castle in San Simeon, spring hikes through the wildflowers of Montana de Oro State Park, the trendy beaches and shopping of Santa Barbara, kids' hands-on museums and zoos, boat cruises out to the Channel Islands, and surfing on the Rincon—or how about the simple pleasures of just hanging out in the 320-plus days of annual sunshine and basking in the waves and smiles from fellow Sunshine State dwellers and visitors? The Central Coast's two main arteries, the magnificent Pacific Coast Highway 1 and the inland U.S. Highway 101, can be your twin pathways to some of the best, and surprisingly most affordable, tastes of your Southern California dream vacation.

San Luis Obispo County

San Luis Obispo County's 3,316 square miles contain the Central Coast's most varied terrain—from windswept beaches to interior lakes, from grass-covered rolling hills to meticulously tended farmlands, plus recurring topographical evidence of seismic shifts along California's main earthquake zone, the San Andreas Fault. There are 85 miles of coastline for exploring.

The climate of San Luis Obispo (San Lewis Oh-bis-poe) features mild summers and winters, with patches of dense seasonal fog along the coast. Temperatures range from coastal lows in the thirties in the winter to inland valley highs in the nineties-plus in the summer. Year-round temperatures average sixty to seventy degrees, with around 22 inches of rain, mostly in the winter.

THE CENTRAL COAST

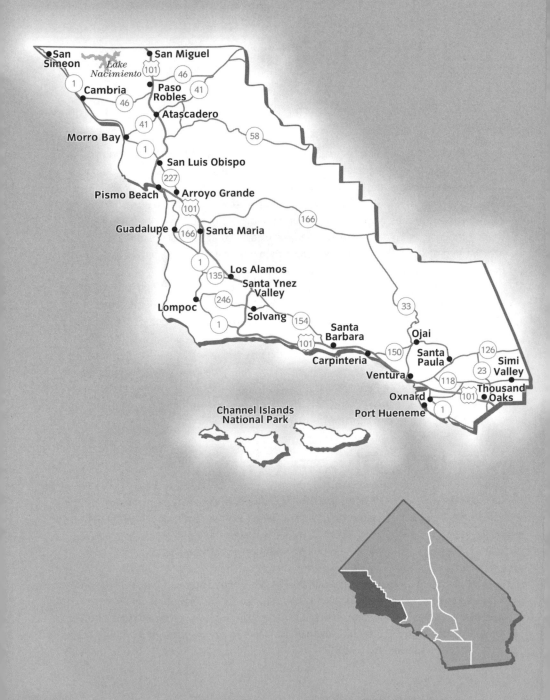

Native Americans occupied the land for thousands of years before its discovery by Spanish explorers in the sixteenth century. Two of California's famous chain of twenty-one missions are here in San Luis Obispo County, preserving the area's Spanish and Mexican heritage. The railroad arrived in the late 1890s, bringing more families and increasing the dominance of agriculture and tourism in the area. Outdoor recreation and historic attractions top the must-see list of county adventures.

For More Information

San Luis Obispo County Visitors and Conference Bureau. 1037 Mill Street, 93401; (805) 541–8000 or (800) 634–1414; www.sanluisobispocounty.com.

San Simeon

Founded in the 1850s by fishermen and whalers, the little seaside village of San Simeon really came into its own in the late 1800s, when most of the area's land was purchased and developed by Sen. George Hearst. His son, William Randolph Hearst, began construction on his fantasy "ranch" in 1919. This incredible estate, and the opportunity to visit it, has put San Simeon on the map. Most of the original village has faded, but Sebastian's General Store and Post Office is fun for kids to explore. The newer tourist town of San Simeon Acres is 4 miles south of Hearst Castle on Pacific Coast Highway 1 and plays host to various motels, restaurants, and a miniature golf course/arcade—facilities to snap you back into modern-day realities.

Hearst San Simeon State Historic Monument (ages 6 and up) 🏛

41 miles north of San Luis Obispo on Pacific Coast Highway 1; (805) 927–2020 or (800) 444–4445 (have your credit card ready to purchase tour tickets in advance); www.hearst castle.org. Open daily, except New Year's Day, Thanksgiving, and Christmas. $$

Don't miss a chance to go on a fascinating tour of publishing baron William Randolph Hearst's real-life fantasy home between 1928 and 1951, officially called Hearst San Simeon State Historic Monument and unofficially called Hearst Castle. See for yourself the lifestyle of someone rich and famous. Advance ticket reservations are strongly recommended.

This is the most popular attraction on the Central Coast, and there are a limited number of tickets and tour times available. If you arrive without reservations, you most likely will have to wait and might find a sold-out/standby situation (especially in the busy summer, weekend, and holiday times).

There are four different guided tours to choose from. Each is seventy-five minutes long, plus a thirty-minute bus ride to and from the castle. For first-timers, **Tour Number 1,** also called the Experience Tour, is the best bet. It includes the National Geographic movie *Hearst Castle: Building the Dream.* When you arrive at the "castle," park **free** at the modern visitor center just off the highway. This family-friendly center has a snack bar, gift shop, restrooms, lockers, and a fascinating **free** exhibition on Hearst himself, which you can visit as you wait for your tour number to be called. You'll then board school buses for the 5-mile, fifteen-minute drive up the hill to see highlights of the 165-room "La Casa Grande"—the main house—plus three separate guesthouses on the 127-acre grounds overlooking the Pacific and the surrounding Santa Lucia Mountains.

There is something for every member of your family to ogle in Hearst Castle, including enormous swimming pools, the lavish dining room (complete with Hearst's favorite Heinz ketchup bottle among the silver and china!), the playroom with billiards and trophy animal heads, incredible art, antiques, tapestries, and collectibles from around the world, plus Hearst's private movie theater with his vintage home movies for your viewing pleasure.

If you want more of a Hearst fantasy fix, take **Tour Number 2** for upper levels of the main house, the libraries, and the kitchen or **Tour Number 3** for the North Wing, gardens, and a special video on the construction of the castle. **Tour Number 4,** for more gardens, the wine cellar, and another private guesthouse, is offered April through October. **Tour 5** is a very special lighted evening tour lasting around two hours on Friday and Saturday from March through May and September through December. The tour lasts one hundred minutes, plus a thirty-minute bus ride. Tour 5 combines the best elements of the above tours at a higher fee, but really is appropriate only for older children, teens, and adults.

For More Information

San Simeon Chamber of Commerce.
250 San Simeon Avenue, 93452; (805) 927–3500; www.sansimeonsbest.com.

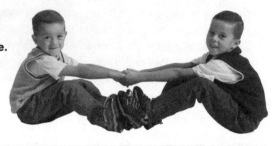

Cambria

Nine miles south of San Simeon and 33 miles northwest of San Luis Obispo on Highway 1 is the quaint, small-town artist's haven of Cambria. This village is a welcome respite from the excesses of Hearst Castle and is a family-friendly place to stay for this part of your coastal explorations. The West Village is adjacent to Highway 1; the East Village, or Old Town, is about a mile inland. Moonstone Beach Drive is right on the Pacific and has many inns and beachcombing spots. Both parts of town are connected by Main Street. Cruise down Main Street and check out the art galleries, antique emporiums, and toy shops. The Soldier Factory in the West Village manufactures and sells detailed miniature combatants and lots of other figures made of pewter. There is a farmers' market every Friday afternoon at the Vet's Hall on Main Street.

Where to Eat

Brambles Dinner House, 4005 Burton Drive; (805) 927–4716; www.bramblesdinner house.com. Opens at 4:00 P.M. most days and has excellent early-bird specials. Located in the East Village, 2 blocks south of Main Street. Choose from multiple dining areas in this rambling English cottage. Friendly servers and a children's menu will make you feel right at home. Superb steaks and prime rib. A great place to unwind after a busy day of touring. $$$

Linn's Restaurant & Bakery, 2277 Main Street; (805) 927–0371; www.linnsfruitbin .com. Open daily for breakfast, lunch, and dinner. Famous for Olallieberry Pie, home-style meals, preserves, and bakery delights. $

Where to Stay

Best Western Fireside Inn, 6700 Moon-stone Beach Drive, Cambria; (805) 927–8661 or (888) 910–7100; www.bestwesternfireside inn.com. You'll find spacious rooms, many with fireplaces and oceanview patios. Other highlights include refrigerators, coffeemak-ers, complimentary continental breakfast, a heated pool, and a whirlpool. Excellent value along the beach. $$$

Cambria Pines Lodge, 2905 Burton Drive; (805) 927–4200 or (800) 445–6868; www.cambriapineslodge.com. A wonderful place for families to stay. Located on a hilltop overlooking the village, the lodge has 125 units, including nice two-room family suites with connecting baths, fireplaces, micro-waves, fridges, and coffeemakers. You'll also enjoy an indoor heated pool, whirlpool, game room, lawn sports, and a restaurant serving California cuisine for breakfast, lunch, and dinner. $$

Moonstone **Beach**

Just north of Cambria, Moonstone Beach is the place to find smooth, milky-white stones and gnarled pieces of driftwood. Don't think about swimming here, because the water is really too cold, but beachcombing is the best! You can often see migrating whales passing by in January and February and hear the cries of sea otters and sea lions year-round. There are several bed-and-breakfast inns, motels, and restaurants along Moonstone Beach Drive if you want to savor the crashing surf.

For More Information

Cambria Chamber of Commerce.
767 Main Street, 93428; (805) 927–3624; www.cambriachamber.org.

Lake Nacimiento

Just over the mountains from Hearst Castle lies Nacimiento, arguably the Central Coast's most beautiful human-made lake. Damming the Nacimiento River created 165 miles of gorgeous shoreline. Fishing, boating, water sports galore, and outstanding hiking make this one of the most popular family recreation destinations in San Luis Obispo County.

Lake Nacimiento Resort

From U.S. Highway 101, take County Road G-14 out of Paso Robles, drive 16 miles north-west; mailing address: Star Route, Box 2770, Bradley, 93426; (805) 238–3256 or (800) 323–3839; www.nacimientoresort.com. $$$

Owned and operated by the Heath family since 1962, the resort is a safe, clean, fun environment, with everything you could possibly want for a great outdoors vacation. There is a full-service marina and dock where you can rent Jet Skis, Wave Runners, canoes, boats (power, paddle, and pontoon), sportfishing tackle, and equipment for diving and wind-surfing.

The lake is famous for its plentiful white bass, waterskiing, and salt-free swimming. Forgot your bathing suit or gear? The fully stocked general store has everything, including provisions for a barbecue or picnic. Lakeshore Cafe serves breakfast, lunch, and dinner during the summer season. Open-air patio dining is available; great views!

Facilities include the boat launch, picnic grounds, playground, volleyball and basketball courts, swimming pool, and hiking trails around the meandering shoreline. Overnight accommodations include nineteen lodge units, one-, two-, and three-bedroom town houses (complete with mini-kitchens and decks) right on the lakeshore; plus forty RV hookups and 270 campsites. Extremely popular April to October, but winter season has mild weather, fewer crowds, and, of course, the same gorgeous scenery.

Paso Robles and Atascadero

Paso Robles (Spanish for "pass of the oaks") is located at the junction of U.S. Highway 101 and State Route 46. The 6.5-magnitude earthquake of December 22, 2003, caused some historic masonry buildings to crumble, but certainly not the friendly, welcoming spirit here. Atascadero (Spanish for "place of much water") is just south of Paso Robles at the crossroads of State Route 41. This area is famous for its stately trees, agriculture, and award-winning wineries and vineyards. Perhaps a taste of the grape for mom and dad before hitting the dusty trail again? (Phone the Vintners and Growers Association at 805–239–8463 for current maps and tasting rooms or access the Web site at www.pasowine.com.) Meanwhile, be sure to explore these area attractions with the entire family.

California Mid-State Fair

Riverside Avenue between 21st and 24th Streets, just off U.S. Highway 101, Paso Robles; (805) 239–0655; www.midstatefair.com.

Call for annual lineup of musical and rodeo events. For two weeks in early August, the annual fair turns Paso Robles into a rockin' and thumpin' western town. Kids will enjoy the 4-H animal exhibits, crafts, art, food booths, carnival rides, and world-class live entertainment (in years past, Kenny Rogers, Diana Ross, Julio Iglesias, and the Beach Boys have appeared).

Pioneer Museum

Riverside Avenue between 19th and 20th Streets, Paso Robles; (805) 239–4556. Open year-round Thursday through Sunday from 1:00 to 4:00 P.M. Free admission; donations welcome.

Young cowpokes can amble over to see the farm equipment from the turn of the last century, while their folks check out home furnishings.

Lake Atascadero Park and Charles Paddock Zoo

South of Paso Robles, Morro Bay/State Route 41, exit off U.S. Highway 101, west 1.5 miles, Atascadero; (805) 461–5080; www.charlespaddockzoo.org. Open 10:00 A.M. to 4:00 P.M.; hours extended in summer and vary by season. $

Thirty-five acres of water and wonder. This very intimate site allows close proximity to some one hundred rare and wonderful species. Among the selection: gleaming black brother-and-sister jaguars from Brazil, a pair of Bengal tigers, furry lemurs, sinewy pythons and boas, strutting pink flamingos, and crested porcupines (can you make them strut their stuff?). Lake Atascadero is next to the zoo. Walk around the 2-mile perimeter of the lake and picnic on benches or dockside at the Lakeside Pavilion's snack bar. Strollers, a gift shop, refreshments, and restrooms all make a visit easier for families.

For More Information

Atascadero Chamber of Commerce.
6550 El Camino Real, 93422; (805) 466–2044; www.atascaderochamber.org.

Paso Robles Chamber of Commerce and Visitors and Conference Bureau.
1225 Park Street, 93446; (805) 238–0506 or (800) 406–4040; www.pasorobleschamber.com.

Morro Bay

Noted for two landmarks—nature's awesome Morro Rock and the human-made trio of smokestacks at the Pacific Gas and Electric power plant—bustling Morro Bay has a busy commercial fishing fleet and is a prized recreational and tourist town. You can't miss the magnificent 578-foot, dome-shaped Morro Rock, a long-extinct volcano, which marks the oceanfront end of the Embarcadero—several miles of waterfront filled with shops, restaurants, motels, and sailing vessels for charter.

Tigers Folly II Harbor Cruises

1205 Embarcadero, near the Harbor Hut restaurant, across the street from the power plant; (805) 772–2257 or (800) 958–4437. $$

This 64-foot stern-wheeler paddleboat offers one-hour bay cruises—a gentle seafaring trip back into yesteryear. Sunday brunches are available seasonally. The bearded captain will delight the kids, especially when he lets them take the helm!

Sub/Sea Tours and Kayaks

699 Embarcadero #9; (805) 772–9463; www.subseatours.com. Call for reservations and current rates.

The company offers forty-five-minute trips in a semi-submersible vessel daily, generally on the hour depending on the tides. Kids love "diving" and seeing kelp forests and marine life. All trips narrated by a naturalist.

Morro Bay State Park

At the south end of town, off State Park Road; (805) 772–2560 or (800) 444–7275. Open daily year-round.

Nearly 2,000 acres along the Pacific shore contain many picnic and camping areas, an eighteen-hole golf course, a marina, a cafe, a primitive natural area, an estuary (great for bird-watching), and boat rentals.

Museum of Natural History

Perched on White Point, overlooking the bay and Morro Rock inside the Morro Bay State Park; (805) 772–2694; www.morrobaymuseum.org. Open daily 10:00 A.M. to 5:00 P.M. except New Year's Day, Thanksgiving, and Christmas. $

Traditional and educational interpretive displays of local marine life, geology, and the history and culture of Native peoples predominate. Video presentations in the auditorium. This is the last remaining blue heron rookery reserve between San Francisco and Mexico. These rare birds can be observed from hiking trails on the museum grounds.

Montana de Oro State Park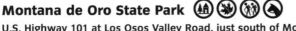

U.S. Highway 101 at Los Osos Valley Road, just south of Morro Bay in the tiny town of Los Osos; (805) 528–0513. Open year-round. Free day use, camping fees vary.

It is considered the Central Coast's premier park for hiking, nature walks, tide-pooling, horseback riding, camping, and shore fishing. The Spanish name means "mountain of gold," referring to the golden fields of poppies, mustard grass, and wildflowers enveloping the hillsides every spring. You can easily spend a day at this incredibly beautiful, 8,000-acre paradise.

Where to Eat and Stay

Harbor Hut Restaurant, 1205 Embarcadero; (805) 772–2255. It's right in the heart of the waterfront action. The seafood is fresh from the trawlers docked in front, making the Hut popular with locals and visitors alike. Lunch and dinner served daily from 11:00 A.M. $$

The Inn at Morro Bay, One mile south on Main Street, right before the entrance to Morro Bay State Park; (805) 772–5651 or (800) 321–9566; www.innatmorrobay.com. Located on the bay, this comfortable ninety-seven-room, full-service hotel has both water- and garden-view rooms. Be sure to ask for a bay view with a balcony or patio to really relax. Enjoy the Wellness Center & Spa as well as complimentary beach cruiser bikes. Two dining rooms offer unobstructed views of the estuary and bay frontage while you are enjoying California cuisine for breakfast, lunch, and dinner. $$$

For More Information

Morro Bay Visitors Center and Chamber of Commerce. 845 Embarcadero Road, Suite D, 93442; (805) 772–4467 or (800) 231–0592; www.morrobay.org.

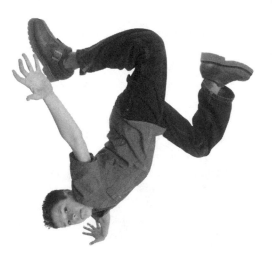

City of San Luis Obispo

This county seat sits in an inland valley ringed by pretty hills. A remarkably friendly municipality of 45,000 that is also home to California Polytechnic State University (known as Cal Poly), San Luis Obispo has a vibrant downtown area filled with historic sites, shopping, and restaurants. The 25-cent downtown trolley runs a circuit that will give you and the kids a chance to take in the sights and sounds.

Mission San Luis Obispo de Tolosa

Chorro and Monterey Streets, in the heart of Mission Plaza; (805) 543–6850; www.old missionslo.org. Open daily 9:00 A.M. to 5:00 P.M. except major holidays. Free admission; donations welcome.

Founded in 1772 and still in operation, the mission is the fifth in the twenty-one-mission chain of parishes founded by Father Junipero Serra. Take a self-guided tour through the Life at the Mission history exhibits and pause in the adobe-brick chapel constructed by the native Chumash people. The mission is named for a thirteenth-century saint, the bishop of Toulouse, often called "Prince of the Missions."

County Historical Museum

696 Monterey Street, opposite the mission; (805) 543–0638. Open Wednesday through Sunday 10:00 A.M. to 4:00 P.M. Closed holidays. Free admission; donations appreciated.

Another trip down memory lane with old photographs and artifacts, all housed in a Romanesque granite, sandstone, and brick building that used to be the city library.

San Luis Obispo Children's Museum

(ages 2 to 12, accompanied by an adult)

1010 Nipomo Street, corner of Monterey Street, downtown (same side of the creek as the mission); (805) 544–6212 for times and admission fees. $

True to its motto of "education through exploration," this is a super, hands-on environment. It gives kids the chance to explore such future careers as news reporter, astronaut, postmaster, or bank teller. Kids can put on their own play, make giant bubbles (way cool!), or run a diner. The creek-side play zone works well for an outdoor picnic break.

Gum Alley
Higuera Street, between Garden and Broad Streets.

Before leaving downtown, you must seek out a relic you'll probably hate and your kids will undoubtedly love. Since the late 1950s, locals (mostly collegians) and visitors alike have been depositing their used gum on the narrow alley walls. Folk art or disgusting nuisance, who's to say, for this representation (it's the one and only) has been featured in *Smithsonian* magazine and on the *Ripley's Believe It or Not* TV show. Care to leave your sticky imprint? Let your taste decide.

Farmers' Market
Downtown, Higuera Street. Every Thursday evening from 6:00 to 9:00 year-round.

Not to be missed is this world-famous farmers' market (a 7-block-long street fair). Kids will love the excitement of musicians, puppeteers, face painters, skate dancers, fire eaters, and, obviously, loads of fresh fruit, veggies, and mouth-watering barbecue. Don't be shy—join thousands of curbside dining families downing tasty ribs, chicken, or beef tri-tip sandwiches. Fantastic people-watching, too!

California Polytechnic State University (Cal Poly)
About 2 miles north of downtown via Santa Rosa Street and Highland Drive; (805) 756–1111 or (805) 756–5734; www.calpoly.edu. Call for general information and to ask about guided inner-campus tours.

Located on more than 6,000 acres at the base of the Santa Lucia Mountain range, Cal Poly is renowned for its agribusiness department and the West's largest schools of engineering and architecture. Visitors and families are always welcome. Hike into Poly Canyon to see experimental architecture and construction or visit the Leaning Pine Arboretum or the Shakespeare Press Museum. Kids of all ages will want to check out the Dairy Unit, where you can buy fresh-made ice cream and other dairy products at the campus store. Yum!

Where to Eat and Stay

Apple Farm Mill House, Restaurant and Inn, 2015 Monterey Street at U.S. Highway 101, just outside downtown San Luis Obispo; (805) 544–2040 or (800) 374–3705 for reservations and **free** video tour; www.applefarm.com. An authentic working gristmill set among gardens and waterfalls. The kids will love watching, and then eating, the results of an intricate series of pulleys, shafts, gears, and water producing fresh apple cider and even ice cream! A family restaurant here serves American favorites. The sixty-nine-unit motor inn is a fun place to stay, too, with rooms that feature early American decor and furnishings. Children younger than 18 stay **free**. $$$

Mission Grill, 1023 Chorro Street; (805) 547–5544. Open daily for lunch, dinner, and Sunday brunch. Early-bird specials. Delicious steak, seafood, and pastas and tasty California cuisine for everyone. Excellent downtown location, indoor and outdoor patio dining overlooking the creek and mission. $$

Madonna Inn, Roadside just south of downtown at U.S. Highway 101 and Madonna Road, San Luis Obispo; (805) 543–3000 or (800) 543–9666; www.madonnainn.com. Not named after the provocative entertainer, this nonetheless hard-to-miss pink-and-white inn was built in 1958 by Alex and Phyllis Madonna. Each of the 109 guest rooms is wackily different. The Caveman Room was carved out of solid rock, for heaven's sake. The men's restroom is world famous for its imaginative waterfalls. The kids will definitely want to check this out! Enjoy freshly baked treats from the Pastry Shop adjoining the Copper Café. The Gold Rush Steak House is over the top in its pink decor (and its prices, too) for basic American fare. Stay if you dare but eat elsewhere. $$$

Pismo Beach Area

The Pismo Beach coastal resort area is actually comprised of the neighboring communities of Oceano, Grover Beach, Pismo Beach, Shell Beach, Avila Beach, and Port San Luis. The area stretches along U.S. Highway 101 and is only ten minutes south of the city of San Luis Obispo. Don't miss the Pismo Monarch Butterfly Grove, where these beautiful creatures congregate each winter (www.monarchbutterfly.org). Tide-pooling is a great family activity at low tide; you never know what marine life or artifact you may find. Outdoor recreation is prime here, including such exciting activities as kite surfing, horseback riding, paragliding, airplane and helicopter rides, and Hummer dune tours.

Oceano Dunes State Vehicular Recreation Area

Call (805) 473–7223 or (800) 444–7275 or visit www.ohv.parks.ca.gov for complete details and entrance fees.

Formerly Pismo Dunes State Vehicular Recreation Area, this is a geologically unique sand-dune complex that is an impressive off-highway vehicular (OHV) playground that also offers activities such as swimming, surfing, fishing, camping, and hiking. Children younger than age eighteen must be accompanied by an adult or take a two-hour state certification safety test to pilot their own buggy.

B.J.'s ATV Rentals

197 Grand Avenue, Grover Beach; (805) 481–5411; www.bjsatvrentals.com. Cost per ATV starting at $40 per hour for adults. Children's machines also available.

The best place to rent your dream machine, with more than 200 to choose from. The staff is really helpful and concerned with your safety.

Clamming

Many families come to Pismo in search of the clams that made it famous around the turn of the last century. It is still known as the Clam Capital of the World. Minus tides are the best for clam digging; the limit is ten, each at least 4.5 inches in diameter. A California state fishing license is required to "catch" this bounty, however. Contact the Chamber of Commerce for current license vendors and more information.

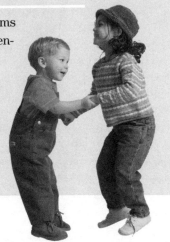

Pismo Pier

In the heart of downtown.

This 1,200-foot pier reopened in 1986. Headquarters for annual celebrations such as the July 4th Fireworks, Clam Festival (October), and Holiday Tree Lighting. Great for strolling or fishing, but beware of nippy winter winds. Or rent some poles and try to catch your family dinner of perch or bass.

Port San Luis

At the very end of Avila Beach Road; (805) 595–5400.

This is a bustling fishing pier and commercial marina. Don't miss the chance to stroll down Harford Pier to find the **free** marine touch tank and look into a fish-processing plant. You'll be amazed how fast sea creatures are transformed into seafood. Tons of salmon, crab, albacore, halibut, cod, shark, and swordfish are brought in here every year by approximately seventy commercial fishing vessels.

Great American Melodrama and Vaudeville Theatre

1863 Front Street (State Route 1), Oceano; (805) 489–2499 for schedule and ticket prices; www.americanmelodrama.com.

Enjoy side-splitting comedy and family entertainment. Don't be put off by the industrial surroundings. Once inside this 260-seat old-fashioned cabaret-style hall, complete with sawdust on the floor, you'll feel completely at home. The theater is owned and operated by Lynn Schlenker and her family. The actors and actresses do triple duty—they serve you food and drinks before they perform, then act on stage, and finally they fraternize with you and other audience members after the show. The best time to attend is definitely during the December holiday season for *A Christmas Carol and Vaudeville Revue*.

Where to Eat

F. McLintock's Saloon & Dining House, 750 Mattie Road, off U.S. Highway 101 between Spyglass Drive and Price Street exits, Pismo Beach; (805) 773–1892; www.mclintocks.com. No visit to this area would be complete without enjoying dinner at this joint. It's easy to avoid the saloon and slip right into the dining rooms (voted as having the best kids' menu in SLO County), where servers will amaze you with their fun attitudes and ability to pour water. (Don't ask, just go and experience this!) The onion rings are a personal favorite, especially dipped in homemade salsa. Open for dinner daily. $$$

Where to Stay

Cottage Inn by the Sea, 2351 Price Street, Pismo Beach; (805) 773–4617 or (888) 440–8400; www.cottageinn.com. The inn has seventy-nine units, all with gas fireplaces, many with ocean views and kitchenettes. You'll also enjoy charming English thatched-roof architecture with all modern amenities, plus **free** deluxe continental breakfast. There's an ocean-view pool and spa, plus beachside access down the cliff stairs. The inn is very friendly to families, with a welcoming staff. Call for specials and package plans. $$$

Spyglass Inn & Restaurant, 2705 Spyglass Drive, Pismo Beach, adjacent to U.S. Highway 101–Pacific Coast Highway 1, between Spyglass and Price Street exits. (805) 773–1892 or (800) 824–2612; www.spyglassinn.com. Located on the cliffs overlooking the Pacific Ocean, this nautical-themed eighty-two-room property is a super family value. Be sure to inquire about seasonal packages and specials. Guest rooms are spacious and many have ocean views. The heated pool and whirlpool make a relaxing destination after a day of "doing the coast." The Spyglass Restaurant, with its outdoor terraced decks, provides stunning ocean views and serves traditional American breakfast, lunch, and dinner daily—at prices that won't shock your wallet. Highly recommended. $$

For More Information

Pismo Beach Chamber of Commerce. 581 Dolliver Street, 93449; (805) 773–4382 or (800) 443–7778; www.pismochamber .com.

Pismo Beach Conference and Visitors Bureau. 760 Mattie Road, 93449; (805) 773–7034 or (800) 443–7778; www.Classic California.com.

Arroyo Grande

"Wide gulch or streambed" is an English translation of this village's Spanish moniker. Founded in 1862, "A-roy-o Grahn-day" was settled in a wide fertile valley on either side of a creek that flows from the Santa Lucia Mountains to the Pacific Ocean. Branch Street is the main thoroughfare, one-quarter mile east off Highway 101. Many of the nineteenth-century buildings, like the Methodist Church, have been restored, and several have been

turned into bed-and-breakfast inns, shops, and restaurants. Access www.arroyograndecc
.com for information on the annual Strawberry Festival (Memorial Day weekend) and
events at the Clark Center for Performing Arts.

Doc Burnstein's Ice Cream Lab

**114 West Branch Street, downtown; (805) 474–4068; www.docburnsteins.com.
Open daily. $**

Famous countywide. Yum! Plus, the trains and toys alone in this old-fashioned ice-cream
parlor are worthy of a stop.

Mustang Water Slides and
Lopez Lake Recreational Area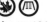

**Outside Arroyo Grande, only 15 minutes off U.S. Highway 101 via Branch Street; (805)
489–8898 or (805) 788–2381 for directions and operating hours; www.slocountyparks.org/
activities/lopez.htm. Open daily.**

There is camping, fishing, picnicking, waterskiing, and windsurfing (this is the favorite local
place) year-round at Lopez Lake with 22 miles of shoreline. The waterslide is open from
May through August. A refreshing good time!

Santa Barbara County

What do space rocket launchers, lemons, avocados, strawberries, Danish pastries, and tri-
tip barbecue have in common? They all are produced in the richly varied domain known as
Santa Barbara County, named after the patron saint of mariners and travelers. With such a
blessing, no wonder people from around the world are drawn here to visit and experience
the joys of life. Santa Barbara County's Pacific sea breezes mean warm days and cooler
nights both along the coast and in the interior valleys. The
average annual temperature in Santa Barbara County is a
mild sixty-two degrees. Very seldom do temperatures drop
below forty in the winter or climb above ninety in the summer.
Such great weather makes visitors as well as plants happy.

The region's colonial history began when Portuguese explorer
Juan Rodriguez Cabrillo sailed along the California coast in 1542 and
claimed everything he saw for the Spanish crown. Sixty years later,
another Portuguese seafarer, Sebastian Viscaino, dropped anchor in the
bay. The day was December 4, the feast day of Saint Barbara, which explains
the name given to the area. Both explorers were greeted warmly by the
native Chumash Indians, who for 10,000 years or so had thrived in the area's
gorgeous climate and year-round growing season. Viscaino's diary records
the first evidence of the vaunted and legendary Santa Barbara hospitality.
Today you can still experience the same warm welcome here with your family.
Start at the Santa Maria River. Here's what you will discover.

Santa Maria

Heading south from San Luis Obispo County on U.S. Highway 101, you will cross into the Santa Maria Valley and find gentle foothills that descend toward the city of Santa Maria. It is surrounded by well-tended farms, where yummy you-can-pick-them strawberries and lots of produce are cultivated. Many award-winning vineyards and wineries are also located here; growers have discovered a micro-climate very similar to that in France. The town's roots are very deep in agriculture and ranching. The twenty-first century has seen dramatic growth in housing and retail shopping.

Santa Maria Valley Discovery Museum

321 Town Center West (located in Mervyn's Shopping Center); Santa Maria; (805) 928–8414; www.smvdiscoverymuseum.org. Open Tuesday through Saturday. Call for seasonal times and fees. $

More than thirty-five activities with eleven permanent exhibits and many rotating displays means you'll always find something fun for kids of all ages. Baby Space stimulates ages eight months to two years with colors, textures, shapes, mirrors, and sounds. In Toddler Territory, ages three to five pretend to be camping, enjoying the faux swimming hole, campfire, lean-to with picnic table, felt storyboard, and puppet theater. Check out the largest exhibit, SEA IT aboard the SS *Discovery*; straddle a life-size John Deere tractor at Ag in the Valley; take a gander at the exotic arthropods in the Bug Zoo; or crawl through the Ocean Tunnel.

Santa Maria Museum of Flight

3015 Airpark Drive; (805) 922–8758; www.smmof.org. Open Friday through Sunday 10:00 A.M. to 4:00 P.M. $

Aviators and wannabe pilots need to gear up for a visit to this exhibit, located next to the (SMX) city airport within two historic hangars. You can see the Fleet Model 2 and Stinson V77-Reliant airplanes, an extensive collection of model planes, and the once-secret Norden bombsight and its accessories.

The History of **Santa Maria–Style Barbecue**

The region's ranching heritage is most evident in the continuing tradition of Santa Maria–style barbecue. This cooking style dates from the Spanish vaquero (cowboy) days, when a special cut of beef was butchered, marinated, and slow cooked over red-hot oak wood. This triangular cut of sirloin, the "tri-tip," is served with special Santa Maria Valley–grown pinquito beans, garden fresh tossed salad, toasted French bread, and spicy salsa. You can find tri-tips sizzling most every weekend in barbecue pits on downtown street corners or marketplaces, presided over by cooks who are generally raising money for local service clubs.

Santa Maria Speedway

One-third mile north of U.S. Highway 101/State Highway 166, Bakersfield exit to Hulton Road; (805) 466–4462 or (805) 922–2233; www.santamariaspeedway.com.

Take your family to the stock-car races in a natural amphitheater surrounded by eucalyptus trees. Every Saturday night April through October. Dedicated family section with no smoking or alcohol allowed. $$

Waller County Park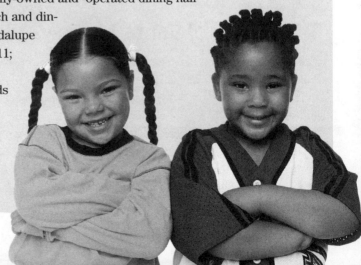

300 Goodwin Road, Orcutt Expressway and Waller Lane; (805) 934–6211 or (805) 937–1302. Open daily.

One hundred-acre park with lake, fountains, a waterfall, fishing, playgrounds, baseball diamonds, and, most important for kids, pony rides. Call for schedule and fees.

Guadalupe **Dunes**

Head 9 miles west out of Santa Maria to the end of State Route 166, and your kids will think you've landed in the Sahara Desert by the Sea—officially known as the **Guadalupe-Nipomo Dunes Preserve.** Up to 500-foot sand dunes stretch for 18 miles along the Pacific Ocean here. More than 1,400 species of animals, including 200 kinds of birds, and 244 species of plants migrate or live in this undisturbed, windswept landscape. To fully appreciate this magnificent work of nature, make your first stop at the **Dunes Visitor Center,** located in a restored Victorian house in downtown Guadalupe at 1055 Guadalupe Street; (805) 343–2455; www.dunescenter.org. This wonderful, family-oriented facility provides entertaining interactive exhibits on dune mammals, birds, plants, and history. (Did you know that Cecile B. DeMille's 1923 film set of *The Ten Commandments* is buried underneath these dunes?) Free maps and tour programs are provided. If hunger strikes, mosey into the **Far Western,** a family-owned and -operated dining hall serving families lunch and dinner daily at 899 Guadalupe Street; (805) 343–2211; www.farwestern tavern.com. Your kids will groove on the rawhide booths and ranching artifacts while you savor the excellent steaks.

YMCA Skateboard Park

3400 Skyway Drive, Santa Maria; (805) 937–8521. Call for fees and operating hours.

Located adjacent to the YMCA facility, this 15,000-square-foot park contains numerous ramps, including quarter pipes, half pipes, boxes, rails, jumps, hills, and a vertical ramp. A special area for beginners is available.

Where to Eat and Stay

Klondike Pizza, 2059 South Broadway, Santa Maria; (805) 348–3667. Open daily from 11:00 A.M. Total family-fun food— pizza, burgers, salads—and **free** roasted peanuts in shells that you're encouraged to throw on the floor. $

Historic Santa Maria Inn, 801 South Broadway, exit Main Street west off U.S. Highway 101, then south on Broadway, Santa Maria; (805) 928–7777. Near Santa Maria Town Center Mall shopping and area attractions, this English-style country inn was built in 1917 and has expanded over the years to include a restaurant serving lunch and dinner, a wine cellar, a gift shop, and newer tower suites for a total of 166 units. Be sure to inquire for current family package plans and special deals. A good choice for value in the area. $$$

For More Information

Santa Maria Valley Chamber of Commerce and Visitor & Convention Bureau. 614 South Broadway, 93454; (805) 925–2403 or (800) 331–3779; www.santamaria.com.

Lompoc Valley

Say Lompoc (Lahm-poke) with me now, and then your entire family can start saying "oooh" and "aahhh" if you visit during the summer, when awesome fields of flowers bloom practically everywhere you gaze. Lompoc is a Chumash Indian word meaning "little lake" or "lagoon." More than 58,000 people call this beautiful valley home now, including the military personnel at Vandenberg Air Force Base. Don't miss the more than sixty murals throughout the city. (Contact the Chamber of Commerce for a map.)

Lompoc Flower Fields

Downtown Lompoc at the corner of Ocean Avenue and C Street; as well as along State Route 246, State Route 1, and Sweeney Road.

This valley produces a good part of the world's flower seeds. More than 1,000 acres are covered with more than 200 varieties of flowers, including marigolds, asters, larkspur, calendula, lavender, and cornflowers. To help "blooming idiots" identify these gems, there is a helpful, fully labeled display garden. The Lompoc Flower Festival is held every June to celebrate this incredible presentation of nature (www.flowerfestival.org).

Lasso-ed into **Los Alamos**

As you travel U.S. Highway 101, midway between San Luis Obispo and Santa Barbara, you'll discover a genuine western town worth your family's visit. Now inhabited by about 1,200 friendly folks, Los Alamos (Spanish for "the cottonwoods") was founded by ranchers in 1876 and became a popular stage-coach and railroad stop—its appearance hasn't changed much since. (Yes, the town still sports two saloons and now two wine-tasting rooms!) For accommodations, check into the hillside **Skyview Motel,** with stunning 360-degree valley views, (805) 344–3770, or the quaint **Alamo Motel** (805–344–2852). The historic 1880 Union Hotel is open only for special events. For foodstuffs, check out the Quakenbush Cafe and Art Gallery, the Twin Oaks Restaurant, or Javy's Mexican Cafe, all on the main drag, Bell Street. Don't miss the antiques stores and the Depot Mall Antique Center in the old railroad station. The town honors its heritage during the last weekend of September with an annual Old Days Celebration. Here's to living history! See www.LosAlamos Info.com.

La Purisima Mission State Historic Park

Three miles northeast of State Route 246 at 2295 Purisima Road; (805) 773–3713; www.lapurisimamission.org. $

See the Americanos' complete and authentic restoration of this important mission back to the way it was in the 1800s. The primitive but effective water system has also been restored and will give kids a fresh appreciation for running *agua.* There are gardens, hiking trails, and picnic facilities. Some scenes from the movie *Seabiscuit* were filmed here in 2003.

Vandenberg Air Force Base (ages 10 and up)

Public Affairs Office, 747 Nebraska Avenue, Room #A103, VAFB, 93437; (805) 606–3595; www.vandenberg.af.mil.

This base, begun in 1941, is located on the outskirts of Lompoc on 99,000 acres of incredibly beautiful Pacific oceanfront property that also includes an ecological preserve. This is the home of the U.S. military's West Coast Space Operations, including research and development. Fully guided base tours may be available. Call for current schedule and details.

For More Information

Lompoc Valley Chamber of Commerce and Visitors Bureau. 111 South I ("Eye") Street, 93436; (805) 736–4567 or (800) 240–0999; www.lompoc.com.

The Santa Ynez Valley

South of Santa Maria on U.S. Highway 101, bordered by the Santa Ynez and San Rafael mountains, lies the Santa Ynez Valley. Many families bypass this magnificent triangle bisected by State Routes 154 and 246, home of more than sixty award-winning wineries and vineyards. Don't you dare miss these five towns that are only forty-five minutes inland from the coastal city of Santa Barbara yet feel like a world away: **Buellton**—home of the original Pea Soup Andersen's Restaurant, the commercial gateway to the valley; **Ballard**—with its continuously operating one-room school; **Los Olivos**—where the movie *Return to Mayberry* was filmed and many artists and galleries reside; **Santa Ynez** itself—a thoroughly western burg; and the largest town of **Solvang**—truly another world, it is Southern California's little bit of Denmark. As the locals say, "Velkommen!"

Solvang means "sunny fields" in Danish. You and your family will find plenty of sunny hospitality in this beautiful village, where the spirit of the founding Danes lives on. Visualize windmills, thatched-roof cottages with dormers and gables, fresh Danish pastries, groaning smorgasbords, kitschy trinket shops, friendly folks, comfortable lodging, and lots of sunshine. More than 300 stores in downtown Solvang will tempt you to open your wallet. You may become laden with goodies, including porcelain figurines, handmade lace, music boxes, jewelry, sweaters, candies, and western wear.

The Honen

Copenhagen Drive near First Street; (805) 686–0022. Daily operations in summer, seasonally on weekends and holidays. $

Turn-of-the-last-century Copenhagen streetcar is pulled by two Belgian draft horses. Twenty-minute ride around town originates from the Solvang Visitor Center.

Hans Christian Andersen Museum

1680 Mission Drive in the Book Loft building; (805) 688–2052. Free.

Andersen was the Danish father of the modern fairy tale. See his books, sketches, paper cutouts, and collages.

Elverhoj Danish Heritage and Fine Arts Museum

1624 Elverhoj Way; (805) 686–1211; www.elverhoj.org. Open Wednesday through Sunday. Free.

Located on a residential street, this attraction lets you discover the origins of Solvang's fascinating history and Danish legacy.

Mission Santa Ines

1760 Mission Drive, right near the village center; (805) 688–4815; www.missionsanta ines.org. $

Number nineteen in the chain of twenty-one missions along the coast. Dedicated in 1804, Mission Santa Ines continues to hold services as well as to provide a museum for original

Indian paintings, seventeenth-century European artworks, and religious vestments. The mission also houses a serene meditation garden in a quadrangle inside the walls. A perfect escape if your family is overdosing on Danish.

Pacific Conservatory of the Performing Arts (PCPA)
In Solvang's outdoor Festival Theater at 420 Second Street; (805) 922–8313 or (800) 549–7272 for tickets and schedules; www.pcpa.org. Open June through October.

Stages world-class Theater Under the Stars, a Santa Barbara County family tradition. Don't miss out on the experience during your visit!

Danish **Food**

No visit to Solvang would be complete without tasting *aebleskivers*—the raspberry-jam-draped, powdered-sugar-coated Danish pancake balls sold throughout the village. This Danish version of the donut is made with a special flour in a unique round cast-iron pan and is definitely delicious. Be on the lookout for *frikadeller* (meat balls), *medisterpoise* (sausages), and *rodkaal* (red cabbage).

Windhaven Glider Rides
Santa Ynez Valley Airport, off State Route 246, near intersection of State Route 154; (805) 688–2517; www.gliderrides.com. Open Wednesday through Sunday for glider plane flights, weather permitting. Reservations highly recommended. Call for fares.

Two-seater planes flown by FAA-certified commercial pilots at approximately 2,500 feet and, pardon the pun, up from there! An incredible experience for older children to share with the folks.

Nojoqui Falls County Park
Seven miles southwest of Solvang on Alisal Road; (805) 934–6123. Open daily 8:00 A.M. to dusk. Free.

This 182-acre site is worth a visit to see the 164-foot waterfall (after a rainy season, of course). Head for the waterfall on the well-marked trail. Plenty of picnic spots, barbecue grills, a playground, and places to savor your Danish treats.

Quicksilver Miniature Horse Ranch
Just east of Solvang on Alamo Pintado Road; (805) 686–4002. Open daily except Thanksgiving and Christmas from 10:00 A.M. to 3:00 P.M. Free.

Has everything from 18-inch newborns to 34-inch mature animals that will be sure to amaze and delight everyone.

Ostrich Land

610 East Highway 246 between Buellton and Solvang; (805) 686–9696; www.ostrich land.com. Open every day. **Free** tours.

This ranch is home to hundreds of the biggest birds in the world, reaching 8.5 feet in height and weighing up to 350 pounds when mature. Impress your children with the fun fact that ostriches run faster than any two-legged animal. How fast? Up to 45 miles per hour!

Santa Ynez Valley Historical Museum and
Parks-Janeway Carriage House

3596 Sagunto Street, downtown Santa Ynez; (805) 688–7889. Open Tuesday through Sunday, closed most major holidays. **Free.** Donations welcome.

You can relive the valley's Old West origins with vehicles, including a full-size, outfitted covered wagon, phaetons, donkey carts, and a stagecoach. Don't miss the farm machinery, implements, saddle collection, and works by famed silversmith Edward Bohlin.

Wining and **Picnicking**

The Santa Ynez Valley is the premier, award-winning wine region of Southern California and home to more than sixty wineries, vineyards, and tasting rooms. Older children may be fascinated by the rituals of grape growing, harvesting, and wine making, but they will have to wait until they are twenty-one to do more than sniff the bouquet. Many vineyards and wineries have lovely picnic areas that make delightful lunch spots for the entire family year-round. Contact the Santa Barbara County Vintners Association at (800) 218–0881 or www.sbcounty wines.com for a **free** map and more information.

Cachuma Lake Recreation Area

Twenty minutes outside Solvang, 18 miles northwest along Scenic State Route 154 over the San Marcos Pass from Santa Barbara; (805) 686–5054; www.sbparks.org/docs/ cachuma.html. $$

This human-made lake (pronounced Ka-choo-ma) takes its name from a nearby ancient Chumash village. The reservoir has a dual purpose as Santa Barbara's water supply, but it is more famous as the winter home of hundreds of bald eagles. The eagle cruises, aboard comfortable pontoon (patio) boats, bring you and your "eagle-eyed" children within 200 yards of the birds' roosting sites. More than 275 other species of birds have been identified on the lake, plus plenty of fish, other wildlife, trees, and plants. Call for schedule and fees.

Forty-two miles of shoreline offer 550 regular campsites and 90 EWS hookups on a first-come, first-served basis. There are hiking, fishing, boating, and other facilities galore, including a general store, Laundromat, snack bar, marina, picnic areas, and barbecues for daytime use year-round. Check out the new yurt camping option. A cross between a tepee and a tent, yurts are on platforms, sleep five to six people, and have gorgeous lake views.

Horsing Around **the Valley**

The Valley is well known throughout the equestrian world for its thorough-bred, Arabian, and Icelandic horse ranches and training and breeding facilities. For periodic shows and events, contact the Santa Ynez Valley Equestrian Association at (805) 688–2224 (ask for Lucy McCarthy) or visit www.syvea.org.

If your family is hankering to ride, check out **Rancho Oso Guest Ranch & Stables,** off Highway 154 and Paradise Road; (805) 683–5110; www.rancho-oso.com. Offering guided train rides to children ages eight and older, camping in covered wagons, cabins, and backcountry grub. Another option is **Circle Bar B Stables and Guest Ranch,** off U.S. Highway 101 at Refugio Road; (805) 968–3901; www.circlebarb.com. Trail rides near President Reagan's former ranch overlooking the Pacific plus lodge, cabins, and dinner theater.

Where to Eat

Cold Spring Tavern, 5995 Stagecoach Road, one-half mile off State Route 154, approximately thirty minutes from Solvang and twenty minutes from Santa Barbara; (805) 967–0066. Make a detour as you go over the San Marcos Pass upon leaving the Santa Ynez Valley and wet your whistle like horse-drawn passengers on the stage-coaches of yesteryear did. Since the 1880s, this historic spot has been serving lunch and dinner and libations daily. Hearty country breakfast on Saturday and Sunday. Kids will love the rustic walls, stone floors, and chance to eat buffalo burgers and venison stew. The tavern is family owned and operated. $$$

Pea Soup Andersen's Restaurant and Motor Inn, 1 block west of junction U.S. Highway 101 and Highway 246 in Buellton; (805) 688–5581. Open from 6:30 A.M. to 10:30 P.M. every day. Home of the original (1924) restaurant serving hearty, bottom-less bowls of split pea soup and other family favorites. This is one of our family's traditional stopovers, no matter what the occasion. The inn has ninety-seven rooms around an attractive central courtyard with a pool, spa, and putting green. Good value for a roadside stopover. $$

Where to Stay

Alisal Guest Ranch and Resort, Two minutes outside the village of Solvang at 1054 Alisal Road; (805) 688–6411 or (800) 4A–ALISAL; www.alisal.com. Rates include dinner and full American breakfast served in the homey Ranch Room. This is a truly one-of-a-kind family-owned and -operated haven after "doing Danish" all day. The resort boasts seventy-three family bungalows with wood-burning fireplaces and no television or telephones in your room. The peace of this 10,000-acre working ranch envelops you immediately upon driving up the tree-lined lane.

Organized family activities and supervised play are featured all summer long. Year-round, you and yours can swim, spa, take in a movie, read in the library, play on one of the Alisal's two golf courses, try your hand at tennis, go horseback riding, or spend a day at Alisal's private 90-acre spring-fed lake for fishing, swimming, canoeing, and sailing.

A two-night minimum stay is required—and worth every moment! Be sure to call for special seasonal packages. Since 1946 the Alisal has been welcoming generations of families with its western hospitality and charm. We recommend you consider starting a family tradition of your own here. $$$$

For More Information

Buellton Visitors Bureau & Chamber of Commerce. 376 Avenue of the Flags, 93427; (805) 688–STAY or (800) 324–3800; www.buellton.org.

Los Olivos Business Organization. Box 280, Los Olivos, 93441; (805) 688–1222; www.losolivosca.com.

Santa Ynez Valley Visitors Association. Box 1918, Santa Ynez, 93460; (800) 742–2843; www.syvva.com.

Solvang Conference & Visitors Bureau. 1511 Mission Drive, 93464; (805) 688–6144 or (800) 468–6765; www .solvangusa.com.

Santa Barbara

If you and the kids want outdoor recreation, nature, scenery, stars, shopping, history lessons, museums, art, culture, great restaurants, and trendy places to hang out, just make your plans for the destination resort of Santa Barbara, the "American Riviera." The city of Santa Barbara was first hailed as a prime tourist stop in 1872 by East Coast travel writer Charles Nordhoff, who said, "Santa Barbara certainly is the most pleasant place throughout the state." The blend of Chumash, Spanish, Mexican, and American cultures has given Santa Barbara an extremely rich heritage—which is visible in the city's lovely buildings with red-tiled roofs and whitewashed adobe walls. Devastated by an earthquake in 1925, downtown Santa Barbara was rebuilt in a Spanish-Moorish colonial motif that is strictly regulated by law.

Along with architecture, locals are proud of their area's well-preserved natural beauty, bounded by the Santa Ynez Mountains and Pacific Ocean to the south. Yes, that's right. All the beaches face south along the Pacific (the only place in the United States where this happens), so when you want to check out the magnificent sunsets, you must look over the mountains behind you, not over the water. This takes some getting used to, so you just might have to stay an extra night to see it again!

Mission Santa Barbara 🏛

2201 Laguna Street, at the corner of Laguna and East Los Olivos Streets, approximately five minutes from downtown; (805) 682–4149; www.sbmission.org. Open daily from 9:00 A.M. to 5:00 P.M. except Easter, Thanksgiving, and Christmas. $

You will definitely want to tour "the Queen of the Missions" and still the longest continuously operating parish among California's renowned chain of twenty-one missions. Founded on December 4, 1786, the feast day of Saint Barbara, and finally completed in 1820, it is one of the best-preserved missions. A fascinating self-guided walking tour that includes artworks, fountains, a courtyard, and a cemetery is recommended.

Santa Barbara Museum of Natural History and Planetarium

2559 Puesta del Sol Road (just around the corner from the Santa Barbara Mission); (805) 682–4711; www.sbnature.org. Open daily (except major holidays). $$. Free to all on the last Sunday of every month.

The museum has exhibits on early Native American tribes as well as animals, birds, insects, plants, minerals, marine science, and geology. The planetarium hosts impressive star shows. Call (805) 682–3224 for a schedule.

Special **Santa Barbara Festivals**

Festivals and celebrations abound in the city of Santa Barbara year-round. Oak Park, on the city's north side, hosts ethnic and cultural festivals in the spring and summer. However, the following two events are worth a special visit for your entire family, from toddler to grandparent.

Summer Solstice Celebration. This is a fantasy fun romp celebrating the arrival of summer on the Saturday closest to the first day of summer. The parade features no motorized floats or amplified music, but almost one hundred "non-floats," including bands, clowns, dancers, and perhaps a rubber sea of sharks, rolling bubble machines, or even a briefcase brigade of lawyers. A different theme is carried out each year. After the parade up State Street from the waterfront, the participants and spectators all congregate at Alameda Park at the corner of Sola and Anacapa Streets. You will love the energy, color, food booths, and vendors at this afternoon, post-parade party. The day concludes with a musical and dramatic program on a stage set up at the Courthouse Sunken Gardens at nightfall. For more information and a detailed schedule of events, call (805) 965–3396; www.solsticeparade.com.

Old Spanish Days (Fiesta). If you visit during the first weekend of August, experience the sights, sounds, and foods of California's early settlers during Old Spanish Days. Commonly known as Fiesta, the celebrations begin with the padre's blessing on the steps of the historic mission on Wednesday evening, followed by performances by the junior (younger than age twelve) and senior (younger than age eighteen) Spirit of Fiesta Dancers. Your family will shout "Viva la Fiesta!" along with the natives during Friday's Annual El Desfile Historico—one of the world's most colorful parades, attracting the most horses and riders in America along with 100,000 enthusiastic spectators.

Your kids can participate in El Desfile de Los Ninos (the Children's Parade) on Saturday morning. During the five-day festival, the entire family can enjoy the *mercados* (marketplaces with traditional foods), carnival rides at the beach, and the family entertainment spectacular, Noches de Ronda, each evening under the stars in the gardens of the courthouse. Call (805) 962–8101 year-round for **free** brochures and schedules; www.oldspanish days-fiesta.org.

Santa Barbara Botanic Garden

1212 Mission Canyon Road, just above the Natural History Museum, about 2 miles into Mission Canyon; (805) 682–4726; www.sbbg.org. Open daily; call for seasonal hours and special exhibits. $

Kids will love exploring the 5 miles of trails through forests and plant life on 65 exquisite acres devoted only to California species. Self-guided and guided tours available daily.

Santa Barbara Historical Museum and Covarrubias Adobe

136 East de la Guerra Street, downtown; (805) 966–1601; www.santabarbaramuseum.com. Open Tuesday through Saturday 10:00 A.M. to 5:00 P.M. **Free.** Donations appreciated.

The Santa Barbara Historical Museum's permanent exhibits include documents, furniture, decorative and fine arts, and costumes from all periods of the area's history. Covarrubias Adobe, circa 1817, may have served briefly as the headquarters of Pio Pico, the last Mexican governor of California.

El Presidio de Santa Barbara State Historic Park

100–200 blocks of East Canon Perdido Street, downtown; (805) 965–0093; www.sbthp.org/presidio.htm. Open daily 10:30 A.M. to 4:30 P.M. except for major holidays. **Free.**

This was the last military outpost built by Spain in the New World, dedicated in 1782. A continuous project restores the actual structures, including El Cuartel, the padre's quarters; the chapel; and the commandant's office. A slide show and guided tours are offered upon request. This is a piece of living history you just can't ignore. Our kids really liked the story of the lost cannon. Ask a docent for the details.

Santa Barbara Museum of Art

1130 State Street; (805) 963–4364; www.sbmuseart.org. Open Tuesday through Saturday 11:00 A.M. to 5:00 P.M., Friday to 9:00 P.M., and Sunday noon to 5:00 P.M. $. Free admission every Sunday.

The museum has important works by American and European artists, including Monet and other impressionists. Displays include American, Asian, and nineteenth-century French art, plus Greek and Roman antiquities and major photographic works. Special exhibits rotate throughout the year. Narrated tours available, usually at 1:00 P.M. The Children's Gallery is outstanding. And don't miss the lovely Cafe and Museum Store.

Karpeles Manuscript Library Museum

21 West Anapamu Street (one-half block off State); (805) 962–5322; www.rain.org/~karpeles/. Open daily 10:00 A.M. to 4:00 P.M. Closed Christmas and New Year's Day. Free.

Houses original manuscripts of great authors, scientists, and leaders from all periods of history, including an original copy of the Declaration of Independence. Rotating exhibits show fascinating glimpses into antiquity.

Book **Zone**

Located along Anapamu Street on opposite sides of State Street, this area is affectionately called "book row." It is anchored by the impressive 225,000-volume Santa Barbara Public Library at 40 East Anapamu; (805) 962–7653. You and your family will discover the joy of finding every type of literature imaginable in the following unique, independent Santa Barbara bookstores. Special events with authors and storytellers abound, so be sure to contact each shop for schedules and hours of operation.

- **Pacific Travellers Supply,** 12 West Anapamu; (805) 963–4438. Guidebooks, maps, and luggage.
- **Metro Comics & Entertainment,** 6 West Anapamu; (805) 963–2168.
- **The Book Den,** 11 East Anapamu; (805) 962–3321. Used, rare, and out-of-print books.
- **Paradise Found,** 17 East Anapamu; (805) 564–3573. Metaphysical books.

Each fall, the **Santa Barbara Book and Author Festival** (805–962–9500; www.sbbookfestival.org) celebrates reading and writing with an inspiring one-day event downtown featuring famous authors, book signings, panels, and awards.

On the **Waterfront**

Stearns Wharf. At the foot of State Street on the waterfront; (805) 564–5518; www.stearnswharf.org. Parking is $2.00 per hour or free with a wharf merchant purchase validation. Built in 1872 to serve cargo and passenger ships, this Santa Barbara historic landmark is now the site of specialty shops, family-friendly restaurants, a small museum, a boat charter dock, and a fishing spot. You can actually drive as well as walk onto the wharf. The kids think it sounds like rumbling thunder when you drive across the wooden planks. Don't worry, it really is quite safe.

Captain Don's Harbor Tours. 219 Stearns Wharf; (805) 969–5217. Call for current schedule and fares. Offers a variety of sunset cruises, coastal excursions year-round, and whale-watching trips in winter.

Santa Barbara Maritime Museum. In the marina, 113 Harbor Way; (805) 962–8404; www.sbmm.org. Open daily 10:00 A.M. to 4:00 P.M. Call for hours and admission fees. Located in the former Naval Reserve Building in the heart of the harbor, the museum illustrates the evolution of nautical technology, starting with local origins in the Chumash culture up to modern-day boats and submarines. Highly interactive exhibits are kid friendly.

Santa Barbara Yacht Harbor, Marina, and Breakwater. West of Stearns Wharf, motor entrance along Cabrillo Boulevard just past Castillo Street intersection. Harbor Master's office phone, (805) 564–5520. More than 1,000 work and pleasure craft rest at Santa Barbara's fascinating yacht harbor and breakwater, home to the city's commercial fishing fleet, which rakes in a catch of more than $6 million annually. Where else can you get "up close and personal" with a spiny sea urchin heading off to market or purchase shrimp, rock cod, and crab fresh from the fisherfolk themselves? Take the older children for a walk along the half-mile breakwater and dodge the incoming surf. Not for the water-timid during high winds or rough seas! Your family's ticket to floating fun can be found right here at the following vendors.

Sea Landing. In the marina; (805) 882–0088; www.condorcruises.com. Call (888) 77–WHALE for current schedules and fares. Hook your own seafood on a fishing expedition charter boat that docks here, or sign up for a dive trip. This is also the home dock of the award-winning *Condor Express*, a 75-foot, 149-passenger high-speed jet-powered catamaran, custom designed and launched in 2002 specifically for naturalist-led whale-watching trips, sunset cruises, and group charters.

Truth Aquatics. In the marina; (805) 962–1127; www.truthaquatics.com. Call for seasonal times, schedules, and fares. Arranges popular sea kayaking, scuba, and diving charters and also acts as official concessionaire for boat trips to the **Channel Islands National Park,** some 20 miles offshore. (See listing in Ventura County section for more details on the park.)

Santa Barbara Sailing Center. In the marina; (805) 962–2826 or (800) 350–9090; www.sbsail.com. Rent a sailboat, there are more than forty to choose from (with or without a skipper). This is the home dock of the *Double Dolphin* catamaran, a forty-nine-passenger sailboat that runs whale-watching trips, sunset cruises, and private charters. The sailing school here offers beginning through advanced instruction. Call about family learn-to-sail packages, including accommodations. How would you like to live aboard a sailboat while learning the ropes and sheets?

Kids World 🛝🏕️
In Alameda Park, at the corner of Micheltorena and Garden Streets, downtown. Free.

Designed by city children and built by them, as well as community volunteers, this two-story wooden playland is truly a kid's dream come to life. A tot lot and sandbox are available for the very young, while older sibs can cruise through tunnels and stride over bridges or clamber up the tree house.

Santa Barbara County Courthouse 🏛️
1100 Anacapa Street, downtown; (805) 962–6464. Open Monday through Friday 8:00 A.M. to 5:00 P.M., Saturday and Sunday 10:00 A.M. to 5:00 P.M. Free.

Most kids would not want to tour a courthouse, except in Santa Barbara, where you can climb the 80-foot clock tower stairs (or take the elevator, for us fogeys) for a stunning panoramic view over the city, all the way to the ocean. The courthouse was built in 1929. You cannot miss the award-winning Spanish-Moorish design from anywhere in the city. Its sunken gardens are perfect for picnicking and are the site of many events during the year, such as Earth Day and Fiesta.

Santa Barbara Zoological Gardens
500 Ninos Drive, 2 blocks from East Beach off Cabrillo Boulevard; (805) 962–5339; www.santabarbarazoo.org. Open daily 10:00 A.M. to 5:00 P.M. except Thanksgiving and Christmas. $$

This is as wild as Santa Barbara gets! The zoo is renowned for its easy accessibility and more than 80 exhibits with 600 child-friendly animals, including big cats, roaring elephants, and gangly giraffes. The huge aviary is a favorite. The zoo, on a former estate overlooking the glittering Pacific, is a must-see. Take a picnic lunch to eat after your morning visit or savor a tasty snack in the **Ridley-Tree House Cafe.** The miniature train that circumnavigates the zoo's beautiful garden setting is a big plus, and so are the dedicated playground and all the services (easy access bathrooms, strollers, guided tours, zoo-camp programs for children, just to name a few).

Chase Palm Park & Carousel

Stretching east from Stearns Wharf along the waterfront on both sides of beachfront Cabrillo Boulevard.

In May 1998, the ten-acre north side of the park opened with a totally festive antique carousel (enclosed in its own pavilion, nominal fee, open daily); a kids-only (toddler through age twelve) Shipwreck Playground with a rubberized deck; grassy knolls and picnic tables; restrooms; a snack bar; and an entertainment zone. "Way cool" characterizes this area—don't miss this park on your tour of the beach area.

The University of California at Santa Barbara (UCSB)

In the neighboring town of Isla Vista, 2 miles south of U.S. Highway 101 via Ward Memorial Boulevard (State Route 217). Free **campus tours; (805) 893–2485; www.ucsb.edu.**

"Take a Vacation **from Your Car!**"

It's easy to do by accessing www.santabaracarfree.org, calling (805) 696–1100, or writing Santa Barbara Car Free Project, Box 60436, Santa Barbara, CA 93160. Discover walking tours, bike maps, bus routes, AMTRAK schedules, free maps, and vacation packages/hotel discounts. **State Street,** Santa Barbara's most famous thoroughfare, begins at the beach and leads into the heart of downtown. It is extremely pedestrian- and family-friendly, with benches, outdoor dining, and plenty of greenery. When you get tired of walking, hop aboard the nifty electric shuttle buses (operated by the Metropolitan Transit District [MTD]; www.sbmtd.gov). Santa Barbara Car Free Project is an award-winning ecotourism partnership sponsored by the County Air Pollution Control District, committed to alternative transportation for cleaner air.

The gorgeous 989-acre, oceanfront campus features the landmark Storke Tower, University Center, and renowned Marine Sciences Institute, home of 18,000 students and 900 faculty, including 5 Nobel Prize winners. During July and August, the UCSB Alumni Association offers the Family Vacation Center, with eight weeklong sessions, providing a fully programmed family resort. Rates include three meals daily, residential-hall living, recreational and social activities, all-day child care, and theme programs. This incredible Santa Barbara family vacation bargain sells out each summer. Visit www.familyvacation center.com or call (805) 893–3123.

South Coast Railroad Museum

300 North Los Carneros Road in adjacent town of Goleta; (805) 964–3540 for track times for the miniature train; www.goletadepot.org. Generally open Wednesday through Sunday. Free.

Budding conductors and engineers will want to explore the wooden Goleta depot. Built in 1901, the depot was in use until 1973, when it was dismantled and moved to its current site. Restoration began in 1981, and the collection of railroad memorabilia continues to grow.

Whale-**Watching**

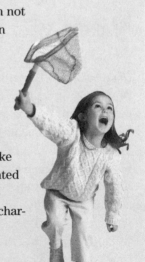

The **Santa Barbara Channel** is becoming well-known not only for the traditional California gray whale migration that occurs annually here between late January and mid-April but also as a year-round whale-viewing and research destination. More than twenty-seven different types of whales inhabit the waters offshore. Blue whales, the largest animals ever to live on earth, have been seen here for the past few summers, apparently feeding on the abundant krill. Humpback whales; minke whales; and orcas, or killer whales, are also often sighted on channel excursions, not to mention porpoises, dolphins, sea lions, and harbor seals. Contact any of the charter boat operators at the harbor or marina for current whale-watching schedules and fees.

Where to Eat

Sambo's on the Beach, 216 West Cabrillo Boulevard, 2 blocks from Stearns Wharf; (805) 965–3269. This is the original and only remaining Sambo's restaurant, founded here in 1957 by two Santa Barbara friends (Sam Battistone and Newall "Bo" Bohnett). Owned and operated by Sam's grandson Chad Stevens, Sambo's dishes up hearty breakfasts featuring its famous pancakes and syrup, and all-American lunches, served seven days a week. $$

Santa Barbara County Certified Farmers Market, (805) 962–5354 for seasonal times; www.sbfarmersmarket.org. The freshest fruits and veggies available. The most popular site is in downtown Santa Barbara every Saturday, at the corner of Cota and Santa Barbara Streets (2 blocks off State) from 8:30 A.M. to 12:30 P.M. Kids will love the musicians, jugglers, and clowns, plus the **free** samples available from generous vendors. Also in Goleta, Carpinteria, and Montecito. $

Woody's Barbecue, 5112 Hollister Avenue, Goleta; (805) 967–3775; www.woodysbbq.com. Dishing up Santa Barbara's favorite barbecue ribs and chicken. Kids' meals start at $2.95, making this a great family value. Don't worry about getting messy—just throw the peanut shells on the floor, slather on the sauce, and clean off in the old bathtub washbasin provided. $

Where to Stay

El Capitan Canyon, 11560 Calle Real, Goleta; (805) 685–3887 or (866) 352–2729; www.elcapitancanyon.com. An ocean-side retreat only 17 miles from downtown Santa Barbara; private, family-owned property on 300 acres featuring cozy cabins and safari-canvas tents. A kids' camp, botanical hikes, massages, swimming pool, campfires, and outdoor summer concerts are highlights, along with bicycling. And it's only a half-mile from the beach for watersports. A grocery store, gift shop, and deli are here, too. Absolutely ideal for families. $$$

Fess Parker's Doubletree Resort, 633 East Cabrillo Boulevard, Santa Barbara; (805) 564–4333 or (800) 879–2929; www.fpdtr.com. Owned in part by local resident Fess Parker (famous for his *Davy Crockett* acting role), this Spanish Mission–style property has all the requirements of a headquarters for your family oceanfront vacation. Located on twenty-three acres across from East Beach, this 360-room resort (Santa Barbara County's largest) has a heated outdoor swimming pool, whirlpool, fitness center, spa, beauty salon, gift shop, putting green, tennis and basketball courts, bicycle and skate rental shop, game room, and full concierge services. Two restaurants and a lounge at the resort include the casual, California cuisine of Cafe Los Arcos for breakfast, lunch, and dinner (best for kids); Rodney's Steakhouse for dinner; and Barra Los Arcos, hosting happy hours and live entertainment (best for adults). Roomy accommodations feature ocean, mountain, or courtyard views—many with patios or decks—great for enjoying the fresh sea breezes. Call for seasonal specials and package plans. $$$$

Upham Hotel & Garden Cottages, 1404 De La Vina Street, just 2 blocks off State Street, downtown; (805) 962–0058 or (800) 727–0876; www.uphamhotel.com. Built in 1871, the Upham is Santa Barbara County's oldest continuously operating hotel. It is located on an acre of eye-catching gardens. You can choose from fifty different Victorian-style rooms or cottages, filled with comfortable, not stuffy antiques. Kids like to play in the garden courtyard, while the older folks enjoy complimentary afternoon wine and cheese. All rates include a deluxe continental all-you-can-eat breakfast buffet, plus Oreo cookies and milk in the evening—a big child pleaser! You can leave your car and walk to all the downtown attractions, or take the electric shuttle bus 14 blocks down to the waterfront. The hotel has always been independently owned and operated and feels like a family home. Call and inquire for special rates and packages. Louie's Restaurant on premises serves lunch weekdays and dinner every night on the veranda. $$$

For More Information

Goleta Valley Chamber of Commerce. 5582 Calle Real, Suite A, Box 781, 93116; (805) 967–4618; www.goletavalley.com.

Santa Barbara Chamber of Commerce Visitor Center. 1 Garden Street at Cabrillo Boulevard, 93101; (805) 965–3021. Walk-up info on the beachfront. Open 364 days per year. www.sbcchamber.org.

Santa Barbara Conference and Visitors Bureau. 1601 Anacapa Street, 93101; (805) 966–9222 or (800) 927–4688 or (800) 676–1266; www.SantabarbaraCa.com.

Summerland

About 5 miles southeast of Santa Barbara is the neighboring antiques, artists', and writers' haven of Summerland. Traveling in either direction along U.S. Highway 101, just exit at the ramp called Summerland and head toward the oceanfront Lookout Park, with its restrooms, volleyball courts, playground, and easy access to a lovely 2-mile stretch of beach. This is the quintessential California beach town, where the 1,200 or so residents enjoy the views from their hillside homes. You and your traveling family can kick back here, too.

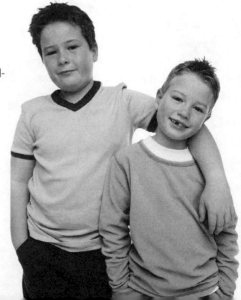

Where to Eat

Big Yellow House Family Restaurant, 108 Pierpont Avenue; (805) 969–4140. Easily visible from U.S. Highway 101, this restored 110-year-old Victorian home has been a roadside landmark since opening as a restaurant in the 1970s. Serving reasonably priced, American fare for breakfast, lunch, and dinner daily, it's popular with locals and visitors for a neighborly, casual atmosphere. Dine in the parlor next to the fireplace or the library upstairs that overlooks the ocean. Don't miss the crispy fried chicken, fresh clam chowder, or a piece of double-chocolate fudge cake. You might be haunted by the house's legendary ghost unless you indulge! $$

Summerland Beach Cafe, 2294 Lillie Avenue; (805) 969–1019. Located in a rambling white clapboard house with a big veranda, this is the place for the best omelets and breakfast fare, as well as lunch, served daily from 7:00 A.M. to 3:00 P.M. The decor is eclectic and sure to hold the family's interest, including some old booths with their own phones. $

Carpinteria

The small seaside community of Carpinteria, about 12 miles southeast of Santa Barbara, down the coast along U.S. Highway 101, was originally a Chumash fishing village and canoe-building spot. It boasts the **Carpinteria State Beach,** aka the "world's safest beach"—a claim justified, perhaps, by a natural reef breakwater that prevents nasty riptides. There are outstanding recreational opportunities and a variety of camping facilities around and inland from the beach. Many flower firms are based here, growing roses, orchids, and mums. Another of Carpinteria's blossoms, a hardy perennial fruit if you will, is celebrated with the popular **California Avocado Festival,** held the first weekend of October downtown on Linden Avenue; www.avofest.com. From April through October, thrill to the sport of kings at the Santa Barbara Polo Club, located in the Carpinteria foothills; www.sbpolo.com.

Carpinteria Valley Historical Society and Museum

956 Maple Avenue; (805) 684–3112; www.carpinteriahistoricalmuseum.org. Open Tuesday through Saturday from 1:00 to 4:00 P.M.; closed holidays. Free; donations welcome.

Check out the valley's heritage from Chumash Indian settlement to today with charming exhibits and knowledgeable docents.

Rincon Point

Just south of Carpinteria along U.S. Highway 101.

At Rincon Point, surfing's legendary mecca, known worldwide as "Queen of the Coast," waves come down the Santa Barbara Channel, hit the corner, and wrap around the shore, creating awesomely "radical" surf, dude! If your kids aren't surfers, they will still enjoy watching the sets and playing along the shore.

Where to Stay

Holiday Inn Express & Suites, 5606 Carpinteria Avenue; (805) 566–9499. This 108-unit property has easy access to U.S. Highway 101, beaches, and local attractions. A nice outdoor pool, a spa, and complimentary continental breakfast buffet are other highlights. Ask about special package rates. $$$

For More Information

Carpinteria Valley Chamber of Commerce. 5285 Carpinteria Avenue, Box 956, 93014; (805) 684–5479 or (800) 563–6900; www.carpchamber.org.

Ventura County

The mighty U.S. Highway 101, known hereabouts as the Ventura Highway (and popularized in the '70s hit song by America), winds south from Santa Barbara County. It is the major artery through such rapidly growing communities as San Buenaventura (Ventura for short), Oxnard, Port Hueneme, Camarillo, Westlake Village, and Thousand Oaks. Exiting this concrete thoroughfare into the interior of Ventura County will reveal such treasures as the artistic and spiritual town of Ojai, rugged Santa Paula, and burgeoning Simi Valley. Embracing its cultural and geographic diversity is a key to enjoying Ventura County. With its mild climate and proximity to Los Angeles, the county offers an affordable getaway less than an hour from the big city. If you have limited time to show your family some California beach living, you can quickly and easily do it in the place Los Angelenos call "up the coast."

Our Fortieth **National Park**

The Channel Islands National Park Visitor Center is located at 1901 Spinnaker Drive in Ventura Harbor Village, (805) 658–5730; www.nps.gov/chis/. It is open daily, except Thanksgiving and Christmas. Less than 20 miles off the coast of Ventura and Santa Barbara Counties, the **Channel Islands National Park** comprises five of the eight offshore Channel Islands: Santa Barbara, Anacapa, Santa Cruz, Santa Rosa, and San Miguel. These islands provide an unparalleled introduction for your family to the flora and fauna of the local marine environment. Nature, unspoiled and unsullied by humans, is the main attraction here; quite frankly, it's the only attraction! Because the balance of nature on these islands and their surrounding waters is so fragile, visitors' activities are strictly regulated. For instance, there are no snack bars or RV campgrounds, and when you tour the area, you must bring (and take back what remains of) your own food, water, and other supplies. Rangers conduct guided hikes on San Miguel and Santa Rosa. Private concessionaires' boats or

Ventura

Wrapped around the east-west ribbons of U.S. Highway 101, the city of Ventura has a historic downtown area that includes the restored Mission San Buenaventura; the Ventura Pier and State Beach, approximately 6 blocks from downtown; and the Ventura Harbor Village, some 2 miles away. Ventura has a population of about 100,000 and is a major agricultural center for citrus and other fruits. Its warm, sunny climate and value-priced accommodations and restaurants make this a very affordable family vacation spot as well as a jumping off point for visiting the Channel Islands National Park.

Ventura Harbor Village

1559 Spinnaker Drive, about 1 mile west of the Harbor Boulevard/Seaward exit from U.S. Highway 101; (805) 644–0169; www.venturaharborvillage.com.

Sailing, fishing, scuba diving, and sightseeing trips can all be arranged at the village. Shops and restaurants abound here, too. Home of the Channel Islands National Park Visitor Center. (See description earlier in this chapter for more information.)

Island Packers Company

1867 Spinnaker Drive, Ventura, adjacent to Channel Islands National Park Visitor Center; (805) 642–1393; www.islandpackers.com.

A tour operator based here since 1968 and offering scheduled charters to all the islands, as well as whale-watching trips and cruises. Call for special packages and itineraries.

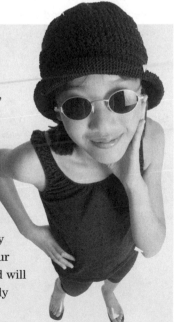

charter craft provide transportation across the channel to specific embarkation points.

The harborside visitor center houses quality exhibits that graphically describe the entire park, including its ecosystem, mammals, and birds. Plus, the center has an indoor tide pool, great for learning about the sea creatures your kids will see en route. There is also a movie and video about the islands shown here. A stairway and elevator lead up to the observation tower that will give you a 360-degree view of the harbor and, on most clear days, all the way to the islands themselves. Taking a day to visit our fortieth national park is well worth the effort and will be a sea journey to another dimension your family won't forget.

Digging into **History**

These three nearby attractions all make for refreshing steps back into early California history. Each is located in downtown Ventura, within easy walking distance, and can be accomplished in a long morning. While you're in the downtown shopping and dining zone, catch some vintage stores and antiques emporiums.

Ventura County Museum of History and Art. 100 East Main Street; (805) 653–0323; www.vcmha.org. Open Tuesday through Sunday 10:00 A.M. to 5:00 P.M. $. Features attractive displays blending local chronicles and illustrations along with the popular George Stuart historical figures, changing exhibits, and a good research library.

Albinger Archaeological Museum. 113 East Main Street; (805) 648–5823. Open Wednesday through Sunday 10:00 A.M. to 4:00 P.M. Free. Museum contains artifacts spanning 3,500 years, all excavated from a single dig site next to the Mission San Buenaventura. Available on request: audiovisual programs describing the labor-intensive process of excavation.

Mission San Buenaventura. 225 East Main Street; (805) 648–4496; www .sanbuenaventuramission.org. Open Monday through Friday 10:00 A.M. to 5:00 P.M., Saturday 9:00 A.M. to 5:00 P.M., and Sunday 10:00 A.M. to 4:00 P.M. $. Founded in 1782 and completed in 1809. The present mission includes a small museum and a restored church that continues to be an active parish.

Skate Street (ages 6 and up)
1954 Goodyear Avenue; (805) 650–1213; www.skatestreet.com.
Open daily (closed major holidays); call for current schedules and special discounts. $$$

One of the newest and most popular indoor skating "theme parks" in Southern California, Skate Street is THE place for in-line, roller, and skateboard enthusiasts. Features include bowls, pipes, half pipes, ramps, and a 12,000-square-foot street course with curbs, benches, planters, and streetlights. (If you have to ask what these features are—you won't enjoy this attraction!) Rental skates, pads, and helmets are available.

Where to Stay

Pierpont Inn & Restaurant, 550 Sanjon Road, adjacent to U.S. Highway 101, northbound exit Sanjon Road, southbound exit Seaward Avenue, Ventura; (805) 643–6144 or (800) 285–4667; www.pierpontinn.com. Children ages twelve and younger stay **free** at this attractive, seventy-two-unit property, established in 1928. Check out the two cottages! Some rooms have fireplaces, and most rooms have ocean views with balconies. Even through you are across the highway from the beach, this property has two heated pools (one indoor). It also has twelve lighted tennis courts and a very friendly, helpful staff. The ocean-view restaurant, Austen's, serves breakfast, lunch, and dinner daily as well as Sunday brunch. $$$$

For More Information

Ventura Convention and Visitors Bureau. 89–C South California Street, 93001; (805) 648–2075 or (800) 333–2989; www.ventura-usa.com.

Ojai

From Ventura, you can take either State Route 150 or State Route 33 inland to reach Ojai, a warm, dry, spiritually inclined artists' colony nestled in a peaceful valley. Say "Oh-high," and you will have mastered the most difficult part of the area. The drive here alone is worth the trip, because of the scenic mountains and lakes. The quaint downtown features **Libbey Park**—home of the annual Bowl Full of Blues concert series and the Ojai Music Festival. The **Ojai Center for the Arts** has displays by California artists and a changing calendar of events. Call (805) 646–1107 for current happenings.

Ojai Valley Museum

130 West Ojai Avenue, located downtown in the historic chapel; (805) 640–1390. Open Wednesday through Friday 1:00 to 4:00 P.M. and Saturday and Sunday 10:00 A.M. to 4:00 P.M. **Free** admission; donations welcome.

Changing exhibits of art, natural history, and local lore. Chumash garden and gift shop provide interesting diversions.

Lake Casitas Recreation Area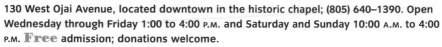

Off State Route 150, approximately 3 miles west of junction of State Route 33, about fifteen minutes from downtown Ojai; (805) 649–2233; www.casitaswater.org. Open year-round for day use during daylight hours. Overnight campsites subject to availability, fees vary.

Set in a valley of its own, this 35-mile-long, irregularly shaped lake is actually a human-made reservoir that provides drinking water for Ventura County. Consequently, there is no swimming in the lake, but the fishing for trout, bass, crappie, and catfish is excellent. Powerboats, canoeing, and sailing are fun here, too, year-round. There is a basic snack bar, small grocery store, boat rental, bait shop, and a large kids' playground. Our advice is to pack a picnic lunch and come kick back here for the day.

Where to Eat

Boccali's, 11675 Santa Paula–Ojai Road, at the corner of Reeves Road; (805) 646–6116. Casual, fun dining inside or outside on the patio. Great pizzas and loads of pastas. Very family oriented, takeout available. Serving dinner seven nights a week and lunch Wednesday through Sunday. $

Where to Stay

Ojai Valley Inn & Spa, 905 Country Club Road, just west of town off State Route 150; (805) 646–5511 or (800) 422–6524; www.ojairesort.com. This magnificent resort nestled in the foothills is a one-stop family fun destination. If you and yours can't find something to keep you happy here, go home! Situated on 220 landscaped acres, the resort offers 207 first-class rooms and suites overlooking gardens, pools, a golf course, and woods. This is the home of the Senior PGA Tour, and the eighteen-hole golf course is very challenging, yet forgiving. Warm up on the putting green, or perhaps try tennis (four courts), horseback riding, a jogging course, hiking, and biking (rentals available). Better yet, let the kids enjoy the petting zoo and incredible supervised children's programs that change with the season. Meanwhile, you can experience the 31,000-square-foot spa facility—featuring a full complement of deluxe services like hydrotherapy, massage, facials, manicures, beauty, toning, aromatherapies, and more. Maravilla Dining Room and Oak Cafe open daily for all meals, but feasting poolside is our favorite. Breakfast buffet ranks right up there, too. Be sure to call for special family packages and rates. A destination resort not to be missed! $$$$

Rose Garden Inn, 615 West Ojai Avenue; (805) 646–1434; www.rosegardeninnofojai.com. A conveniently located, very moderately priced eighteen-unit motel with two spacious cottages. Highlights include lovely gardens, a large swimming pool, a steam sauna room, a whirlpool, and a playground. You'll also enjoy **free** continental breakfast plus **free** popcorn in the evening. Neighborly welcoming staff. $$

For More Information

Ojai Valley Chamber of Commerce and Visitors Bureau. 150 West Ojai Avenue, 93023; (805) 646–8126; www.the-ojai.org.

Santa Paula and Fillmore

Exiting Ventura Highway 101 onto State Route 126 leads you through citrus groves and ranches to the pretty villages of Santa Paula and Fillmore. The **Santa Paula Airport** at Santa Maria and Eighth Streets has an extensive collection of privately owned antique, classic, and homebuilt aircraft. Call the chamber of commerce for a current schedule of tours and air shows.

California Oil Museum of Santa Paula

1001 East Main Street; (805) 933–0076; www.oilmuseum.net. Open Wednesday through Sunday; closed holidays. **Free** admission; donations appreciated.

The museum depicts the history of oil exploration in California through relics, photos, computer games, and videos. Thinking about a career in oil or gas?

Fillmore & Western Railway

Central Park Plaza, downtown Fillmore; (805) 524–2546 or (800) 773–TRAIN; www.fwry.com. Runs Saturday and Sunday, but not major holidays. Times change seasonally. $$$

This antique train offers one-hour scenic sightseeing trips between Fillmore and Santa Paula. Vintage cars include a 1920s Pullman and restored dining, sleeper, and parlor carriages. Train workers dress in period costume. Theme parties and dinners are popular, especially the Christmas tree trains. Call for a current schedule and fares.

For More Information

Santa Paula Chamber of Commerce.
Santa Barbara at 10th Street, 93060; (805) 525–5561; www.santapaulachamber.com.

Fillmore Chamber of Commerce. 275 Central Avenue, 93015; (805) 524–0351; www.fillmorechamber.com.

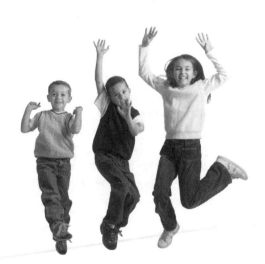

Oxnard

What could you possibly find to do, see, or enjoy in a place with the funny name of Oxnard? The town got its name from entrepreneur Henry T. Oxnard, a visionary who foresaw that the fertile plain just north of the Conejo Hills would be an excellent place to raise sugar beets. In 1899 he built the $2 million American Sugar Beet Company processing plant, which remained in operation until 1959. Legend has it that the all-powerful Henry wanted to name his company town Sakchar—the Greek word for "sugar." Fortunately or not, when the day came in 1903 to register the name with the clerk in the state capital of Sacramento, Henry had a bad phone connection and decided to settle for his surname, Oxnard. Sweet history aside, Oxnard has grown into a culturally and economically diverse community, with business parks, sandy beaches, and a fine marina, just 60 miles north of Los Angeles.

Heritage Square

Downtown at 715 South A Street; (805) 483–7960. Open every day during daylight hours. **Free.**

The square reflects the area's past, with its faithful restoration of a late-1800s church, water tower, pump house, and eleven vintage homes. The buildings were moved from various parts of Oxnard to this single block. Be sure to call for guided tours and frequent special events.

Gull Wings Children's Museum (ages 2 to 12)

418 West Fourth Street, downtown, a bit off the beaten path in the old USO Hall; (805) 483–3005; www.gullwingsmuseum4kids.org. Open Tuesday through Saturday from 10:00 A.M. to 5:00 P.M. $

Children will find plenty to do and dream about here. Indoor sports abound at this innovative museum, from a variety of hands-on exhibits (can you find the fossil?) to a medical room with cutaway models to a stage to do a rock-and-roll show on video and see yourself on the screen to a simulated campground and farmers' market. How about that apparatus for making giant soap bubbles? Can you do it?

Carnegie Cultural Arts Center

424 South C Street; (805) 385–8157. Open Thursday through Saturday 10:00 A.M. to 5:00 P.M. and Sunday 1:00 to 5:00 P.M. $

A dozen art galleries are scattered about like candy waiting to be unwrapped for the arty family unit. Carnegie Art Museum is housed in an imposing, two-story structure built in 1906 as a library. The museum's permanent collection focuses on twentieth-century California painters. Ever-changing exhibits highlight photography, sculpture, oils, watercolors, and some humorous displays.

Channel Islands Harbor & Visitor Center

2741 South Victoria Avenue, Suite F; (805) 985–4852; www.channelislandsharbor.org.

Fisherman's Wharf, Harbor Landing, and the Marine Emporium Landing (www.marine emporiumlanding.com) have shopping, fine dining, and plenty of sailing and fishing options as well. Twenty-six hundred working and pleasure craft call this bustling port home. There are plenty of parks, a swimming beach, and the Maritime Museum. The Channel Islands Water Taxi, with its painted-on smiling face, is the best way to see the seafront. Call (805) 985–4677 for current schedule and fares.

Ventura County Maritime Museum

2731 South Victoria Avenue, just past Channel Islands Boulevard; (805) 984–6260. Open daily 11:00 A.M. to 5:00 P.M. Closed major holidays. **Free.**

You and your mates will find a collection of ship models, made with materials ranging from bone to wood to metals, that reflect maritime history from ancient to modern times. Changing exhibits deal with maritime commerce, art, Channel Islands history, whaling, and shipwrecks.

Oxnard Farmers' Market 🔒 🍴

At the corner of B and Fifth Streets, downtown; (805) 483–7960. Open Thursday from 9:00 A.M. to 1:00 P.M. year-round.

This market is a sure hit for fresh fruit and veggies—perfect ingredients for a picnic lunch at the beach.

Where to Eat and Stay

Casa Sirena Marina Resort & Lobster Trap Restaurant, 3605 Peninsula Road, at Channel Islands Harbor, exit Victoria Avenue off Highway 101, to Channel Islands Boulevard; (805) 985–6311 or (800) 447–3529; www.casasirenahotel.com. This is a value-priced family-fun place to stay right at the marina, with 273 rooms including 26 two-bedroom units. There is so much to see and do right from your patio overlooking the marina or gardens. Try to stay in the main hotel instead of the nondescript north wing. Some rooms are being renovated in 2004, so focus on the view and the feeling of being in the heart of the marina activity. There is a pool, whirlpool spa, tennis court, exercise room, sauna, gift shop, coffee shop, and the Lobster Trap Restaurant for lunch, dinner, and Sunday brunch. Select the children's menu; casual attire is fine. $$$

Embassy Suites Mandalay Beach Resort & Capistrano's Restaurant, 2101 Mandalay Beach Road on the beach, just off Channel Islands Boulevard; (805) 984–2500; www.mandalaybeach.emb suites.com. All 250 units here are two-room, two-bath suites, just perfect for family accommodations. You will love the deluxe amenities in every suite—fridge, microwave, coffeemaker, two TVs, plus a **free** cooked-to-order hot breakfast every morning and **free** beverages and refreshments every evening in the garden courtyard. This resort is right on the sand, with its own beach, and you can rent boogie boards, bicycles, beach chairs, snorkeling gear, and the like. Or just kick back in the serpentine pool. Dine at Capistrano's on fresh seafood and pasta. $$$$

For More Information

Oxnard Convention & Visitors Bureau. 200 West Seventh Street, 93030; (805) 385–7545 or (800) 2–OXNARD; www.oxnardtourism.com.

Port Hueneme

In 1941 the U.S. Navy took advantage of the only natural deepwater harbor between Los Angeles and San Francisco to build its Construction Battalion (known as CB or Seabee) in Port Hueneme (pronounced Why-nee-me). Named after a Chumash settlement, Weneme, that occupied the site, this town of 20,000 actually was plotted in 1869, but its prominence today is its military importance as the home base of the U.S. Navy Civil Engineer

Corps (CEC). These skilled construction experts have actively fought in military engagements around the world. It is also the only commercial port for international shipping between Los Angeles and San Francisco. Access www.huenemechamber.com.

CEC/Seabee Museum

U.S. Naval Construction Battalion at Ventura Road and Sunkist Avenue, within the gates of the Naval Base Ventura County; www.seabeehf.org. Call ahead to confirm hours and current accessibility to civilians at (805) 982–5165. Children younger than age sixteen must be accompanied by an adult. Free.

You can see models of equipment, actual weapons, and uniforms of the Civil Engineer Corps (CEC) and U.S. Navy Seabees.

Simi Valley

The Simi Valley lies on a plateau at around 800 feet above sea level, about twenty minutes inland from Oxnard. State Route 118 (also known as the Ronald Reagan Freeway) bisects the valley, connecting it to State Route 23 with access to U.S. Highway 101 along the coast. With a population of more than 100,000, this area is a popular bedroom community for adjacent Los Angeles County. It is worth a visit to see Ronald Reagan's legacy at his presidential library.

Ronald Reagan Presidential Library & Museum

40 Presidential Drive. Five miles inland from U.S. Highway 101 at Simi Valley off State Highway 118 (follow the signs); (805) 522–2977; www.reaganfoundation.org. Open daily 10:00 A.M. to 5:00 P.M.; closed New Year's Day, Thanksgiving, and Christmas. $$

Located in a Spanish Mission–style building constructed around a courtyard and set on a hilltop, this site provides you with an incredible view of the rolling hills leading down to the Pacific Ocean including the late president's memorial site and final resting place. Within the library's museum are photographs and memorabilia of President Reagan's entire life (1911–2004), gifts of state he received during his administration, and a replica of the Oval Office. Perhaps most impressive to the younger generation is a piece of the crumbled Berlin Wall. This facility provides all generations with a compelling look at "The Great Communicator" and his legacy as the fortieth U.S. president. Set to open in 2005, the Air Force One Pavilion will house the former president's Boeing 707 airplane, which will be available for boarding and tours.

Where to Eat and Stay

Grand Vista Hotel, 999 Enchanted Way, exit First Street off State Route 118, only 2 miles from Reagan Library, Simi Valley; (805) 583–2000 or (800) 455–7464; www.grandvistasimi.com. Very spacious 195-room, full-service hotel with two swimming pools (one heated) and the Vistas Restaurant ($$$). Complimentary continental breakfast will get your family off to a good start. $$$$

Thousand Oaks and Westlake Village

The adjoining communities of Thousand Oaks and Westlake Village are located just off U.S. Highway 101 in the southernmost section of Ventura County. Originally part of a Spanish land grant called Rancho El Conejo (co-nay-ho), today this lovely residential area still has plenty of open rangeland, parks, and things for your family to take pleasure from. Access www.towlvchamber.org. Conejo Valley Days is an annual spring festival with parades, a rodeo, and a carnival. Visit www.conejovalleydays.com.

Stagecoach Inn Museum

51 South Ventu Park Road, off U.S. Highway 101, Newberry Park; (805) 498–9441; www.stagecoachmuseum.org. Open Wednesday through Sunday 1:00 to 4:00 P.M.; closed holidays. $

First opened in 1876, this Monterey-style structure, now faithfully restored, was a major stopover on the stage route between Los Angeles and Santa Barbara. The carriage house, pioneer house, adobe, and ever-changing exhibits will give the kids a great taste of western life in the 1800s.

Thousand Oaks Civic Arts Plaza

2100 East Thousand Oaks Boulevard, Thousand Oaks; (805) 449–2787; www.toaks.org/theatre/.

Performance art in every shape and form takes place here year-round. This complex has beautiful sculpture, fountains, an 1,800-seat auditorium, a 400-seat theater, and a seven-acre park. Be sure to call for a current schedule of events. There is always something happening here for families.

Where to Eat and Stay

Westlake Village Inn, 31943 Agoura Road, Westlake Village, exit Westlake Boulevard South off U.S. Highway 101; (805) 496–1667 or (800) 535–9978; www.wvinn.com. This beautifully landscaped, full-service property has 140 rooms and 18 suites to house your family in luxury. Relax from your travels in the pool/whirlpool spa area or play golf (eighteen holes), practice on the putting green, play tennis (ten courts), or merely stroll around the pretty lake. Package plans and special rates for families abound at this deluxe oasis in the tony community of Westlake. Le Café ($$$$), overlooking the lake and gardens, serves breakfast, lunch, and dinner daily in an elegant atmosphere, best suited for older children and teens. $$$$

Greater
Los Angeles

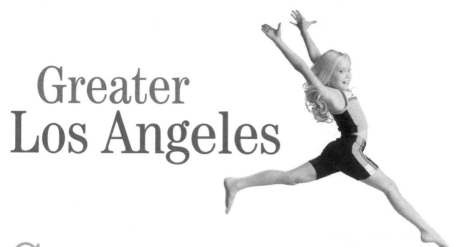

S ay it like a native—L.A.—and you're already on the road (or freeway, as it were)
unlocking the mystique of one of the most fascinating places on earth. For L.A. is
many different things to many millions of ethnically diverse people. For some, the
city is synonymous with Hollywood and the legends of glamour that go along with it. For
others, it is the leading metropolis of the Pacific Rim, a cutting-edge capital of culture and
industry where culture happens be a thriving industry unto itself.

For just about everyone, L.A. means paradise. Palm trees, beaches, and the best
darned weather in the world. In recent years Los Angeles has suffered more than its fair
share of issues, both sociological and geological. But more impressive than the scope of
these setbacks is the furious pace at which the city rebounds. The vaunted laid-back
mind-set of Los Angelenos belies their determination to make L.A. as livable as it can possibly be. Creativity, hard work, and frequent trips to the beach help make civic aspirations
come alive.

The size of the city provokes inspiration or consternation, depending on your point of
view. On a clear day—of which, contrary to popular belief, there are many—one gets a
sense of its general proportions. The core of Los Angeles, city and county, is a vast, level
basin studded with palm trees and laced with freeways. (By the way, always remember the
name and the number of the freeway you are on or looking for, as both locals and road
signs use them interchangeably. Thus "the 5" is also the Golden State, "the 101" is also
the Hollywood, which turns into the Ventura, etc. Radio traffic reports generally refer to
freeways by their names.) The L.A. basin is flanked on all sides by foothills and mountains,
many of which are snowcapped in winter. In the city itself, the higher up in the hills you
go, the bigger the mansions get. These are actually the Santa Monica Mountains, an
enchanting urban oasis with miles of hiking trails, scenic drives, and, after a good rain,
even a waterfall or two. Of course L.A. is prime beach country: In the land where Beach
Blanket Bingo was born, there are 72 miles of county coastline, from Malibu in the north
to Long Beach in the south. Oldies radio stations have an unabashed bias for Beach Boys
hits. But despite its reputation for sunshine and stars, L.A. County also boasts a vast array
of stellar cultural attractions.

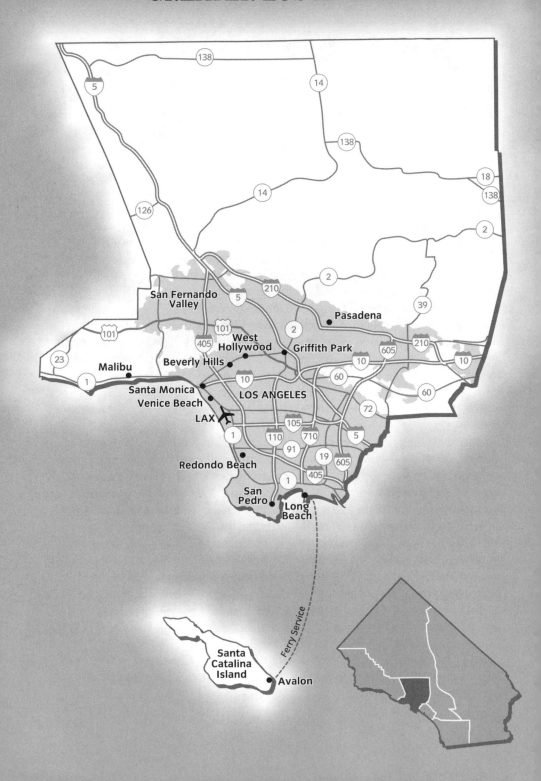

GREATER LOS ANGELES

Over the years, a patchwork of quite separate cities and towns in the L.A. basin was incorporated into the City of Los Angeles, creating a sprawling urban tapestry of contrasting colors and textures. Even if you're superparents, you won't be able to explore all 4,083 square miles of Los Angeles County, or even the City of Los Angeles's 467 square miles. No matter, because the most interesting things to see and do are relatively concentrated in five major areas: downtown; Hollywood; Westside and Beverly Hills; the valleys—San Fernando (including Burbank), San Gabriel (including Pasadena), and Santa Clarita; and coastal Los Angeles County–from northernmost Malibu heading south through Santa Monica, Venice Beach, Marina del Rey, LAX, Redondo Beach, the port of LA/San Pedro, and Long Beach. By East Coast standards, things are still very spread out, but that merely adds to the adventure, even for natives. Equipped with a reliable car—an absolute necessity—a full tank of gas, and the stamina to tackle the world's most extensive network of freeways, you and your family are prepared for experiencing a great deal of the excitement this pocket of the world has to offer.

Downtown Los Angeles

Start at the center. That's as good a rule as any for those unfamiliar with the greater L.A. area. Downtown Los Angeles has been the commercial and cultural core of this sprawling city since it was merely a pueblo. Downtown gives the city a focus, and many central district attractions are perennial favorites. You will instantly recognize downtown by its cluster of skyscrapers. There are seven major districts in downtown L.A.: the **Fashion District,** between Broadway and Wall Street, Seventh Street and Pico Boulevard, designer-wear at a discount anchored by the historic California Mart and Cooper Building at Ninth and Los Angeles Streets; the **Jewelry District,** on Hill Street between Sixth and Seventh Streets, where you'll find discount diamonds, gold, and bangles galore; the **Toy District,** bordered by Third, Fifth, Los Angeles, and San Pedro Streets, and a mecca for wholesale toys and children's clothing; **Little Tokyo,** between Central Avenue, First, Fourth, and San Pedro Streets; **Chinatown,** between North Broadway and North Hill Streets, for Chinese shopping, dining, galleries, and cultural festivals; the **Theatre District,** on Broadway between Third and Ninth Streets, where you'll find architecturally amazing theaters such as the Orpheum; and **Bunker Hill,** bordered by First, Fifth, Flower, and Olive Streets, and featuring the Music Center, Disney Hall, and performing-arts venues.

The *Los Angeles Times* (ages 10 and older for tours)
202 West First Street, right across the street from City Hall; (213) 237–5757 or (800) 528–7637 (tour info); www.latimes.com.

The *Los Angeles Times* is the nation's biggest metro daily newspaper. Kids love to see the newsroom and printing facility, with its mesmerizing, rapid-fire machinery that churns out more than a million newspapers each day. **Free** 35-minute "editorial" tours of the original plant as well as the Olympic, San Fernando Valley, and Orange County facilities. Tour hours vary. Call in advance for a schedule. Tour participants must be at least ten years old.

Music Center
135 North Grand Avenue; (213) 972–7211; www.musiccenter.org.

Tours are **free** at this world-class performing-arts complex that includes the Dorothy Chandler Pavilion (LA Opera); the Mark Taper Forum, the Ahmanson Theatre, and now the Walt Disney Concert Hall. The striking, stainless-steel $247-million Disney Hall, designed by Frank O. Gehry, premiered in October 2003 as the new home of the LA Philharmonic and LA Master Chorale (www.laphil.com). Get your kids interested in arts and architecture with a self-guided audio tour, available daily for a nominal fee. Call (323) 858–2000 for schedule and times, or visit www.disneyhall.com. The Hall also features REDCAT (Roy & Edna Disney CalArts Theatre—www.redcatweb.org for an eclectic performance) as well as gardens, a dedicated children's outdoor amphitheater, five restaurants, an art gallery, and an underground parking garage.

Grand Central Market
317 South Broadway; (213) 624–2378; fax (213) 624–9496; www.grandcentral square.com. Open Monday through Sunday 9:00 A.M. to 6:00 P.M.

Opened in 1917, Grand Central Market is L.A.'s oldest and largest food market. Here you can sample not just a cross-section of L.A.'s ethnic diversity but some of the country's best Mexican and Asian food as well. Locals come here to bargain for bananas, try authentic burritos, or indulge in raspberry guava smoothies at the all-natural exotic juice bar. You may hear more Spanish than English, but that's half the fun, and *gracias* is really all the Spanish you need to know anywhere in Los Angeles.

Museum of Contemporary Art (MOCA)
250 South Grand Avenue, in California Plaza; (213) 626–6222; fax (213) 620–8674; www.moca.org. Open Thursday through Monday. Call for seasonal times. $$

Kids will find the often outrageous and totally unexplainable artwork here to be, well, mysterious. Many people do! The eclectic, always changing, never boring collections range from the cute to the controversial. Kids can roam at will through the museum to see an artistic show, including enormous multimedia sculptures, unpredictable creations of various shapes and sizes, and monochromatic paintings of nothing much at all. **Free** on-site children's workshops are offered. And stop by the museum's cafe, Patinette, for an imaginative California-style salad or pasta. After placing your order, you can sit inside or on the patio.

Cathedral of Our Lady of the Angels
555 West Temple Street; (213) 680–5200; www.olacathedral.org.

Whether you're Catholic or not, you can't miss this twenty-first century architectural wonder that opened in September 2002. Its concrete angularity and lighting is awe-inspiring inside and out. Open daily to the public for self-guided tours. **Free** guided tours Monday through Friday at 1:00 P.M. Gardens, artwork, sculpture, fountains, a cafe, and a gift shop on the plaza surround this home of the Roman Catholic Archdiocese of Los Angeles. Daily masses in English and Spanish as well as other liturgies. Call for current schedule and times.

The Museum of Neon Art

501 West Olympic Boulevard; (213) 489–9918; www.neonmona.org. Open Wednesday through Saturday 11:00 A.M. to 5:00 P.M., Sunday noon to 5:00 P.M. Second Thursday of the month: 11:00 A.M. to 8:00 P.M. Closed Monday, Tuesday, and major holidays. Free parking available underground in Renaissance Tower. $. Children age twelve and younger, free.

Here's the place to gaze upon a glowing collection of electronic-media neon signs. Nostalgia lovers will enjoy the exhibits of the neon signs their grandparents grew up with.

Wells Fargo History Center

333 South Grand Avenue, 2 blocks south of the Music Center; (213) 253–7166; fax (213) 686–2269; www.wellsfargohistory.com. Open Monday through Friday 9:00 A.M. to 5:00 P.M. Free.

Chronicles 130 years of western history. Step into a stagecoach! Free concerts are frequently held at noon and in the evening on the plaza; call (213) 687–2159 for schedule information.

Exposition Park Area

Just south of downtown Los Angeles, bounded by Figueroa Street, Vermont Avenue, Exposition Boulevard, and Martin Luther King Jr. Boulevard.

This has been a civic, cultural, and recreation area since the turn of the twentieth century. Here you'll find the Coliseum, Sports Arena, Natural History Museum, the California Science Center, and the California African American Museum, as well as a seven-acre Rose Garden containing 16,000-plus specimens of 190-plus varieties. Free and open daily until sunset. Adjacent to the park is the world-famous urban campus of the University of Southern California (USC); www.usc.edu. Across the Harbor Freeway is the new retail and entertainment complex Mercado La Paloma; www.mercadolapaloma .com.

DASH

Around downtown L.A., hop on one of the 25-cent DASH shuttle buses and visit all the city's districts without having to hassle with expensive parking. Children age four and younger ride for free! Customer Service: (213) 808–2273; www.ladottransit.com.

Natural History Museum of L.A. County

900 Exposition Boulevard, Exposition Park; (213) 763–DINO (3466); fax (213) 763–4843; www.nhm.org. Open Monday through Friday 9:30 A.M. to 5:00 P.M., Saturday and Sunday 10:00 A.M. to 5:00 P.M. Closed major holidays. $. Children younger than age five, free. First Tuesday of every month, free admission for all.

Kids love the museum because of its lifelike dinosaur replicas, animal habitat dioramas, insect zoo, Native American Cultures exhibit, plus the Halls of Birds, Gems & Minerals, and Marine Life. The Discovery Center is awesomely interactive. Well worth your time!

The California Science Center

700 State Drive, west of the 110 Freeway; (213) 744–2019; fax (213) 744–2934; www.casciencectr.org. Open 10:00 A.M. to 5:00 P.M. daily. Closed Thanksgiving, New Year's Day, and Christmas. Free.

Popular for its fun, innovative, and interactive exhibits, including the Air and Space Gallery with NASA capsules and a real jet fighter plane. The Explore Store is enlightening while shopping. There is also a wide-screen IMAX theater here. For current IMAX production schedule and admission fees, call (213) 744–2019. Don't leave the Science Center until you meet Tess, the 50-foot animatronic woman. She is the star of a show that uses videos, sound effects, and pulsating strobe lights to explain how the body works. Wonder Woman, watch out!

California African American Museum

600 State Drive; (213) 744–7432; www.caam.ca.gov. Open daily except major holidays.

History, culture, and art are featured in ongoing and special exhibitions.

Los Angeles Memorial Coliseum

3911 South Figueroa Street; www.lacoliseum.com.

First opened in 1923 and refurbished extensively in the 1990s, this 92,516-seat stadium hosted the 1932 and 1984 Olympics, two Super Bowls, and NFL football teams, and it is currently home to the USC Trojan football team. The adjacent, indoor Sports Arena opened in 1959 and hosts an incredible variety of events and concerts.

Hungry?

Try the **Pacific Dining Car,** 1310 West Sixth downtown; (213) 483–6000; open twenty-four hours. Just look for the revolving cow. If the kids want a big breakfast, L.A.-style, this is the place. Dinner is expensive, but the lunch menu is good family fare. Kids will like the railway car ambience reminiscent of the good old Union Pacific days.

Thomas Bros.—**A Good Travel Companion**

Welcome! You'll be joining thousands of travelers taking to the roads to explore the scenic highways and byways (and freeways) of Southern California. Get off on the right foot by investing in the full-color *Thomas Bros. California Road Atlas and Driver's Guide*. Your family will benefit from the useful mileage charts, the index of cities, state highway maps, street details, metropolitan area maps, and a separate foldout map. We especially liked the driving tours and points of interest for the Greater Los Angeles area, the deserts, Orange County, the Inland Empire, and the Central Coast—all part and parcel of the *Fun with the Family Southern California* guide. To obtain your copy, try any bookstore or visit **Thomas Brothers Maps and Books,** 521 West Sixth Street, downtown Los Angeles; (213) 627–4018 or (888) 277–6277. The soft-bound, wire-ringed book (the navigational bible to Southern Californians) costs $34.95. And it's worth every penny.

After all, in 2004 alone, there were hundreds of new streets in Los Angeles and Orange Counties! You'll find the guide to be indispensable, with its foldout maps and easy-to-read index. With your trusty Thomas Guide in hand, you can navigate L.A. like a native—from "the 5" to "the 10" and beyond! Visit www.thomas.com.

Little Tokyo
Between Central Avenue, First, Fourth, and San Pedro Streets.

This is the social, cultural, and economic center of Southern California's Japanese-American community. The twenty-one-story New Otani Hotel (see Where to Stay), the Japanese American Cultural and Community Center, and the Japanese American National Museum are here, along with great restaurants and shops for your family to explore—Village Plaza, Little Tokyo Plaza, and Weller Court.

Japanese American National Museum
369 East First Street; (213) 625–0414 or (800) 461–5266; fax (213) 625–1770; www.janm.org. Open Tuesday through Sunday 10:00 A.M. to 5:00 P.M., Thursday 10:00 A.M. to 8:00 P.M. $$

The museum, set in a remodeled Buddhist temple, chronicles the history of Japanese immigration to and life in the United States.

Chinatown
Generally bordered by North Broadway and North Hill Streets and Cesar Chavez Avenue (near Union Station).

Chinese shops and restaurants line the "Street of the Golden Treasures" or Gin Ling Way.

Spectator **Sports**

There is a sport for all seasons in greater L.A., and this town knows how to put on a show. If your family likes to watch professional sports action, here's where to go.

Auto Racing. NHRA drag racing takes place at Pomona Raceway at the L.A. County Fairplex; (800) 884–6472. NASCAR races run at California Speedway in Fontana; (800) 944–7223. Stock cars, midgets legends, and trucks hit the track at Irwindale Speedway; (626) 358–1100.

Baseball. Head downtown for Chavez Ravine and Dodger Stadium, home of the MLB National League Los Angeles Dodgers; (323) 224–1448.

Basketball. The multi-winning NBA Championship Los Angeles Lakers (www.nba.com/lakers/), the sibling NBA Los Angeles Clippers (www.nba.com/clippers/), and the WNBA Los Angeles Sparks all play round ball at the sparkling Staples Center, 1111 South Figueroa Street; www.staples center.com. For ticket information, call (213) 742–7340.

Football. The Arena Football League (AFL) Los Angeles Avengers take to the turf at Staples Center; www.laavengers.com.

Hockey. The Staples Center ices down and plays host to the NHL's Los Angeles Kings; www.lakings.com.

Soccer. The Los Angeles Galaxy take to the new field at The Home Depot Center, on the campus of California State University Dominguez Hills. For tickets, call (877) 342–5299. The Home Depot Center is also the U.S. Soccer Federation–National Team Training Headquarters. Visit www.homedepot center.com.

The Chinese Chamber of Commerce coordinates parades, festivals, and other events. Call (213) 617–0396 for information.

El Pueblo de Los Angeles Historic Monument/Olvera Street
At the heart of El Pueblo de Los Angeles Historic Park, 125 Paseo de la Plaza; (213) 628–1274; www.olvera-street.com. Open Monday through Saturday 10:00 A.M. to 3:00 P.M. (to 8:00 P.M. in the summer). Shops open 10:00 A.M. to 7:00 P.M.

This is an authentic L.A. experience that is ideal for the family. Kids will love the wide variety of brightly colored piñatas—splendid, reasonably priced souvenirs. Don't ask us how you'll get one on the plane or in your trunk. This forty-four-acre cluster of shops and landmark buildings is the birthplace of Los Angeles. Every day seems to be Cinco de Mayo at El Pueblo, located at the site of a Spanish farming village founded in 1781. Kids and adults alike may be surprised to learn Los Angeles was actually a Mexican city from 1835 (when

Spain ceded it to Mexico) until 1847, when it became American. Nowhere in the city is the proud Spanish heritage kept alive to the extent it is here.

The effect is like making a detour to Mexico without a passport. More than twenty historic buildings line the colorful streets of El Pueblo. One is the Avila Adobe, built in 1818, today the oldest house still standing in Los Angeles. At the center of El Pueblo is La Placita (the Plaza), where the rich Spanish influence is visible in art and architecture. Kids love the old-fashioned candy shops and the sound of mariachi music in the Mexican marketplace. Everyone loves the aroma of Mexican food and the unparalleled sombrero-buying opportunities. Not even Disneyland has atmosphere like this.

Where to Eat

Ciudad, 445 South Figueroa Street, Suite 100; (213) 486–5171; fax (213) 486–5172; www.millikenandfeniger.com. As long as you are downtown, make it a point to visit this colorful (yellow interior!), noisy, and always busy restaurant. It has an exciting Latin-inspired menu for adults and a pretty good one for the kids created by MarySue Milliken and Susan Feniger, known around these parts as the Two Hot Tamales.

Among the seven choices for the little ones (para los niños) are el Cubanao Wedges with roasted pork, ham, Swiss cheese, and pickles, served with fries at $4.50. The desserts, such as cookies and flan, made in-house, have charmed the most jaded L.A. restaurant critics. You can make reservations via their Web site. $$

The Original Pantry, 877 South Figueroa Street, downtown Los Angeles; (213) 972–9279. This historic institution in Los

Experience **L.A. without a Car!**

Downtown L.A. is undergoing an urban renaissance that can be seen in its cultural activities, dining, and nightlife—and easily experienced with its re-emergence as a transportation hub. The center of that hub is Union Station, handling long-distance AMTRAK trains (Coast Starlight, Southwest Chief, Sunset Limited, Texas Eagle; www.amtrak.com); Pacific Surfliner trains running north to San Luis Obispo and south to San Diego; Metrolink trains to Ventura, San Bernardino, Orange County, Riverside, and other destinations (www.metrolinktrains.com); and Los Angeles' subway and light-rail systems (Metro Rail Red, Gold, Blue, and Green lines; 800–COMMUTE or www.metro.net or) and DASH shuttles.

Now it's easier than ever before to experience Greater Los Angeles without a car. For complete information on where to go and how to get there, visit www.experienceLA.com.

Union **Station**

First opened in 1939, Union Station, 800 North Alameda Street; (213) 683–6875; www.wgn.net/~elson/larail/, is an architectural gumbo of Spanish Mission, art deco, and Streamline Moderne styles that somehow fit together. The waiting room has marble floors, wood-beamed ceilings more than 50 feet high and stunning art deco chandeliers. Huge archways lead to patio areas laced with flowering trees. Needless to say, it's been featured in many films, including *The Way We Were*, *Bugsy*, and *Blade Runner*. It has all been scrubbed, polished, and reupholstered, and is once again a pleasure to visit.

Angeles is owned by a former mayor of Los Angeles, Richard Riordan. His slogan is "Never closed. Never without a customer!" The restaurant has an incredibly diverse menu. Cash only—no credit cards. $–$$

Philippe The Original, 1001 North Alameda Street; (213) 628–3781; www.philippes.com. If the kids' taste buds don't blossom over the prospect of a platter of sushi or a bowl of bird's nest soup, you might stroll over to Philippe's, the city's best-known place for roast beef sandwiches. Arrive early (before noon) to secure one of the roomy booths (we old-timers called them "booths") and dig into a classic Philippe's roast beef sandwich, a heaping portion of coleslaw, and a juicy baked apple. Yum! Remember that there are no hamburgers served here. An added perk: **Free** parking adjacent to the restaurant and across the street. $–$$

Where to Stay

Holiday Inn City Center, 1020 South Figueroa Street; (213) 748–1291; www .hicitycenter.com. Newly renovated 195-room full-service hotel locally owned and

operated with friendly staff. Great location across the street from Staples Center and the L.A. Convention Center. Emerald Grill for all-day dining.

New Otani Hotel & Garden, 120 South Los Angeles Street; (800) 273–2294; fax (213) 622–0980; www.newotani.com. This 434-room hotel is ideal for families interested in exploring the downtown neighborhood. Three restaurants serve excellent cuisine: Azalea (breakfast and lunch buffets), Garden Grill (teriyaki, steak, and seafood), and Thousand Cranes (Japanese, sushi, and tempura). $$$

For More Information

L.A. Inc.—The Convention and Visitors Bureau/Visitor Center. 685 Figueroa Street, 90071; (213) 689–8822; www.visit LAnow.com.

City of Los Angeles. For civic information and assistance, dial 3-1-1 inside city limits or (866) 4–LACITY in Southern California; www.lacity.org.

Hollywood

Movie stars, glamour, palm tree–lined streets, and excitement in the air—hooray for Hollywood! If downtown is the city's historic center, Hollywood is its heart. For millions around the world, Hollywood is Los Angeles, an illusion promoted by movie studios that remain very much alive in these quarters. Although the "Golden Age" of Hollywood is long gone, the 50-foot-high HOLLYWOOD sign still proclaims it to be the entertainment capital of the world. With the exception of the beaches, Hollywood is probably where your kids will have the most fun in Los Angeles. For that reason we suggest you spend at least two full days here.

Hollywood & Highland Entertainment Complex 🍴 🛍️

Corner of Hollywood Boulevard and Highland Avenue; www.hollywoodandhighland.com.

Located in the thumping heart of Hollywood, you can't miss this enormous complex sure to please everyone in your family somehow! This signature project for Hollywood's revitalization opened in 2001 to worldwide acclaim. It features the modern 640-room Renaissance Hollywood Hotel, more than sixty world-class retail shops and restaurants, a multiplex cinema, and the Kodak Theatre, a live-broadcast performing-arts center and permanent home of the annual Academy Awards Ceremony.

Kodak Theatre

6801 Hollywood Boulevard, anchor of the Hollywood & Highland Entertainment Complex; (323) 308–6300, (323) 308–6363 (box office and guided-tour information); www.kodak theatre.com. Daily thirty-minute guided tours from 10:30 A.M. to 2:30 P.M. (subject to change depending on events scheduled). $$. Be sure to call for tickets in advance since tours fill quickly, with only twenty people allowed per group.

Since opening in November 2001, the theater has hosted a range of prestigious artists and events, including the Academy Awards Ceremonies, Celine Dion, Prince, Elvis Costello, Barry Manilow, American Ballet Theatre, ESPY Awards, and even the American Idol finals. Be sure you don't miss this super chance to step behind the velvet rope and personally experience the glamour of the permanent home of the Oscar ceremonies. During your tour, you'll see an Oscar statuette, visit the exclusive George Eastman VIP Room (where stars party), view twenty-six Academy Awards images, learn where this year's Oscar nominees sat (and maybe sit there, too), and gain an insider's view of behind-the-scenes production from friendly, knowledgeable actor/tour guides.

Walk of Fame

Hollywood Boulevard from Gower Street to La Brea Avenue and along Vine Street from Yucca to Sunset Boulevard.

In Hollywood even the sidewalks have stories to tell. This is most visibly apparent on the Walk of Fame. There is no admission charge to stroll along sidewalks with more than 2,000 terrazzo-and-brass stars etched into them. Some stars' famous sidewalk addresses are: 1644 Hollywood Boulevard (Marilyn Monroe), 1719 Vine Street (James Dean), 1750 Vine Street (John Lennon), and 6777 Hollywood Boulevard (Elvis Presley).

El Capitan Theatre

6838 Hollywood Boulevard; (323) 468–8262; www.elcapitantickets.com.

Disney and Pacific Theaters restored this historic theater in 1989, now on the National Register of Historic Places. Originally built in 1925, it is now where Disney previews all of its movies. The recently restored 4/37 Wurlitzer pipe organ—known as the "Mightiest of the Mighty Wurlitzers"—is just one of the jewels of this architectural masterpiece. It is across the street from Mann's Chinese Theatre.

Mann's Chinese Theatre

(formerly known as Grauman's) 6925 Hollywood Boulevard; (323) 461–3331; http://mann.moviefone.com. $$

Hollywood doesn't get any more Hollywood than at the unofficial emperor of Hollywood Boulevard. Both the young and young at heart revel at the sight of what looks like the entrance to a Chinese imperial palace. But the main attractions here are in the theater's forecourt, where the handprints, footprints, and signatures of Hollywood celebrities dating from 1927 are quite literally cast in stone. "Gee, Mom, did Rita Hayworth really have such tiny feet?" The proof is in the pavement.

On busy street corners along Hollywood Boulevard and particularly in front of Mann's Chinese Theatre, you might spot tanned young men and women wearing sun visors and holding clipboards. If they don't approach you, make a point of approaching them: They have passes for movie previews at area studios, and sometimes you are paid to see them. It's a way the studios get audience feedback before films are released and a way for you to learn about an important, if little known, aspect of the entertainment industry.

Hollywood Guinness World Records Museum

6764 Hollywood Boulevard; (323) 463–6433. Open daily 10:00 A.M. to midnight. $$

The museum showcases offbeat testimonials to a wide variety of facts, feats, and incredible achievements. It is located in Hollywood's first movie house, The Hollywood, which is now a national historic landmark. Hands-on exhibits include technology, space adventures, and natural phenomena.

Hollywood **Celeb Homes**

If you want a guided tour past Hollywood celeb homes, here are some choices:

- **Hollywood Tours,** 7095 Hollywood Boulevard #705; (800) 789–9575; www.hollywoodtours.us. Air-conditioned minivans or open-air trolley.

- **Starline Tours,** (323) 463–3333 or (800) 959–3131; www.starlinetours.com. Has two-hour tours in Beverly Hills and Bel Air. The company promises forty celebrity homes and offers excellent value on more than twenty other Hollywood/L.A. itineraries.

Hollywood Wax Museum

6767 Hollywood Boulevard; (323) 462–8860; fax (323) 462–3953. Open Sunday through Thursday 10:00 A.M. to midnight, Friday and Saturday until 1:00 A.M. $$

The wax museum has 220 life-size renditions of celebrated film stars, political leaders, and sports greats. Park at the rear of the building and visit all the museums at one stop. For a discount, purchase one ticket for both the wax museum and the Guinness museum.

Hollywood Entertainment Museum

7021 Hollywood Boulevard; (323) 465–7900; www.hollywoodmuseum.com. Open Tuesday through Sunday 10:00 A.M. to 6:00 P.M. $$

This museum, which opened in 1996, is the Smithsonian of the film and television world, a la L.A. gaudy, brassy, and neon-lit. It's a monument to Hollywood's glitzy and glamorous past and provides a behind-the-set look at the nuts-and-bolts mechanics of the movie and TV industry, from sound effects to scenery. There are high-tech and multimedia exhibits, too. Small-group tours are available with savvy guides. *Star Trek* lovers will go ballistic over the props and sets from that series.

Ripley's Believe It or Not! Odditorium (ages 5 and up)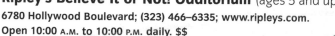

6780 Hollywood Boulevard; (323) 466–6335; www.ripleys.com. Open 10:00 A.M. to 10:00 P.M. daily. $$

No problem finding the place; there's a giant *Tyrannosaurus rex* poking his mighty head and substantial torso out of the rooftop. The Odditorium claims to have the world's most outstanding collection of the bizarre and unusual, and it probably does. Kids love the innovative special effects, which actually help them learn some quirky facts of history they'd really have to dig for in schoolbooks.

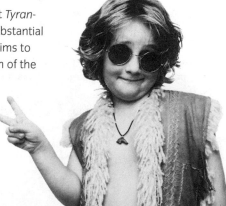

Hollywood **CityPass**

CityPass is the best way to enjoy Hollywood at one low price (up to 40 percent savings off tickets purchased separately). With CityPass, you get admission tickets to famous attractions, including Universal Studios Hollywood, Kodak Theatre, Hollywood Entertainment Museum, Starline Tours, and the Hollywood Museum in the Historic Max Factor Building. CityPass is good for thirty days from first day of use. Access www.citypass.com.

Capitol Records
1750 North Vine Street; www.hollywoodandvine.com.

This landmark building is one of Hollywood's most recognized icons. The light on its rooftop spire flashes "Hollywood" in Morse code. In the lobby gold albums of many Capitol recording artists, such as John Lennon and Garth Brooks, are displayed.

Hollywood Toys and Costumes
6600 Hollywood Boulevard; (323) 464–4444; www.hollywoodtoys.com. Open daily.

Here's where kids can find that monster mask they won't find back home or that conversation starter costume perfect for next Halloween. There are tiaras in all shapes and sizes and novelties too numerous to describe. In town since 1950, this has to be the biggest supermarket of Hollywood-inspired memorabilia and trinkets.

Hollywood Bowl and Hollywood Bowl Museum
2301 North Highland; (323) 850–2000; fax (323) 617–2017; www.hollywoodbowl.org. Visit the museum (it's **free!**) October through June, Tuesday through Saturday 10:00 A.M. to 4:30 P.M. and July through September, Tuesday through Saturday 10:30 A.M. to 8:30 P.M.

The summer home of the Los Angeles Philharmonic Orchestra, the bowl is a terrific place to take in a concert. Pack a picnic to get the most out of an outdoor performance at this gleaming Los Angeles landmark.

Samuel French Inc. Bookstore
7623 Sunset Boulevard; (323) 876–0570; www.samuelfrench.com. Open Monday through Friday 10:00 A.M. to 6:00 P.M., Saturday 10:00 A.M. to 5:00 P.M. Parking on Stanley behind the building.

This is the ultimate bookstore for entertainment-industry-related publications. It has a wide selection of books for kids—along with an extensive selection of works on the theater, movies, television, and the other performing arts. This is your chance to add a serious and educational dimension to the pomp and puffery purveyed by Hollywood's ubiquitous PR spin doctors.

Hollywood's **Rock of Fame**

Hollywood's Rock of Fame, 7425 West Sunset Boulevard, in the outer lobby of Hollywood's Guitar Center; (323) 874–1060. Open Monday through Friday 10:00 A.M. to 9:00 P.M., Saturday 10:00 A.M. to 6:00 P.M., and Sunday 11:00 A.M. to 6:00 P.M. Inductees include Black Sabbath, Elvis Presley, Johnny Cash, Bo Diddley, the Doobie Brothers, Jimi Hendrix, and Eddie Van Halen, just to name a few.

Where to Eat

Musso & Frank Grill, 6667 Hollywood Boulevard; (323) 467–5123. Closed Sunday and Monday. A Hollywood institution where movers and shakers have "done deals" over filet mignon steaks and chicken potpies since 1919. Whether you go for the atmosphere or the food, you simply must go to say you've been! $$

Pink's, 709 North La Brea Avenue (corner of Melrose and La Brea); (323) 931–4223. You can't miss the line that has wrapped around this pink building since it opened in 1939, where they serve probably the best chilidog in L.A. Chilidogs, chili fries, chiliburgers, turkey dogs, burrito dogs— every imaginable presentation of the wiener can be found here. No matter what time of day or night, you will find yourself standing in line with tourists, corporate climbers, and celebrities. Cash only. $

For More Information

Hollywood Chamber of Commerce. 7018 Hollywood Boulevard, 90028; (213) 469–8316; www.hollywoodcoc.org.

The LACVB Hollywood Visitor Information Center. 6541 Hollywood Boulevard, 90028; (213) 461–4213; www.visitLA now.com. Open Monday through Friday 8:30 A.M. to 5:00 P.M. Pick up the **free** handy pocket guides on dining, shopping, and entertainment in Los Angeles County.

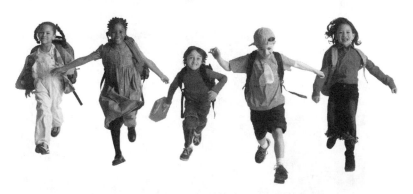

Griffith Park

With its 4,000-plus acres, this park has some of L.A.'s most renowned attractions.

Los Angeles Zoo
Griffith Park, Golden State Freeway at Ventura Freeway, downtown; (323) 644–6400; fax (323) 662–9786; www.lazoo.org. Open daily from 10:00 A.M. to 5:00 P.M. $$.

Let your kids run wild in this parklike setting where wildlife from around the world now resides. Be sure to spend at least two hours here before proceeding to other area attractions, such as the inimitable Autry Museum.

Gene Autry Western Heritage Museum
4700 Western Heritage Way; (323) 667–2000; fax (323) 660–5721; www.autry-museum.org. Open Tuesday through Sunday 10:00 A.M. to 5:00 P.M. Open Thursday until 8:00 P.M. $$. Second Tuesday of the month free.

More than 4,000 Old West artifacts and hands-on exhibits are here, including many designed with children in mind. Special exhibits explore America's western heritage such as Native American culture, early tourism, and weaving.

Travel Town
Griffith Park, 5200 Zoo Drive; (323) 662–5874; fax (818) 247–4740. Open weekdays 10:00 A.M. to 4:00 P.M., weekends 10:00 A.M. to 5:00 P.M. Free parking.

Kids love this outdoor transportation museum with steam locomotives to scramble over and Live Steamers, a large collection of miniature trains.

Universal City

Universal City is home to some of the best attractions for movie lovers.

Universal Studios Hollywood
100 Universal City Plaza (Universal Center Drive or Lankershim Boulevard from the 101 Hollywood Freeway); (818) 622–3801 or (800) UNIVERSAL; www.UniversalStudiosHollywood .com. Open weekdays 10:00 A.M. to 6:00 P.M. and weekends 9:00 A.M. to 6:00 P.M.; expanded hours for summer and holidays. $$$$

Universal Studios is an integral part of L.A.'s history. And while another version is now in Florida, for Southern Californians there is but one Universal Studios. The movie theme links all rides and attractions, making this the quintessential L.A. theme park. And like many legends, it just gets better with age. Recent additions include the cutting-edge roller-coaster Revenge of the Mummy—the Ride; the Waterworld live-action show (where you can get wet); Terminator 2:3-D; Shrek 4-D; The Blues Brothers; Animal Planet Live!; Backdraft; Back to the Future—the Ride; and the latest Jurassic Park ride (you will get soaked!).

But it's the classics that make Universal a genuine hoot for both kids and adults. The staple is the forty-five-minute tram ride (catch one every five to ten minutes), during which Hollywood history and special effects cast their magical spell. You're whisked past the Norman Bates House (from the movie *Psycho*), over a collapsing bridge, into a Mexican village that falls prey to a flash flood, and through a Red Sea that parts just for you. Then there's a landslide and a simulated fishing village where the naughty shark from the movie *Jaws* surfaces with a vengeance. Adults fidget nervously when this happens; kids go wild. The tram ride also takes visitors past enormous studio back lots, reminding you that this is the world's biggest film and television studio. Something is almost always in production, and chances are you'll catch a bit of the action.

Universal CityWalk

1000 Universal Center Drive, Universal City; (818) 622–4455. Open 11:00 A.M. to 9:00 P.M. Monday through Thursday, 11:00 A.M. to midnight Friday and Saturday, and 11:00 A.M. to 10:00 P.M. Sunday.

An eclectic outdoor pedestrian promenade with an atmosphere made to resemble a studio back lot. There are actually two streets lined with palms and joined by a central courtyard area with fountains. But all is not so sedate: A mammoth King Kong clings to the facade of one building, and a huge photographic likeness of Wayne Gretzsky adorns a sports memorabilia emporium. Get the picture? There are many theme restaurants here, including Gladstones, B.B. King's Blues Club, and a Hard Rock Cafe. CityWalk is adjacent to the Cineplex Odeon, which houses—count 'em—eighteen movie theaters and connects to Universal Amphitheatre, an outstanding concert and performance venue with no seat more than 150 feet from the stage. Visit www.hob.com/venues/concerts/universal.

Universal Studios **VIP Experience Tour**

For the ultimate insider's perspective on the world's largest movie and television studio as well as genuine hospitality and personal special treatment—treat yourself and your family to the "VIP Experience" tour. You will have your own private tour escort (with encyclopedic knowledge) for the entire day (only fifteen people per group) and enjoy front-of-the-line admission and the best views and seating at all attractions and rides. Plus your tour escort will take you deep into the "Back Lot," where you'll have special access to soundstages—many in use by your favorite stars. Best of all, instead of the huge tram you'll have a private trolley bus that can stop and let you out to take pictures (how about the steps of the *Psycho* house or *Back to the Future*'s courthouse). Feel like a movie star yourself. It's expensive but worth the truly VIP experience!

Filmed before a **Live Studio Audience**

Hollywood is the place to see the television industry in action. Live studio audiences are always needed and tickets are **free!** With some advance planning, you could be part of the audience for your fave show! Here are some of the best sources for tickets. **Audiences Unlimited, Inc.**; www.tvtickets.com. More than forty sitcom, pilot, and talk-show tickets available. Tickets are offered online starting approximately thirty days prior to show date. This is an excellent Web site and a good source of information about what to expect, along with maps on how to reach the studios. **HollywoodTix.com.** This easy-to-navigate Web site offers tickets to a wide variety of game shows, talk shows, specials, and sitcoms. You can search by date and/or the show you want to see—and print out your ticket selection right away. **Paramount Pictures,** 5555 Melrose Avenue; (323) 956–5000; http://paramount.com/studio/. Visit this Web site for current ticket availability. This is the only remaining "big name" studio lot still located and operating in Hollywood. If you're up for a non–theme park and want to look at a real working studio, Paramount is the place. Tickets to TV tapings are given out on a first-come, first-served basis five days in advance at the Paramount Visitor Center as well as via their Web site, but be forewarned, little taping is done during the summer months because shows are on hiatus.

There are age requirements for attending most TV show tapings. Most sitcom tapings require audience members to be at least age eighteen, but game shows and children's variety shows sometimes set the age requirement at age twelve. This rule is strictly enforced, so be sure to check in advance. Not all shows use audiences (e.g., *ER* is a closed set, as are most soaps). The more popular the show, the harder it is to get tickets. Comedies shoot a few times a month, usually from September to March. Besides having to show up early to get through security, most tapings last three to six hours, so allow yourself plenty of extra time. Soundstages generally have bleacher-type seating, and it's sometimes hard to see the action even though you're right in front of the stage, so most stages have video monitors that show what's going on. Most scenes are shot several times, and this can get boring for kids (and us adults, too!). To help pass the down times between shooting, a comic often entertains the audience. Soundstages are notoriously cold so bring a sweater—the lights only heat up the actors! Tickets may also be available outside of Mann's Chinese Theatre. Don't ever pay for TV taping tickets. They are given out **free,** always by production companies and studio representatives.

Where to Stay

Sheraton Universal, 333 Universal
Hollywood Drive, Universal City; (818)
980–1212 or reservations (800) 325–3535.
A high-rise landmark since 1969. Enjoy 436
recently redone rooms and suites with
views of the studio. Excellent packages for
families. You'll appreciate the shuttle service to Universal Studios. $$$$

Sportsmen's Lodge Hotel, 12825 Ventura Boulevard, Studio City; (818) 769–
4700 or (800) 821–8511; www.slhotel.com.
This triple-A-rated hotel, with 193 country-
style rooms and three restaurants, offers
free Universal Studios shuttle services
and discount tickets for guests.

West Hollywood

Pop-culture types regard West Hollywood (incorporated in 1984), while small by Los Angeles standards (just 1.9 square miles), as the creative center of L.A. This enclave, bordered
by Beverly Hills on the west, is a trendy one that will appeal to older, more "cool con-
scious" kids. Unpredictable and irreverent, West Hollywood-ites work and play by their
own rules (of which there aren't many). The cast of TV's *Queer Eye for the Straight Guy*
would feel right at home here.

Few drives in Los Angeles are as exhilarating as **Sunset Boulevard.** Originating downtown, Sunset winds up at the Pacific Ocean. Zipping along its famous curves in Beverly
Hills, you'll see stunning mansions and gorgeous gardens at every turn. But the most
famous stretch, hands down, is the **Sunset Strip,** directly after Beverly Hills in West Hollywood. The heart of the action, the 1.2-mile portion between numbers 8221 and 9255, is
the mecca of L.A. nightlife. Celebrities are sighted so often here that they hardly raise eye-
brows. After cruising Sunset (preferably in a convertible), park your car **free** at number
8600, **Sunset Plaza,** an open-air mall. From here, you can see the entire city of L.A. teem-
ing and (if it's nighttime) twinkling below. And your musical tweens will want to hit the
original Tower Records (8801 Sunset; 310–657–7300).

Where to Eat

House of Blues, 8430 Sunset Boulevard;
(323) 848–5100; www.hob.com. Take the
kids to dinner at the ultimate Sunset hot
spot. Great southern cooking, a wild decor,
and daily live blues performances will
make for an unforgettable evening. Try the
popular Sunday Gospel Brunch (served at
9:30 A.M., noon, and 2:30 P.M.) or, to save
the whopping valet parking fee, stop for
lunch Monday through Saturday. The menu

features "eclectic southern fare" such as
barbecue chicken and ribs.

The House of Blues is the best compro-
mise if you wish to steer the kids clear of
the area's irresponsibly loud and obscenely
crowded evening concerts. To enjoy the
decor (recycled bottle caps, auto license
tags, etc.), take your time. Don't leave
without pigging out on a hefty slab of
banana cream pie laced with chocolate
fudge and caramel. Afterwards, work off
those calories by simply strolling along the

boulevard's trendy boutiques, sidewalk cafes, and record stores—all aglow under a sea of neon lights. $$

Tail O' The Pup, 329 North San Vicente Boulevard; (310) 652–4517. A Los Angeles landmark. Predating drive-ins, this giant hot-dog stand is actually shaped like a hot dog, bringing smiles to kids' faces even before they order. For those who don't mind dining in the midst of the traffic, take your place in line. Dogs start at $2.50 and go up, depending on what you find to stuff the bun. $

For More Information

West Hollywood Convention and Visitors Bureau. 8687 Melrose Avenue, Suite M-38, 90069; (310) 289–2525 or (800) 368–6020; www.visitwesthollywood.com.

Westside

In this immense, loosely defined swath of the city, punctuated by estates and eateries, museums and boutiques, trendiness reigns supreme. Here you may quite acceptably judge your neighbors according to where they "do lunch." You're more apt to bump into a celebrity in the Westside than in Hollywood, and if you spend only five minutes driving around tony Beverly Hills, you'll find out why. There is one (perhaps only one) rule in these parts: If you've got it, flaunt it—and preferably in style. And the sheer amount of wealth people have here simply must be seen to be believed.

But not all of the Westside is given over to ostentation and glitz. Here it must be said that, to an Angeleno, certain areas of L.A. defy easy geographical classification. One of these is **Melrose Avenue,** which is neither part of the Westside nor quite part of anything else, either.

Melrose Avenue, now immortalized by the hit TV series *Melrose Place,* actually begins (or ends, depending on your point of view) in Hollywood. The hippest sections begin at La Brea and branch out toward the west. But the street is as much a state of mind as it is a chunk of asphalt. This is a place with a carnival-like atmosphere, where anything goes. Find a parking spot (keep looking, you'll find one) and simply drift. Whatever boutique, gallery, or cafe you settle into is not as important, though, as the simple act of "doing" Melrose, which affords a close-up look at what makes Los Angeles tick. An hour or two or three here, and you'll begin to understand the triple L.A. creed: creativity, individuality, and sunshine. You'll love it.

Museum Row

Stretching along the "Miracle Mile" of busy Wilshire Boulevard, "Museum Row" is the home of a singularly fun and educational selection of family-worthy museums.

George C. Page Museum of La Brea Discoveries
5801 Wilshire Boulevard; (323) 934–7243; fax (323) 783–4843; www.tarpits.org. Open Monday through Friday 9:30 A.M. to 5:00 P.M. and Saturday, Sunday, and holidays 10:00 A.M. to 5:00 P.M. Free admission on the first Tuesday of the month. $$

The Page Museum can be found at the La Brea Tar Pits, a black and slightly malodorous lake of ancient goo that trapped thousands of Ice Age creatures. More than 100 tons worth of their fossilized remains have been extracted from the pits, and new discoveries are always being made. Dozens of saber-toothed tiger and wolf skulls, woolly mammoth skeletons, and other specimens are on display. This is educational, unadulterated magic for adults and the under-twelve crowd.

Los Angeles County Museum of Art
5905 Wilshire Boulevard; (323) 857–6000; fax (323) 931–7347; www.lacma.org. Open Monday, Tuesday, and Thursday noon to 8:00 P.M., Friday noon to 9:00 P.M., Saturday and Sunday 11:00 A.M. to 8:00 P.M.; closed Wednesday. $$

The anchor museum for Museum Row, it now spans the world of art and artifacts from prehistory to the present. If you manage your time right, you can sweep through in two hours or less and still be able to visit other museums in the neighborhood. Music, film, and educational events happen year-round, and there's a good chance something is happening during your stay. The information desk is accommodating, so just ask. While you're here, be sure to step over to the legendary La Brea Tar Pits. Your kids might recall the pits erupting in the film *Volcano*. Don't worry, the site is perfectly benign. The only thing you have to fear around these parts is the horrific traffic on Wilshire Boulevard.

Petersen Automotive Museum
6060 Wilshire Boulevard; (323) 930–2277; www.petersen.org. Open Tuesday through Sunday 10:00 A.M. to 6:00 P.M. $$. Children age five and younger, free.

This museum, opened in 1997 and already a landmark by virtue of its striking, futuristic design, celebrates L.A.'s icon, the automobile—its history and role in the development of Southern California. In its 300,000 square feet of exhibition space, you'll find more than 200 cars and motorcycles, plus loads of fascinating automotive memorabilia.

Original Farmers Market
6230 West Third Street, a few footsteps north of Museum Row; (323) 933–9211; www.farmersmarketla.com. Open Monday through Friday 9:00 A.M. to 9:00 P.M., Saturday 9:00 A.M. to 8:00 P.M., and Sunday 10:00 A.M. to 7:00 P.M. Free entrance.

This is the Westside's answer to downtown's Grand Central Market, with seventy restaurants, produce stands, and retail stores thriving since 1934.

No tour of the Westside would be complete without visiting Westwood Village, a vibrant neighborhood just west of Beverly Hills bounded by Wilshire Boulevard, the 405 (San Diego Freeway), and the UCLA (University of California, Los Angeles; www.ucla.edu) campus, where you can enjoy visiting the Botanical Garden, the Sculpture Garden,

Museum of **Tolerance**

At the **Simon Wiesenthal Center.** Simon Wiesenthal Plaza, 9786 West Pico Boulevard, between Century City and Beverly Hills; (310) 553–8403; www .wiesenthal.com. Open Monday through Thursday 10:00 A.M. to 4:00 P.M., Friday 10:00 A.M. to 3:00 P.M. and Sunday 10:30 A.M. to 5:00 P.M. Closed Jewish holidays, January 1, July 4, Thanksgiving, and December 25. Some exhibits recommended for kids age twelve and older.

Inside a shimmering $55 million building are a series of high-tech exhibits dedicated to the promotion of understanding among people from all backgrounds and walks of life. Interactive exhibits chronicle the history of racism in American history and the events and consequences of the Holocaust. The presentations have been crafted with historical precision and much sensitivity. Both children and adults will leave the museum enlightened and moved by history and the dangers of forgetting it.

the Hammer Museum—a cutting-edge arts institution, and the Fowler Museum of Cultural History. UCLA's presence imbues Westwood with a youthful air. It is an ideal area for walking around, browsing in record stores, or simply "hanging out" at a cafe or ice-cream parlor. College students aside, it's movies that really make Westwood tick. Movie theaters are everywhere, and these are not your ordinary theaters. Screens are enormous. Seats are plush and tilt back. Popcorn is fresh and usually made with real butter. We're talking cinematic heaven here.

Westside Pavilion Shopping Center

10800 West Pico Boulevard (at the intersection of Westwood Boulevard); (310) 474–6255; www.westsidepavilion.com.

This is a *very* Los Angeles mall, with more than 180 shops, restaurants, and movie theaters.

The Skirball Cultural Center and Museum

2701 North Sepulveda Boulevard; (310) 440–4500; fax (310) 440–4595; www.skirball.org. Open Tuesday through Saturday noon to 5:00 P.M. and Sunday 11:00 A.M. to 5:00 P.M. Closed Monday. Children younger than age twelve admitted for **free.** $$

This museum highlights the experiences of American Jews as they transitioned from the Old World to the New World. The goal of the Skirball Center is to bring people of all backgrounds together. The museum enjoys a tranquil setting along the Sepulveda Pass near the Getty Center, so you can plan a full day of museum touring while in this vicinity.

Exhibits here follow the ebb and flow of Jewish immigration; displays include fragments of original Ellis Island wooden benches and a sectional reconstruction of an archaeological

Getty **Center**

1200 Getty Center Drive; (310) 440–7300; www.getty.edu. Open Tuesday through Thursday and Sunday 10:00 A.M. to 6:00 P.M. and Friday and Saturday 10:00 A.M. to 9:00 P.M. Closed Monday and major holidays. Admission is **free.** Parking $5.00. It is essential that you call ahead for a parking pass.

This landmark complex on a dramatic hilltop location commands breathtaking views of Los Angeles, the Santa Monica Mountains, and the Pacific. Its vast collection of art defies imagination. The 110-acre complex, designed by Richard Meier, is designed as a nexus for families and neighbors, as well as scholars and students. It all begins with a tram ride to the summit, where your family will be awed by panoramic views of the L.A. area. The center will fascinate every family member, even the two-year-olds in strollers with microscopic attention spans. At the central plaza, you'll find gardens, terraces, and dramatic architecture.

Start your exploration by viewing the orientation film so you can best decide how to spend the next few hours. There are five two-story pavilions around an open courtyard. Each gallery pavilion has an information room: Stop here to watch an artist carve a block of marble or have your kids handle a piece of wood. These hands-on experiences are accentuated by ongoing films, concerts, and demonstrations. Try to visit on the weekends when family festivals give you and your kids "new ideas about the cultures and people behind the art."

Just to give you a hint of the magnitude of the collection, there are fourteen galleries of French furniture and decorative arts, including four eighteenth-century paneled rooms. After an hour or so of visiting the galleries, we suggest stopping off at the courtyard at the Museum Cafe for a snack. The center houses such masterpieces as *Adoration of the Magi*, by Andrea Mantegna; *Irises*, by van Gogh; *Spring*, by Sir Lawrence Alma-Tadema; and Middle Ages miniatures by various painters. Plus there are sculptures, manuscripts, and photographs. After all this, you'll be ready for time in the Family Room for a look at activity guides and game boxes for children and adults. Arrive when the center opens (10:00 A.M.). The "Getty experience" should generate enthusiasm to ignite your children's appreciation of art—they may just want to return again!

dig. For lunch, Zeidlers, at the museum entrance, can't be beat. Cuisine is light, fresh, and imaginative. Salads, sandwiches, and desserts are reasonably priced, and the ambience is family-friendly. The gift shop has an impressive range of books covering the Jewish experience, with an excellent selection of books for children. Count on two hours, including lunch.

Where to Eat

Apple Pan, 10801 West Pico Boulevard; (310) 475–3585. Closed Monday. Here's a diner of sorts that has been feeding hungry Angelenos since the 1940s. The layout is simple: a long, three-sided countertop with a kitchen in the center. Wait for a vacant stool (there are no tables) then move in for the kill: The burgers served here are so divine they have been known to reconvert vegetarians. Many visit for the apple pie (it's the Apple Pan, after all), but the banana cream is also really luscious. $

Eiger Ice Cream, 124 East Barrington Place, off Sunset Boulevard and North Barrington Avenue; (310) 471–6955. Hours vary daily. The decor is minimalist; the ice cream is not. With an 18 percent butterfat content, we're talking ice crème de la crème here. Most flavors, including the ever-popular dark chocolate and raspberry combo, taste surprisingly light because of the purity of the ingredients. No wonder Eiger is a favorite snack spot for quality-conscious Westside families. Cash only. $

Beverly Hills

If you continue west on Wilshire Boulevard, you will enter the heart of Beverly Hills. The chief appeal of this city (population 33,000) for many families will be strolling up and down **Rodeo** (row-DAY-oh) **Drive,** a scaled-down version of New York's Fifth Avenue—with palm trees. It's fun to do a little window shopping at the most exclusive boutiques in Los Angeles. This is the center of the Golden Triangle district, framed by Crescent Drive and Wilshire and Little Santa Monica Boulevards, which represents the crème de la crème of Beverly Hills shopping. **Via Rodeo,** a new addition to Rodeo Drive, is a cobblestoned cache of shops and eateries at the Wilshire Boulevard end that resembles a charming European village.

After the price tags make you wonder who in the world can afford all of this stuff, hop in your car and find out. The gracefully curving palm- and jacaranda-lined streets between Santa Monica and Sunset Boulevards are home to affluent Mediterranean-style villas and many an elegant English Tudor–style manse. North of Sunset, however, especially in the exclusive **Bel Air** neighborhood farther west on the boulevard, is where the real estate truly boggles the mind.

Beverly Center

(310) 854–7616; www.beverlycenter.com.

A megamall with 160-plus shops and a sixteen-screen cineplex, where Beverly Boulevard meets La Cienega. Here you will find the original Hard Rock Cafe, easily recognizable by the automobile projecting from the rooftop. Show your hotel room key at Guest Services or the California Welcome Center and receive special treatment and discounts.

Beverly Hills Trolley

Leaves from the corner of Dayton Way and Rodeo Drive; (310) 285–2438; www.beverly hills.org. Open Tuesday through Saturday noon to 4:00 P.M. $

If you'd rather leave the driving to someone else for a while, park your car at one of Beverly Hills's numerous two-hour **free** parking lots and head for the Beverly Hills Trolley, a San Francisco–style cable car that takes visitors on forty-minute guided tours of the area's historical landmarks and residential areas. In a city where Rolls Royce Silver Clouds seem to outnumber Toyotas, the trolley is a welcome bargain.

Museum of Television and Radio

465 North Beverly Drive; (310) 786–1000; www.mtr.org. Open Wednesday through Sunday noon to 5:00 P.M.; closed on January 1, July 4, Thanksgiving, and Christmas. Free admission. Donations are welcome and suggested.

More than 120,000 archived broadcasts (duplicating the first museum founded in New York City) reside in this museum, which opened in 1996. Everything you and your family want to know about eighty-plus years of broadcasting is here. Special exhibits and screenings year-round. For example, "Re-creating Radio" workshops are held on Saturday mornings for families with children age nine and older. Call for schedules and times.

Where to Eat and Stay

Nate 'n Al Delicatessen Restaurant, 414 North Beverly Drive; (310) 274–0101; www.natenal.com. Open daily 7:00 A.M. to 9:00 P.M. Since 1945, serving top-notch smoked fish, cured meats, and matzo ball soup for hungry locals, visitors, celebrities, and families in a bustling, joyous atmosphere. Don't miss the matzo Brie, potato latkes, corned beef brisket, and anything made with pastrami.

Beverly Pavilion–a Best Western Hotel, 9360 Wilshire Boulevard; (310) 273–1400; www.beverlypavilion.com. Located just 3 blocks from world-famous Rodeo Drive shopping and dining and minutes from the Beverly Center, Melrose, and downtown Los Angeles. The excellent location and eighth-floor rooftop swimming pool give you the feeling of staying luxe without the high price.

Regent Beverly Wilshire, 9500 Wilshire Boulevard; (310) 275–5200. www.regent hotels.com. This world-class hotel is an oasis of elegance and impeccable service located at one of the world's most famous intersections—Wilshire Boulevard and Rodeo Drive (this place was featured in the movie *Pretty Woman,* starring Julia

Roberts, remember?). When making your reservation, tell the reservationist the ages of your kids and they will receive welcome gifts—stuffed animals, toys, robes—and cookies and milk at bedtime. Family packages are also available.

For More Information

Beverly Hills Chamber of Commerce. 239 South Beverly Drive, 90212; (310) 248–1000.

Beverly Hills Conference and Visitors Bureau. 239 South Beverly Drive, 90212; (800) 345–2210; www.beverlyhillsbe here .com.

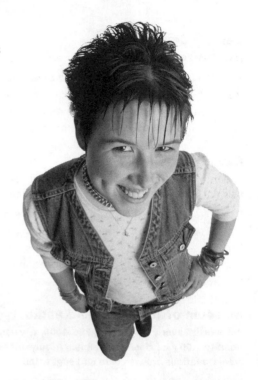

The Valleys

Did you think a trip to L.A. would be, like, complete without a visit to the valleys? Think again, dude (or dudette). The valleys are worlds unto themselves.

When you hear people talk about "the Valley," they are referring the **San Fernando Valley**, home of more than a million people and bigger than metropolitan Chicago. You can get an overview of the valley from serpentine **Mulholland Drive,** which bisects the Santa Monica Mountains, the natural topographical separator of the Los Angeles Basin from the vast valley floor.

If you have time for an outdoor interlude, by all means explore the **Santa Monica Mountains National Recreation Area.** These chaparral-covered slopes, which stretch 55 miles from Griffith Park all the way to Point Mugu in Ventura County, have provided the backdrop for many a Hollywood movie. For instance, *M*A*S*H* (movie and TV show) was filmed at **Malibu Creek State Park** (alongside Las Virgenes Road/Malibu Canyon) and at **Paramount Ranch,** Agoura Hills, 1813 Cornell Road; (805) 370–2301. The latter, once owned by Paramount Studios, still has the fabricated western town used in dozens of films and TV shows. Horseback riding and nature walks through the canyons covering 2,400 acres also make for refreshing mini-escapes from the city's bustle.

If you have more time, explore the stretch of miles-long **Ventura Boulevard,** which bisects Encino and Sherman Oaks. Together with U.S. Highway 101 (the Ventura Freeway), "the Boulevard" is the valley's main artery. Of the two, Encino has the more upmarket sections, whereas Sherman Oaks (along Ventura Boulevard) has a myriad of Melrose-like establishments.

The **Canyons**

Coldwater Canyon (which connects Beverly Hills to Studio City) and, about 10 miles to the west, **Topanga Canyon** (connecting Malibu to Woodland Hills) are sights to see. *Topanga* is a Chumash Indian word meaning "mountains that crash down to the sea." You'll see what the Chumash meant if you drive the length of the canyon. If you park your car along any of the turnouts along the road and look closely at the exposed mountain sides, you may well see fossils of ancient sea creatures—proof positive the whole area was once under water.

The intersection of Topanga and Old Topanga Canyon Roads is marked by the village of—no surprise here—Topanga, with its health-food stores, hippie feel, and more. One place you'll want to visit is the **Will Geer Theatricum Botanicum,** an open-air ancient Greek-style amphitheater that features first-rate performances of Shakespearean works and other classics and a children's concert series, 1419 North Topanga Canyon Boulevard, 5 miles from U.S. Highway 101; (310) 455–2322; fax (310) 455–3724; for schedule, (310) 455–3723; www.theatricum.com. Open in May, this outdoor theater offers more than culture. It occupies a natural setting with a youth drama camp, youth classes, and a variety of plays. Call ahead for schedule.

Burbank

Among the largest cities in California (population 100,000-plus) is Burbank, known as the home of major film and television studios, a bustling airport, and shopping malls. Many jokes have been made by television shows that emanate from here about "beautiful downtown Burbank," but you and your family will want to visit those studios.

Warner Bros. Studio VIP Tour (ages 8 and over)

4301 Olive Avenue, Gate 3; (818) 972–8687 or (818) 846–1403. http://wbsf.warnerbros.com/ home.html. Tours generally Monday through Friday 9:00 A.M. to 3:00 P.M., with expanded hours in summer. Call for schedule. Reservations are required. $$$

This is an insider's look at a very busy and famous motion picture and television studio—past and present. The tour begins with a short film highlighting the movies and television shows created by Warner Bros. talent. Then, via electric tour carts to the Warner Bros. Museum and from the museum, you visit back-lot sets, soundstages, and craft/production shops. Routes change from day to day to accommodate production on the lot, so no two tours are exactly alike. Tours last approximately two and a half hours.

NBC Studios (ages 5 and over)
3000 West Alameda Avenue; (818) 840–3537.

Escorted walking tours are generally available on a first-come, first-served basis Monday through Friday, every hour on the hour between 9:00 A.M. and 3:00 P.M. If you're lucky you might see Jay Leno or his famous Studio 3. Call for current tour schedules and fees.

Where to Stay

Hilton Burbank Airport Hotel & Convention Center, 2500 Hollywood Way; (818) 843–6000; fax (818) 842–9720; www .burbankairport.hilton.com. Located across the street from the Burbank Glendale Pasadena Airport, the airport closest to Hollywood, Universal Studios, CityWalk, and Six Flags Magic Mountain. **Free** air-

port shuttle service. Renovated in 2001, 488 comfortable guest rooms and suites. Excellent "home base" for exploring greater L.A. $$$

For More Information

Burbank Chamber of Commerce. 200 West Magnolia Boulevard, 91502; (818) 846–3111; www.burbankchamber.org.

Santa Clarita Valley

Just twenty-five minutes north of Hollywood, discover Valencia—home to the Six Flags California Entertainment Complex, a not-to-be-missed area for your thrill-seeking family!

Six Flags Magic Mountain—The Xtreme Park
26101 Magic Mountain Parkway; (661) 255–4111; www.sixflags.com. The complex is located off Interstate 5, from the Magic Mountain Parkway exit, thirty minutes north of downtown Los Angeles. Open daily from March through September; weekends and holidays rest of year. Call for exact schedule and opening and closing hours. $$$$

In 2003, The Xtreme Park opened SCREAM, the park's "Sweet 16" roller coaster, shattering its own Guinness Book world-record status as the theme park with the most coasters on the planet! Known worldwide as a thrill-ride haven, the 260-acre theme park features more than one hundred rides, games, and attractions for the entire family. Enjoy such exciting thrill rides as X—the world's first and only four-dimensional roller coaster; Deja vu—the world's fastest and tallest suspended, looping boomerang coaster; Goliath—the coaster GIANT among GIANTS; The Riddler's Revenge—the world's tallest and fastest stand-up roller coaster; Superman The Escape—towering 415 feet in the air; Colossus; Batman The Ride; Viper; and many more. For younger guests there is Bugs Bunny World, featuring rides and attractions that provide real thrills for kids and adults alike. In addition, meet your favorite Looney Tunes characters—Bugs Bunny, Daffy Duck, Yosemite Sam, and Sylvester. ALL this in one day!

Six Flags Hurricane Harbor

Located next door to Six Flags Magic Mountain; (661) 255–4100. Open weekends May through August and daily Memorial Day through Labor Day. Call for exact schedule and times. $$$

This tropical-themed water-park attraction features more than twenty-two slides and attractions, including Black Snake Summit, with two of the tallest enclosed speed slides in Southern California; Lizard Lagoon, a 7,000-square-foot pool for teen and adult activities; Bamboo Racer, an exciting 45-foot-tall, six-lane racing attraction; Castaway Cove, an exclusive children's water-play kingdom; Shipwreck Shores, with water-play activities for the entire family; the Forgotten Sea wave pool; and The River Cruise lazy river. Way cool fun!

For More Information

Santa Clarita Valley Tourism Bureau.
23920 Valencia Boulevard, Suite 300, Santa Clarita, 91355; (661) 255–4318 or (800) TOUR–395; fax (661) 259–8125; www.visit santaclarita.com.

Pasadena

Pasadena is the shining star of the San Gabriel Valley, just northeast of downtown L.A. While the annual **Tournament of Roses Parade** (626–449–4100; www.tournamentof roses.com), held every January 1 since 1890, and **Rose Bowl Stadium** (626–577–3100; www.rosebowlstadium.com) have made the city famous, the charm is in Old Pasadena with its Spanish Mission–style buildings, many of which are listed on the National Register of Historic Places.

Huntington Library Art Collection and Botanical Gardens

1151 Oxford Road, San Marino (2 miles from Pasadena); (626) 405–2100; fax (626) 405–0225; www.huntington.org. Open noon to 4:30 P.M. Tuesday through Friday and weekends 10:30 A.M. to 4:30 P.M.; closed Monday. $$

At the 150-acre Huntington, you can walk through perfectly manicured gardens on your way to view a precious scrap of Emily Dickinson poetry or other historical documents and manuscripts. The library is home to many first-edition books, including a Gutenberg Bible. The wonderful exhibits bring history into perspective, reminding us how people managed to communicate before computers and faxes. The oil paintings, furniture, and decorative accessories are elegantly displayed. There's a restaurant, the Rose Garden Cafe (enjoy an English tea) (626) 683–8131, and an excellent bookshop. Opened in 2004, the Helen and Peter Bing Children's Garden offers one acre of kinetic sculptures and activities for children ages two through seven.

Santa Anita Park (Home of Seabiscuit)

285 West Huntington Drive, Arcadia; (626) 574–7223; www.santaanita.com.

Located just a few miles east of Pasadena, Santa Anita Park is more than just a racetrack.

The architecture is art deco and the cuisine is outstanding. Thoroughbred racing is the main event at the track, but this park is relaxing, exquisitely landscaped, and worth the trip. New in 2003 is a Seabiscuit tram tour that includes riding by Seabiscuit's barn, looking at the locations where the movie *Seabiscuit* was filmed, observing the daily activities of the stable area during training, discovering the receiving barn, and having a "never-before-permitted" look inside the jockeys' room, the saddling paddock, and more, all with detailed explanations. Visit the *Seabiscuit* and *George Woolf* statues in the Paddock Gardens. Tours depart from the new tram boarding area across from the receiving barn at 8:30 A.M. and 10:00 A.M. every Saturday and Sunday during racing season only.

Raging Waters

111 Raging Waters Drive (take the Raging Waters Drive exit off Interstate 210), San Dimas (east of Pasadena) where the 10, 210, and 57 freeways meet; (909) 592–1457, 24-hour information line (909) 802–2200; fax (909) 592–1457; www.ragingwaters.com. Open daily June 1 through late September; weekends in May. It is essential you call in advance as hours and days of operation constantly change. $$$$

The fifty-acre park, the largest water-theme park west of the Mississippi, houses fifty million gallons of water and more than thirty-five water attractions for aquatic thrillseekers, including the Vortex, a four-story tower with two enclosed, 270-foot-long, spiral body flumes; and the world's highest headfirst water ride, the High EXtreme. For those not inclined to plunge from such heights or velocities, there are tamer options, including a children's activity pool and play area. New for 2004 is the Dragon's Den, a 45-foot drop down an enclosed flume. OutRAGEous!

Where to Stay

The Ritz-Carlton, Huntington Hotel and Spa, 1401 South Oak Knoll Avenue; (626) 568–3900 or (800) 241–3333; www.ritz carlton.com. Located in Pasadena, fifteen minutes from downtown Los Angeles, this lovingly restored historic landmark first opened in 1907 and recalls the grace and elegance of a past era. The hotel has two restaurants, a full-service spa, twenty-three acres of gardens and grounds, and eight guest bungalows with working fireplaces. Special packages are available. $$$$

For More Information

Pasadena Convention and Visitors Bureau. 171 South Los Robles Avenue; (626) 795–9311 or (800) 307–7977; fax (626) 795–9656; www.PasadenaCal.com.

Coastal Los Angeles

After a few days spent driving, museum hopping, driving, stargazing, driving, shopping, and driving some more, you and the kids may begin to feel a little antsy. If you're starting to think "L.A.'s great, but . . ." then it's high time you hit the beach. Whereas in cities like Boston or New York there are only gradations of stress—it never totally dissipates—in

L.A., stress can be lowered to tolerable levels thanks to the proximity of a long and stunning coastline and the beach. And when it comes to beaches, you're truly spoiled with choices in Southern California. Three areas are absolute must-sees for families on vacation: Venice Beach, Santa Monica, and Malibu. While there are other beaches, none bear the singular L.A. signature as indelibly as these. (The Long Beach area is discussed separately.)

Venice Beach and Marina del Rey

Venice Beach lies due south of Santa Monica. Venice is sort of like Melrose Avenue (see Westside, earlier) meeting the sea: Anything goes, but with copious amounts of suntan oil.

While L.A. beaches are endowed with more than 22 miles of bicycle paths, the most colorful swath is **Oceanfront Walk** in Venice, where bikers, roller skaters, and zany in-line skaters all compete with pedestrians for maximum mobility. Add street performers—from jugglers and mimes to musicians and comedians—and you'll get an idea of the carnival-like atmosphere permeating the place. People come to Venice Beach not so much for the beach, which is actually quite nice, but to watch other people. A serious amount of body spotting goes on at **Muscle Beach,** a section of the sand where bodybuilders work out in the sun and flex their Schwarzenegger deltoids, pectorals, and biceps. If your kids are needling you for souvenirs, this is the place (and remember that when buying trinkets on the beach, tackiness is a virtue).

Marina del Rey lies adjacent to Venice Beach, on the shore of the Pacific Ocean, 4 miles north of Los Angeles International Airport (LAX) and 3 miles south of Santa Monica. Boasting the world's largest man-made marina (more than 5,000 vessels), every conceivable type of water sport is offered here, from boats and watercraft you pedal, paddle, sail, or drive to windsurfing, sunbathing, swimming, and surfing. Other water-based options include boat charters, harbor cruises, whale-watching, and ocean fishing. From "the Marina," bike, skate, walk, or run along a 26-mile coastal path that stretches from Malibu at the northern end through the marina and south to Palos Verdes. Kid-friendly **Mother's Beach,** as the name implies, is a must for families; as is **Fisherman's Village,** a quaint area of shops, restaurants, and charter/cruise boat docks.

Where to Eat and Stay

Jody Maroni's Sausage Kingdom, 2011 Ocean Front Walk, Venice Beach; (310) 822–5639. Open, thankfully, every day. This zany beach is the perfect place for this eclectic stand that brings sausage to a new level. Just try the Mexican Jalapeño and you'll understand why! Open for breakfast, too. Check out the Family Special.

Tony P's Dockside Grill, 4445 Admiralty Way, Marina del Rey; (310) 823–4534; www.tonyps.com. Totally family-friendly waterfront casual dining. Open daily for lunch and dinner and on Saturday and

Sunday for an all-American breakfast. Generous portions of steak, fresh seafood, pasta, and burgers at reasonable prices. The "Dinghy Club" kids' menu is one of the best we've seen for ages ten and younger—all meals $3.95! Every kid gets a gift bag of little toys, including a compass. What kid can resist a non-alcoholic "FooFoo drink" such as a Pina Colada or Strawberry Margarita? If kids clean their plate, they get a **free** dessert.

Best Western Jamaica Bay Inn, 4175 Admiralty Way, Marina del Rey; (310) 823–5333; www.bestwestern-jamaicabay.com. Forty-two spacious guest rooms right on the sand (private beach) with stunning views of the bustling marina. Casual, laid-back atmosphere; great for relaxing but close to so many attractions you want to visit. The Beachside Café serves breakfast and lunch daily around the pool. Great values; ask for family packages.

For More Information

Marina del Rey Convention and Visitors Bureau. 4701 Admiralty Way, 90292; visitor information line (310) 305–9545; www.VisitTheMarina.com.

Santa Monica

Santa Monica has been a favorite family hideaway since the early 1930s when wealthy Easterners came for winter respites and never left. Just 8.3 square miles and surrounded on three sides by Los Angeles (and the fourth side by the Pacific Ocean), the city's safe, eco-friendly environment is easy to navigate. Most of the major hotels, attractions, shopping, and dining outlets are conveniently located within a 14-block radius. Be sure to check out **Palisades Park,** a cliff-top twenty-six-acre greenbelt overlooking the Pacific with miles of lush greenery and shady palms for walking, resting, jogging, picnicking, and bicycling. Three miles of coastline, two excellent beaches, historic Santa Monica Pier, hike-friendly mountains, and year-round warm weather in which to enjoy it all!

Santa Monica Pier and Pacific Park

The oldest pleasure pier on the West Coast, Santa Monica opened in 1909. The pier also features Heal the Bay's Santa Monica Pier Aquarium, the historic Hippodrome, and a handcrafted carousel (circa 1922) with forty-four handpainted wooden horses. Here you'll discover dining, amusement games, shops, and a fresh fish market. Year-round live entertainment is offered.

Pacific Park (310–260–8744; www.pacpark.com) is a traditional small, family amusement park. Hours vary by season so be sure to call in advance. Admission to the park is free, with all twelve rides and dozens of games on a "pay-as-you-go" basis, or you can buy an all-day wristband for unlimited rides. The world's first solar-powered Ferris wheel offers stunning views from its nine-story height. A special Kiddy Zone has pint-size rides for kids less than 42 inches tall. Of course, there are bumper cars, a roller coaster, minigolf, a nine-story plunge tower, and a flying swing for us big kids.

Bergamot Station Arts Center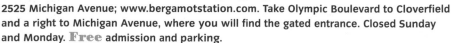

2525 Michigan Avenue; www.bergamotstation.com. Take Olympic Boulevard to Cloverfield and a right to Michigan Avenue, where you will find the gated entrance. Closed Sunday and Monday. Free admission and parking.

Check your street map because this enclave of forty eclectic art galleries exhibits a range of art. This is a light industrial area, so galleries have metallic roofs, high ceilings, and lots of wall space. From sculpture and wearable art to paintings, photography, and prints, this is a wonderland of creativity. Recent artists seen here include Frank Stella, Robert Mother-well, and David Hockney. There is a schedule listing each gallery, openings, and current exhibits. The Gallery Cafe is a good place to stop first and take a moment to plan your gallery stops. The **Santa Monica Museum of Art** has changing exhibits as well, and kids will find it a friendly place to start their art exploration. Plan to spend about an hour. Parking is free. For information on the Santa Monica Museum of Art, call (310) 586–6488 or fax (310) 586–6487; www.smmoa.org. Hours are Tuesday through Saturday 11:00 A.M. to 6:00 P.M.

Third Street Promenade

In Santa Monica, some of the best times await families just a few blocks from the sand. Here you can shop in the sunshine or at night until midnight at this ultra-lively spot that begins at Broadway (actually at the Santa Monica Place mall) and stretches north to Wilshire Boulevard along Third Street. Now one of the hippest areas in L.A., the prome-nade (www.thirdstreetpromenade.com) overflows with shops, restaurants, entertainment centers, and street performers. Wander and enjoy.

Magicopolis

1418 Fourth Street; (310) 451–2241; fax (310) 451–2341; www.magicopolis.com. $$$

This new 350-person, two-theater club welcomes all ages to ninety-minute magic shows Tuesday through Sunday. World-class magicians entertain at evening performances (8:00 P.M.) and weekend matinees (2:00 P.M. and 7:00 P.M.).

Museum of Flying

2772 Donald Douglas Loop North; (310) 392–8822; fax (310) 450–6956; www.museumofflying.com. Call for schedule and hours. $$

Visitors often forget that, like Beverly Hills, Santa Monica is a separate municipality from L.A., even though L.A. surrounds it. So it should not be too surprising that Santa Monica has its own airport. But what makes it such a Southern California air-port is that, in addition to the usual runways and airplanes, it has the Museum of Flying.

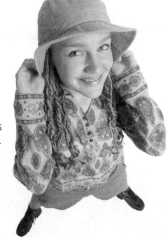

Where to Eat

Cora's Coffee Shop, 1802 Ocean Avenue; (310) 451–9562. This great institution is a leftover from the 1930s. This tiny diner serves marvelous daily specials, a terrific steak salad, and fresh-baked pies, such as pear and peach. A real find. Limited **free** parking. $$

Typhoon, 3221 Donald Douglas Loop South, at the edge of the Santa Monica Airport; (310) 390–6565; www.typhoon-restaurant.com. Kids can watch the airplanes land between bites of Pan-Asian cuisine, such as Vietnamese spring rolls, fried rice, and puffy *bao* buns. New on the menu are insects! Yes, there are crunchy crickets, stir-fry crickets, giant mountain ants, and Thai-style crispy scorpions. Now that's a mouthful! Celebrities such as John Travolta have been known to fly their private planes to Typhoon, so be prepared for a stellar dining experience. $$$

Where to Stay

The Georgian Hotel, 1415 Ocean Avenue; (310) 395–9945 or (800) 538–8147 (toll-free reservations); www.georgian hotel.com. This distinctive turquoise and gold art deco gem, built in 1933 as a seaside getaway for the exclusive Hollywood set, was beautifully restored and refurbished (even Nintendo games and WiFi) in 2001. Choose from fifty-six spacious rooms and twenty-eight suites overlooking the city and Santa Monica Bay. Great for families. $$$$

Loews Santa Monica Beach Hotel, 1700 Ocean Avenue; (310) 458–6700; fax (310) 458–6761; www.loewshotels.com. Operating since 1989 in an unbeatable location adjacent to Santa Monica Pier overlooking the Pacific, with excellent beach access out the back ground-floor doors. This casually elegant 342-room luxury property has an outstanding children's program that includes lending-game libraries, special menus, tours, welcome gifts for children younger than age ten, and supervised recreational programs. Children younger than age eighteen stay **free** in same room as parents. Also ask about "generation g," a program for grandparents and grandchildren traveling together with adjoining rooms at half price (subject to availability), a photo memory album, a handy phone card to call home, matching luggage tags, and a **free** movie with popcorn. The spa, fitness suite, ocean-view pool, and whirlpool are perfect for relaxing after a hard day's touring. $$$$

For More Information

Santa Monica Convention and Visitors Bureau. 1114½ South Cloverdale, 90019; (800) 544–5319; www.santamonica.com.

Santa Monica Walk-in Visitor Centers. Santa Monica Place, 2nd Floor, Suite 203 and 1400 Ocean Avenue; (310) 393–7593.

Malibu

Malibu is Beach Boys country, where a dozen or so beaches beckon alongside the Pacific Coast Highway (PCH) at the foot of the Santa Monica Mountains. Although part of Los Angeles County, Malibu is actually a separate city—and a funny-shaped one at that. Because of the area's geography, Malibu is barely 1.5 miles wide but some 27 miles long. PCH is the lifeline of this seaside community and the commuting route to Hollywood for the hundreds of celebrities who live in seaside villas and estates here. You might even bump into one or two on the beach—it happens all the time.

One of the finest stretches of sand is **Malibu Beach,** on either side of the **Malibu Pier** (you can't miss it). White sand, pounding surf, sun-bronzed lifeguards with fluorescent-colored zinc oxide on their noses—yes, this is Malibu. Even in summer, the beach is not as crowded as those in Santa Monica and Venice, and there is less emphasis on people-watching. Malibu-ites know what's really important in life: surfing.

Actually, the best surfing beach is **Zuma Beach,** 5 or 6 miles farther up PCH.

Where to Eat

Dukes at Malibu, 21150 Pacific Coast Highway; (310) 317–0777. Lunch and dinner daily. Named after Duke Kahanamoku, the "father of surfing," this is the ideal place for your family to get the feeling of the Malibu lifestyle, thanks to the magnificent stretch of windows overlooking the beach. The prices are reasonable, and the kids will like the exhibit of surfing memorabilia. You might remind them about the Beach Boys and all of those surfing movies from the 1960s. $$

Granita, 23725 Pacific Coast Highway; (310) 456–0488. A nifty lunchtime stop, Granita is the brainchild of super-chef Wolfgang Puck (of Spago fame). It resembles a temple in Atlantis from the outside and a futuristic aquarium on the inside. Named for an Italian dessert of flavored, shaved ice (always available), Granita offers a California eclectic menu, and the desserts are deliciously inventive. Granita is located in a shopping center with a variety of trendy Malibu boutiques. Pick up a **free** copy of the local newspaper, the *Malibu Times,* for a look at what's happening around town. $$$$

For More Information

Malibu Chamber of Commerce. 23805 Stuart Ranch Road, Suite 100, 90265; (310) 456–9025; www.malibu.org.

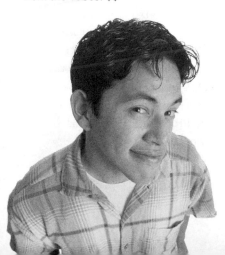

Long Beach

As its name indicates, life in Long Beach centers around things of a coastal nature, with more than 50 miles of sandy beaches and shorelines. Settled by the Spaniards in 1784, Long Beach has been a visitor-friendly place ever since. Real live guides are at visitors' disposal in the animated downtown area. Though close to downtown Los Angeles, Long Beach has a distinctly different, somewhat lower-key feel. If you have the time, give yourself two full days here.

In Long Beach, you will find an array of peaceful beaches that invite sunbathing and sand-castle building. Thanks to a human-made breakwater, the beaches of Long Beach do not experience high surf and are therefore ideal for families with small children.

Long Beach offers countless ways to spend a pleasant morning or afternoon. The 15-block stretch of Second Street in the **Belmont Shore** area has swimming, lots of boutiques, and restaurants that range from Indian to Chinese to New York–style bagel shops. A mile and a half away, down Ocean Boulevard, downtown activity hustles and bustles along revitalized Pine Avenue.

Gondola Getaway

5437 East Ocean Boulevard; (562) 433–9595; www.gondolagetawayinc.com. Open daily from 11:00 A.M. to 11:00 P.M. Children younger than age two ride free. **$$$$**

Locally famous, the Getaway features Venetian-style gondolas that cruise through narrow canals in the "backyards" of affluent home owners. They started plying the waters in 1982. Ten gondolas seat from two to fourteen people each. Cruises last fifty minutes. Your family will be enchanted!

Queen **Mary**

There are many fun family attractions in Long Beach, but none so famous as the majestic *Queen Mary*. The world's largest luxury liner is permanently docked in the fifty-five-acre **Queen Mary Seaport,** located at the end of the 710 Freeway. There are many hotels in Long Beach, but if this is your first visit, try the **Hotel Queen Mary,** 1126 Queens Highway; (562) 435–3511 or (800) 437–2934; fax (562) 437–4531; www.queenmary.com. The ship has been converted into the 365-stateroom hotel. While aboard, you can take a Behind the Scenes guided tour or dine in one of the ship's restaurants. The **Chelsea** serves lunch and dinner. Here you'll also find the **Piccadilly Circus,** the boat's original shopping center. If you can't stay on the ship for a night or two, be sure to indulge in a tour. Add a tour of the Russian Foxtrot Submarine *Scorpion* or the Ghosts and Legends Show. $$$

On the **Water**

Alfredo's Beach Rentals. (562) 434–6121. Boogie boards? Skates? Bikes? All of the equipment you couldn't get on the plane and in your car can be rented from Alfredo! Also in Redondo Beach and Manhattan Beach.

Star Party Cruises. (562) 799–7000. Offers a 300-passenger, 100-foot motor cruiser.

Rainbow Rocket. (562) 43–ROCKET; www.rainbowrocket.net. 124-passenger 200 HP speedboat. Fast fun for everyone!

Long Beach Sport Fishing. (562) 432–8993.

Off Shore Water Sports. (562) 436–1996.

Bay Boat Rentals. (562) 598–BOAT or (562) 433–9595.

Shoreline Village Cruises. (562) 495–5884. Sail aboard a 90-foot motor yacht. All tours include narration, and Shoreline guarantees whale sightings or a second trip is **free.**

Latin American Art Museum

628 Alamitos Avenue; (562) 437–1689; fax (562) 437–7043; www.molaa.com. Open Tuesday through Friday 11:30 A.M. to 7:00 P.M., Saturday 11:00 A.M. to 7:00 P.M., and Sunday 11:00 A.M. to 6:00 P.M. Call ahead for calendar of events. Children younger than age twelve admitted **free.** Friday is **free** to everyone.

This facility in downtown Long Beach is the only museum in the country that focuses on Latin American art and culture. The 20,000-square-foot building was built in 1920 and houses the Robert Gumbiner Foundation collection of Latin American art, galleries for temporary showings, Viva Cafe and Museum Store, a research library, and a performance area.

Long Beach Aquarium of the Pacific

100 Aquarium Way; (562) 590–3100; www.aquariumofpacific.org. Open daily 9:00 A.M. to 6:00 P.M. $$$

When you see the full-scale model of a blue whale, you'll know you're at the Long Beach Aquarium, a 156,000-square-foot facility that covers five acres and includes 550 species and 12,000 specimens. After you've checked out the wonderful exhibits, including Sea Lion/Seal Tunnel, Baja Gallery, Wetlands Discovery Lab, Pacific Gallery, Coastal Corner, Live Coral Discovery, Lorikeet Aviary, and the Shark Lagoon, head for Kid's Cove. A playground of the Pacific Ocean, Kid's Cove is a hands-on interactive aquarium experience for kids of all ages. The focus is on feeding habits, family structures, and the lives of the exhibit specimens. Dine at the Bamboo Bistro or Cafe Scuba.

Where to Eat

King's Fish House/King Crab Lounge,
100 West Broadway at Pine Avenue; (323)
423–7463. Here are the ingredients for a
popular family restaurant: friendly service,
comfortable wood booths, and fair prices.
It all adds up to our favorite seafood
restaurant in Long Beach. $$

Parker's Lighthouse, 435 Shoreline Drive,
Long Beach; (562) 432–6500; www.parkers
lighthouse.com. Serves lunch and dinner
daily. Your best bet is the Sunday brunch.
Just look for the lighthouse to find this
family-friendly restaurant. The view is ter-
rific from the patio: the *Queen Mary* and
harbor. The down-to-earth menu includes
fresh fish, mesquite-grilled with a choice of
side sauces. And don't forget to save room
for a slice of key lime pie. $$$

Where to Stay

Dockside Boat & Bed, Long Beach, Rainbow Harbor; (562) 436–3111; www.boat
andbed.com. Four private moored yachts
to stay aboard overnight. All boats fully furnished; continental breakfast basket provided. Next to Aquarium of the Pacific and
Shoreline Village. A highly recommended
unique family-lodging experience. $$$$

For More Information

**Long Beach Area Convention and Visi-
tor's Bureau.** 1 World Trade Center, Third
Floor, 90831; (562) 570–3170 or (800)
452–7829; fax (562) 435–5653; www.visit
longbeach.com.

San Pedro—Port of Los Angeles

Originally settled as a commercial fishing village in the 1800s, today San Pedro is home to
the Port of Los Angeles, one of the world's largest deepwater commercial seaports. Here
you also will find the **World Cruise Center** (located at Berths 91, 92, and 93A/B), point of
embarkation for more than 1.1 million passengers sailing on vacations to Mexico, Alaska,
Hawaii, and beyond onboard ships from Royal Caribbean Cruises, Crystal Cruises, Holland
America, and Princess Lines. Located at the end of the 110-Harbor Freeway, San Pedro
offers value-priced lodging, restaurants, and shopping options. It is easy to explore the
attractions via the 25-cent San Pedro Electric Trolley, which runs every fifteen minutes
(Thursday through Monday) from the World Cruise Center/Catalina Air & Sea Terminal to
the Maritime Museum and Ports O'Call Village.

Los Angeles Maritime Museum

**Berth 94, at the foot of Sixth Street; (310) 548–7618; www.lamaritimemuseum.org. Open
Tuesday through Sunday 10:00 A.M. to 5:00 P.M. $1 donation requested.**

Built in 1941, this "Streamlined Moderne" building was the base for an auto ferry. Saved
and beautifully restored, it now houses the largest maritime museum in California. This
75,000-square-foot facility features more than 700 ship and boat models, a variety of navigational equipment, and an operating amateur radio station. Try your hand at tying any of
the sixty-four types of seaman's knots on display.

Cabrillo Marine Aquarium

3720 Steven White Drive; (310) 548–7562; (310) 548–2649; www.cabrilloaq.org. Open Tuesday through Friday noon to 5:00 P.M., Saturday and Sunday 10:00 A.M. to 5:00 P.M. Parking is $6.50 per car. **Free** but a donation of $2.00 for adults and $1.00 for children appreciated.

Featuring thirty-five aquaria, these innovative exhibits will teach kids about the plant and animal life of Southern California. The simulated "tide pool touch tank" is a good place to start this aquatic journey. In addition, there are whale trips organized from December through March focusing on the Pacific gray whale. This museum predated the Long Beach Aquarium by sixty-five years. Here's where it all started, and that's no fish story.

SS *Lane Victory*

Berth 94 off Harbor Boulevard; (310) 519–9545; www.lanevictory.org. Open for tours daily 9:00 A.M. to 4:00 P.M. except for six Saturday daylong cruises each summer. $

This operational World War II cargo ship with wartime armament was built in 1945 and saw service in WWII, Korea, and Vietnam. Decommissioned and fully restored, her 455-foot length and 10,000 tons are a marvel to behold. If your family is visiting the Los Angeles area in the summer, make every attempt to secure reservations on one of the six-day cruises, where the seamen's lives will come alive as you sail. You will even be buzzed by attacking biplanes. This ship is a living memorial to all Merchant Marines.

For More Information

San Pedro Peninsula Chamber of Commerce. 390 West Seventh Street, 90731; (310) 832–7272 or (888) 447–3376; www.sanpedrochamber.com or www.sanpedro.com.

Port of Los Angeles. 425 South Palos Verdes Street, 90731; (310) SEA–PORT; www.portoflosangeles.org.

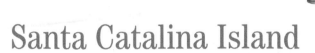

Santa Catalina Island

Sail away to Mediterranean-like Santa Catalina Island, a relaxing 22-mile (one-hour) boat trip from Long Beach or San Pedro Harbor. You might want to spend a couple of days on this enchanted isle, where you won't need a car for a change. The best way to get to Santa Catalina is aboard the *Catalina Express,* (310) 519–1212; fax (310) 548–8425; www.catalinaexpress.com. You'll arrive in sun-splashed **Avalon.** With its restaurant- and boutique-filled streets and a population of around 3,000, it's Catalina's biggest town. Your headquarters for fun.

On the **Wild Side**

Catalina now has a four-hour off-road tour that is ideal for families. Visiting the "wild side" of the island on the **Cape Canyon Tour,** passengers ride in a four-wheel-drive vehicle driven by a Catalina Island Conservancy–trained guide. The tour features a scenic drive along a ridgeline overlooking coves of west Avalon, a guided tour of the American Bald Eagle Habitat at Middle Ranch, and a ride in Cape Canyon for stunning views of the Catalina outback. Lunch is included at the famous Catalina Airport-in-the-Sky. Reservations required, (310) 510–2000; www.scico.com.

Catalina Casino

You can't miss this red-roofed Avalon landmark as you approach the harbor. Never actually used for gambling, the casino is famed for its ballroom and the Avalon Theatre, the first theater designed for sound movies. Art deco murals of stylized underwater scenes grace the theater, which also has a full-scale pipe organ with 250 miles of wire. Call (310) 510–2414 for information.

Santa Catalina Island Company's Discovery Tours

(310) 510–2500 or (800) 626–1496; www.scico.com/html/discovery_tours.html.

Operating since 1894 and departing from Avalon and Two Harbors; celebrated an incredible milestone in 2004. Discovery Tours by Land include the Avalon Scenic Tour, Casino Tour, Skyline Drive Tour, and Inland Motor Tour (the most comprehensive at four hours). Discovery Tours by Sea include Undersea Tour, Glass Bottom Boat Trip, Seal Rocks Cruise, Sundown Isthmus Cruise, and the Flying Fish Boat Trip. Money-saving combinations are the best way to tailor the tours to your family at a 25 percent discount off regular pricing. Reservations are recommended, especially during the busy times of weekends, holidays, and the summer season.

Catalina Adventure Tours

(310) 510–2888; www.catalinaadventuretours.com.

Tours via modern air-conditioned buses include the Avalon Explorer, City Passport, City Botanical, and Inside Adventure (the most popular). On the water, tours include the SS *Nautilus* (a semi-submersible sub), *Sea View* (glass-bottom boat); Seal Rock Explorer Cruise; and a Scenic Harbor cruise. Village Walking tours are also offered.

Kid **Cuisine**

The **Blue Parrot** at Metropole Market Place, Avalon (310–510–2465; www.blueparrotcatalina.com), is priced right. This second-floor restaurant has a terrific view of Avalon Bay, and the burgers are among the best in town. For dessert, walk over to the **Catalina Cookie Company** at 205 Crescent Avenue (310–510–2447) for an Eclipse, a fudge cookie dipped in white chocolate. It's just another delicious day in Catalina!

Where to Stay

Pavilion Lodge, 513 Crescent Avenue, Avalon; (310) 510–2500 or (800) 626–1496; www.scico.com. Seventy-three newly renovated rooms in a central location perfect for families. Excellent values and packages. Beach lovers will like the Pavilion Lodge— it's just "14 steps from the beach." $$

For More Information

Catalina Island Visitors Bureau and Chamber of Commerce. On the Green Pleasure Pier in the center of town, P.O. Box 217, Avalon, 90704; (310) 510–1520; www.visitcatalina.org or www.catalina .com.

Santa Catalina Island Company. P.O. Box 737, Avalon, 90704; (310) 510–2000 or (800) 626–1496; www.scico.com. Owners of Discovery Tours, Pavilion Lodge, Hotel Atwater, Banning House Lodge, Catalina Country Club, Descanso Beach Club, and other services.

Leave the Driving to **Someone Else**

Riding the rails—it's the alternative to driving on your trip through Southern California. AMTRAK has excellent routes in the West, and it's the best way to circumvent the traffic! The train that does it best in Southern California is called the Pacific Surfliner, with daily service between San Diego, Los Angeles, Santa Barbara, and San Luis Obispo.

Among the attractions along the route are Disneyland, the missions at San Juan Capistrano, Sea World, the beaches of Santa Barbara, and bustling Los Angeles, with connections to the MTA light-rail and subways.

Children's discounts offer savings for families. Kids ages two to fifteen are entitled to a 50 percent discount every day, any day when traveling with an adult paying full fare. Plus, book tickets online and save an additional 5 percent. Call AMTRAK at 800–USA–RAIL; www.amtrak.com.

Redondo Beach

Known as the South Bay (because the area is south of Long Beach), Redondo Beach is within a forty-five-minute range of Disneyland, Knott's Berry Farm, Universal Studios, Six Flags Magic Mountain, the La Brea Tar Pits, Catalina Island terminals, and the *Queen Mary*. Redondo has the Galleria at South Bay (with 150 stores), superb sportfishing, and charters at the Redondo Beach King Harbor Marina.

Where to Eat and Stay

Captain Kidd's, 209 Harbor Drive; (310) 372–7703; www.CaptainKidds.com. Open for breakfast, lunch, and dinner daily. Fresh-from-the-market fish and crab are prepared grilled, Cajun-style, charbroiled, or deep fried and come with two generous side dishes. Check the Captain Kid's menu for seafood specialties. $$

The Fun Fish Market & Restaurant/Fun Factory Amusement Center, 121 International Boardwalk; (310) 374–9982. The Redondo Pier has an amusement center, which is good, but even more appealing around lunch- or dinnertime is Fun Fish, where fresh fish is served any way you like it. Kids will like selecting their fish from a tank. And don't forget the chowder! $$

Versailles, 1000 North Sepulveda Boulevard, Manhattan Beach; (310) 937–6829. Fine examples of Cuban cuisine. Share with the kids as the portions are huge. Nothing on the menu is over $10.95 except for the fresh lobster. $–$$

Portofino Hotel and Yacht Club, 260 Portofino Way; (310) 379–8481 or (800) 468–4292; www.hotelportofino.com. If you should base the family here, you'll have the best of both worlds—the atmosphere of a small, seaside village and the accessibility of most of Greater L.A.'s attractions. The oceanfront location places you but 6 miles from LAX and within walking distance of King Harbor, Seaside Lagoon, and a 27-mile-long coastal walking and biking path passing through Venice, Santa Monica, and Malibu. The Portofino's 163 rooms include 90 with views of the Pacific. Fifty-six rooms are smoke-free. An assortment of complimentary family amenities is provided, from "baby joggers" and snugglies to high chairs and diapers.

For More Information

Redondo Beach Chamber of Commerce and Visitors Bureau. 200 North Pacific Coast Highway, 90277; (310) 376–6911; fax (310) 374–7373; www.redondochamber .org.

Orange County

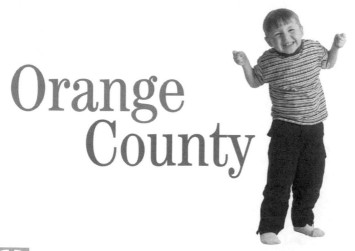

The land on which the visionary Walt Disney built his Magic Kingdom in 1955 was discovered more than 150 years earlier by a Spanish explorer. Gaspar de Portolá gazed upon the magic river bringing life to the fertile valleys and fields leading to the Pacific Ocean and named it Santa Ana. In 1857, German immigrants bought portions of the area, at the time a Spanish land grant, for a mere $2.00 an acre. They called their new settlement Anaheim, which means "home of the Ana." With cuttings from their native Rhineland, the settlers began growing California's first grapes and making wine. In the late 1880s, the vineyards of California's wine capital in Anaheim were devastated by blight. So the settlers decided to plant oranges instead, and the current name Orange County was created.

Today's fastest-growing crops in the area are neither grapes nor oranges but amusement parks, sports attractions, and a galaxy of animated stars from Disney—all ready and waiting for the picking by you and your fun-starved entourage. If oranges thrive in this climate, so will you! Wintertime highs of 65 degrees rise to but 79 degrees in summer, and overnight lows—even in winter's darkest hours—rarely dip below 45 degrees. December through February is what passes for the area's "rainy season," although total annual rainfall is only 13 inches. Days are sunny and mild, nights clear and cool—that's the forecast for your Orange County visit.

Casual clothing is the way to go for 90 percent of your family fun here. Be sure to pack shorts, T-shirts, cotton pants, skirts, and really comfortable walking shoes or sandals. Bring a sweater or light jacket for evenings—along the waterfront it may get nippy. Don't forget your bathing suit and shades (but never fear, you can always buy the latest beachwear and gear at one of the numerous malls or gift shops).

Your family can still visit the city of Orange itself, with its historic district featuring a nineteenth-century soda fountain; relax on the beaches of Newport and Laguna; check out the world-class surfing at Huntington Beach; shop 'til you drop in Costa Mesa; and see the swallows in Capistrano and the marine life in Dana Point. By popular kid demand, however, you will doubtless make your first Orange County stop in Anaheim at "Uncle Walt's place"—the unparalleled Disneyland Resort, which includes the original Disneyland and the new Disney's California Adventure parks, plus the Downtown Disney District.

ORANGE COUNTY

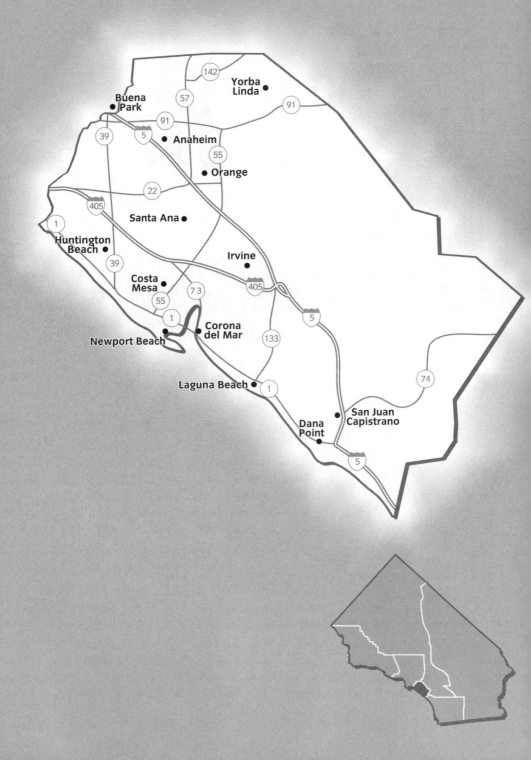

Anaheim Resort Area

From Los Angeles, drive south on Interstate 5 to the city of Anaheim and vicinity, the family fun center of Orange County. Using Disneyland Resort as your Orange County starting point makes much sense geographically and economically. Family-style lodging and restaurants are plentiful and very affordable in Anaheim and neighboring Buena Park. Make room reservations as far in advance as you can, especially for summertime and holiday periods, since Anaheim attracts 20-million-plus visitors every year, including many who visit at the West Coast's largest exhibition center, the Anaheim Convention Center. Many hotels and motels provide package plans that include Disneyland Resort tickets (passports) as well as **free** breakfasts and transportation services.

Disneyland Park

1313 Harbor Boulevard, at the intersection of Interstate 5; (714) 781–4565; www.disneyland.com. $$$$

Hours: During the fall, winter, and spring, hours are generally Monday through Friday 10:00 A.M. to 8:00 P.M., Saturday 9:00 A.M. to midnight, and Sunday 9:00 A.M. to 10:00 P.M. Summertime hours are usually 8:00 A.M. to midnight every day. Extended hours are in effect during holiday periods. Very Important Note: Hours are subject to change, so call ahead for exact opening and closing times on your preferred days to avoid disappointment.

Directions: Follow the signs to designated parking areas. Trams are provided to the main entrance. (Parking is $8.00 per car per day).

The magic of Disneyland exists in eight "themed lands." Begin with your entrance on Main Street USA, a composite of America in the 1900s. Move along to Adventureland, housing Tarzan's Treehouse, one of our favorites; the Indiana Jones Adventure; and the Jungle Cruise. New Orleans Square features the classic Pirates of the Caribbean and Haunted Mansion. Critter Country has the wettest ride—Splash Mountain—and Many Adventures of Winnie-the-Pooh. Fantasyland is highlighted by Sleeping Beauty's Castle, King Arthur's Carousel, Mr. Toad's Wild Ride, Peter Pan's Flight, and the breathtaking Matterhorn Bobsleds. Next comes Frontierland, with the cool Big Thunder Mountain mine ride. The Fantasmic! special-effects show is presented nightly each summer and on weekends. Mickey's Toontown is base camp for all your young ones' favorite Disney characters. See Mickey's and Minnie's residences and Goofy's Bounce House, and ride Roger Rabbit's Car Toon Spin. Tomorrowland is the launching pad for space-age attractions. Here you will thrill to classics such as Star Tours and Space Mountain, plus the Astro Orbitor, Rocket Rods, Innoventions, an interactive water fountain, and 3-D "Honey I Shrunk the Audience."

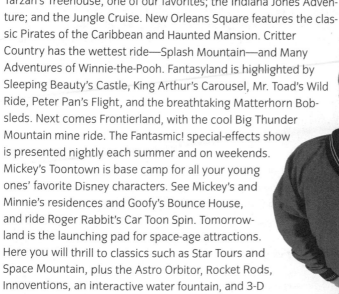

Doing **Disneyland**

With three attractions—the original Disneyland, the new Disney's California Adventure, and the Downtown Disney District—this trip can be a visual and physical overload for you and your family. We advise a minimum two-night stay and three days to really enjoy all the fun available. (It's practically impossible to do both parks in one day; even one overnight and two full days can be tricky, depending on your stamina.) For first-timers, begin with the original Disneyland early in the day. Take a short break midday for lunch and naps, then return for the afternoon and evening shows (such as the fireworks over the Magic Castle). You'll need a second full day to really explore DCA (Disney's California Adventure) because many of the activities are live stage shows and movies presented at specific times. On the third day, revisit favorite attractions at either park and get in some shopping at Downtown Disney. Always check park operating hours and plan your visit around your kids' eat-sleep schedule. The best time-saving option is the FASTPASS, a computerized ticketing system that allows you to reserve a time slot for the most popular rides. When you arrive at your designated time period with your computer-generated pass, you'll go to a special line and get on within minutes. Highly recommended!

Disney's California Adventure Park

1313 Harbor Boulevard, at the intersection of Interstate 5 (you can also exit at Disneyland Drive); (714) 781–4565; www.disneyland.com. Open year-round, generally Monday through Friday from 10:00 A.M. to 8:00 P.M., Saturday from 9:00 A.M. to 10:00 P.M., and Sunday from 9:00 A.M. to 10:00 P.M. Extended hours during the summer and holiday periods. Note: Hours are very subject to change; call ahead for exact opening and closing times on your preferred days to visit. Admission fees are also subject to change. Many special packages and promotions are offered throughout the year. $$$$

Opened in February 2001 with much fanfare and continually adding new rides and shows, this newer fifty-five-acre theme park celebrates the great state of California—from Disney's imaginative perspective. You'll enter the park, affectionately known as DCA for short, from the promenade area under a replica of San Francisco's Golden Gate Bridge to explore four distinct lands. Paradise Pier recreates a beachfront amusement zone reminiscent of Santa Monica Pier or the Santa Cruz boardwalk. Check out California Screamin'—a superfast steel roller coaster that loops you upside down around a Mickey Mouse head icon. The 150-foot Sun Wheel Ferris wheel, Orange Stinger, Jumpin' Jellyfish, and Golden Zephyr rides get family fun points here, along with plenty of concessions and food vendors along the midway.

The second land, dubbed the Hollywood Pictures Backlot, has huge soundstages that hold attractions such as Jim Henson's *Muppet Vision* 3-D movie; Hyperion Theater's live hip musical/dance performances; the Superstar Limo ride; and the Animation Center, with its five separate options to discover the magic behind cartoons and films. In May 2004 the Twilight Zone Tower of Terror began dropping guests thirteen stories faster than the speed of gravity.

The Golden State land features the must-do Soarin' Over California experience, where you will hang with feet dangling as you fly like an eagle—visually—around an 80-foot dome-shaped motion-picture screen filled with an amazing view of the best California scenery. Don't miss Grizzly River Run, a white-water-rafting ride that swirls you down two waterfalls; Bountiful Valley Farm with its demonstration veggie and fruit gardens; Robert Mondavi's Golden Vine Winery (with wine tasting for us adults); Pacific Wharf, where you can watch Boudin's Bakery make sourdough bread and mission tortillas pop out; and a movie starring Whoopi Goldberg in the Golden Dreams Theatre.

October 2002 saw the opening of "A Bug's Land," a fourth area including five attractions inside Flik's Fun Fair. Plenty of food and beverage options inhabit DCA, and be prepared to spend some gold nuggets to enjoy the diverse range of fare, ranging from traditional burgers, dogs, and fries to sushi, chowder, pizza, and Chinese and Mexican cuisine. Disney's California Adventure certainly embraces Walt's original promise: "Disneyland will never be complete as long as there is imagination left in the world."

Disneyland **Turns 50!**

Launching on May 5, 2005, and continuing for eighteen months, the "Happiest Celebration on Earth" pays tribute to Walt Disney's original dream of Disneyland. For the first time ever, the ten Disney theme parks around the world will join for one glorious celebration, each premiering new shows and attractions in honor of this fiftieth-anniversary event. At Disneyland Resort itself, the "Happiest Celebration on Earth" is the "Happiest Homecoming on Earth." In Disneyland Park, premiering May 5, 2005, Sleeping Beauty's Castle will be transformed and topped by five regal turret "crowns"; the new "Walt Disney's Parade of Dreams" will feature one of the largest casts of Disney characters and performers ever assembled; and the all-new fireworks spectacular "Remember . . . Dreams Come True" will ignite the sky. An attraction titled "Disneyland—The First 50 Years" will showcase never-before-seen artwork, models, and designs, including rare film footage. At Disney's California Adventure, starting May 5, 2005, the "Block Party Bash" will be a celebratory free-for-all with wacky entertainment and irresistible music, where guests will suddenly find themselves surrounded by one of five instant celebrations starring Mickey, Minnie, the Muppets, the crew from *Monsters, Inc.*, Lilo and Stitch, and Flik and Princess Atta from *A Bug's Life*. This is a fiftieth birthday party you and your family do not want to miss!

Disneyland Resort
Fun Facts

21,000 men and women are employed as cast members at the peak of summer season.

7,000 gallons of paint are used each year to spiffy up the park.

150,000 lightbulbs are used to brighten up the park.

More than 7,500 trees, 50,000 shrubs, and 900 species of plants can be found here. It takes a 110-person landscaping staff to maintain it all.

Park guests buy in one year: 4 million hamburgers, 1.6 million hot dogs, 3.4 million orders of fries, 1.5 million servings of popcorn, and 1.2 million gallons of soft drinks to wash it all down.

Annual trash totals approximately 27 million pounds. However, Disneyland does recycle 5 million pounds of cardboard, 1 million pounds of office paper, and 14 million pounds of aluminum cans every year.

Edison International Field
2000 Gene Autry Way, Anaheim. Baseball season runs April through September; call (714) 634–2000 for a schedule and ticket prices; www.angelsbaseball.com.

The 70,000-seat stadium is home to baseball's Anaheim Angels (2002 World Series champions) and a variety of other sporting events, concerts, and festivals.

Arrowhead Pond of Anaheim
2695 East Katella Avenue, Anaheim; (714) 704–2400; www.arrowheadpond.com.

This 18,900-seat enclosed arena hosts many events and concerts and is home to the National Hockey League's Mighty Ducks, who skate from October through March (714–704–2701). Call for ticket prices and event schedules.

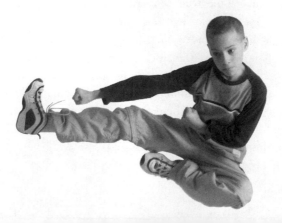

Glacial Garden Ice Arena

1000 East Cerritos Avenue, Anaheim; (714) 502–9185; www.glacialgardens.com. Open daily, with varying times and fees for open figure skating, instruction, and hockey matches.

This is the place to go if your family would rather participate than watch ice sports. Head over to this dual-rink facility, complete with a pro shop, snack bar, locker rooms, and skate rentals.

The Anaheim Family Fun Center

1041 North Shepherd off the 91 Riverside Freeway; (714) 630–7212 for times and current fees. Open daily. Note: Height restrictions apply to all rides and activities.

This huge complex has batting cages, bumper boats, go-karts, roller-skating, and an arcade and snack bar.

Adventure City (ages 2 to 12)

1238 Beach Boulevard between Cerritos Avenue and Ball Road, on the outskirts of Anaheim; (714) 236–9300 for current operating hours or check the Web at www.adventure city.com. Generally open daily in summer from 10:00 A.M. to 10:00 P.M. and in winter from Friday through Sunday, but hours are subject to change without notice. $$$

Opened in August 1994 by the Ansdell family, Adventure City, "the Little Theme Park Just for Kids," resembles a storybook village designed and proportioned for children ages two to twelve. For a wonderfully relaxing experience, consider visiting this two-acre park with

Downtown **Disney District**

Opened in January 2001, this 20-acre dining, shopping, and entertainment area is located between the original Disneyland and the new Disney's California Adventure and encircles three Disneyland Resort hotels. The district is **free** and open to the public year-round. It features nicely landscaped gardens and promenades interspersed with 300,000 square feet of retail shops, restaurants, and twelve movie theaters. Some highlights: excellent pastries and espresso at La Brea Bakery; wood-fired pizza at Naples Ristorante; tapas at Catal Restaurant; Ralph Brennen's Jazz Kitchen for Cajun food; the House of Blues for live entertainment (the Sunday gospel brunch is inspiring!); Y Arriba! Y Arriba! for Latin cuisine and dance shows; Rainforest Cafe for tropical treats; and the ESPN Zone for a fantastic sports fix (live sports broadcasts, interactive games, and food at the Studio Grill). Shopping includes the ubiquitous World of Disney store, plus plenty of other gift, souvenir, music, jewelry, and fashion emporiums. For more information, contact (714) 300–7800 or www.disneyland.com.

its sixteen kid-size rides that are quiet yet still zoom and thrill, as well as hourly puppet shows, a 25-foot climbing wall, live theater, storytelling, and face painting. Parent-child interaction is made easy here because the atmosphere is very casual and low-hype. There are plenty of park benches for us parental units to sit and relax on while the kids go brave the Kid Coaster or the carousel.

Hobby City

1238 Beach Boulevard between Cerritos Avenue and Ball Road, on the outskirts of Anaheim, adjacent to Adventure City; (714) 821–3311; www.hobbycity.com. $

This minitown was founded in 1955 by Bea DeArmond and her husband (the grandparents of the creators of Adventure City). The nine-acre parcel contains twenty-three different hobby and collectible shops—most remarkably, a half-scale reproduction of the White House that shelters the Doll and Toy Museum. Browse the Cabbage Patch Kids Official Adoption Center, complete with doctors and nurses. Visit the American Indian Trading Post, located in a log cabin, and find your new favorite stuffed animal at the Bear Tree.

Children's Museum at La Habra (ages 2 to 10)

301 South Euclid Avenue, La Habra, approximately 30 minutes from Disneyland; (562) 905–9793; www.lhcm.org. Open 10:00 A.M. to 5:00 P.M. Monday through Saturday and 1:00 to 5:00 P.M. on Sunday; closed major holidays. $

Opened in 1977 as California's first children's museum, this facility is located in a renovated 1923 Union Pacific train depot. It contains fifteen permanent exhibits including a nature walk, science station, dino dig, kids on stage, and preschool play park. Temporary exhibits change at least three times a year.

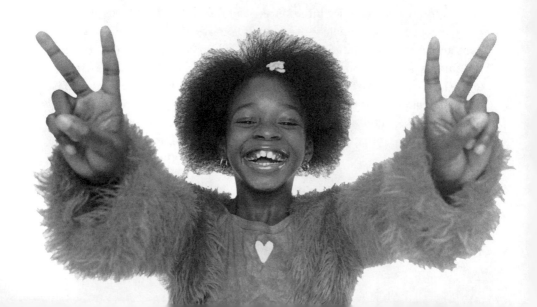

Getting in **the Swing**

The ever-popular **Golf N'Stuff** is conveniently located across the street from Disneyland at 1656 South Harbor Boulevard (714–778–4100) and has two beautifully landscaped eighteen-hole miniature golf courses and an arcade center open seven days a week. Real golf enthusiasts can swing out under the instruction of PGA pros at the **Islands Golf Center,** 14893 Ball Road (714–630–7888), on eighteen acres of practice tees, greens, and a fairway. There are more than twenty other Orange County golf options, including **Pelican Hill Golf Club,** in Newport Beach (949–759–5103 or www.pelicanhill .com) and the **Tustin Ranch Golf Club** in suburban Tustin (714–730–1611). Call for tee times and directions.

If your family wants to swing out with a racket, you can choose from twelve championship hard-surface tennis courts at the **Anaheim Tennis Center Inc.,** located at 975 South State College Boulevard (714–991–9090). The center is open year-round and offers computerized, self-loading ball machines as well as professional instruction. More than fifty tennis courts can be found at hotels and in Orange County's public parks. Call (714) 771–6731, ext. 220; www.ocparks.com for information.

Crystal Cathedral of the Reformed Church in America

13280 Chapman Avenue, Garden Grove. Call the visitor center at (714) 971–4000 to check tour times or (714) 544–5679 to reserve tickets for the extremely cherished holiday pageants; www.crystalcathedral.org. Free tours are generally available daily, but times are subject to change due to church services and events. Donations appreciated.

For some religious and architectural history, visit the dramatic, all-glass sanctuary designed by Philip Johnson, considered a dean of American architects. This incredible place features 10,000 glass panes covering a weblike steel frame resembling a four-point star. The 2,890-seat cathedral hosts the annual Glory of Christmas and Glory of Easter pageants, with live animals, flying angels, and incredible special lighting reflected from the twelve-story glass walls and ceilings.

Richard Nixon Presidential Library, Museum, and Birthplace

18001 Yorba Linda Boulevard, Yorba Linda. From Anaheim, take the Riverside Freeway Route 57 northbound and exit Yorba Linda Boulevard, then travel about 5 miles east to the library, on the left-hand side (watch carefully for signs); (714) 993–5075 or (800) 872–8865; www.nixonfoundation.org. Open Monday through Saturday from 10:00 A.M. to 5:00 P.M. and Sunday from 11:00 A.M. to 5:00 P.M. $$

Be sure to schedule at least half a day to let your family experience a view of political and world history depicted at the nine-acre site. This was the first presidential library and museum built using no tax dollars. The user-friendly, well-thought-out facility was first opened and dedicated on July 19, 1990. It features a self-guided tour, beginning with the twenty-eight-minute film *Never Give Up: Richard Nixon in the Arena.* Propaganda? Let your taste decide! Continue through galleries focusing on "The Road to the Presidency" and "The Wilderness Years," life-size statues of world leaders, a portion of the Berlin Wall, a re-creation of the White House's Lincoln sitting room, gifts from supporters, the Watergate years, and personal memorabilia. The exhibits portray America's thirty-seventh commander in chief right up until his death on April 22, 1994. Both President and Mrs. Nixon are buried here in the tranquil First Lady's Garden. You may visit the grave site, the reflecting pool, and the white clapboard farmhouse where Nixon was born on January 9, 1913. It remains precisely as it was when Nixon and his family lived there, right down to the bed where he was born. The intimate museum store on the premises contains commemorative souvenirs, postcards, and a selection of Nixon's books.

In late 2004, adding more than 47,000 square feet, the Katherine B. Loker Center will nearly double the size of the Nixon Library and include a full-size replica of the White House East Room, a 4,100-square-foot rotating exhibit gallery, a new entrance court, and staff offices.

All-Suite Hotels **Near Disneyland**

Like California wildflowers, an amazing variety of all-suite hotels have sprung up near the park in recent years. This trend really is a boon for traveling families like us, who like to have a private bedroom for the adults and a multi-function living room/dining area with hide-a-bed arrangements for the kids. Each suite hotel has varying amenities such as **free** breakfasts, kitchenettes, pools, and spas. However, all feature **free** shuttle buses to Disneyland and **free** parking. You might want to investigate the **Castle Inn & Suites** (714–774–8111), the **Peacock Suite Resort** (714–535–8255), or **Anaheim Portofino Inn and Suites** (714–782–7600).

Where to Eat and Stay

Disney's PCH Grill at Disney's Paradise Pier Hotel, 1717 Disneyland Drive; (714) 999–0990. Open daily for breakfast, lunch, and dinner. Hours vary seasonally. PCH stands for Pacific Coast Highway, California's prime and celebrated coastal route.

Dining in the PCH Grill for lunch and dinner celebrates all the foods and beverages that make up California cuisine. Menu maps plot your meal course by course and feature fresh seafood, pastas, oak-fired pizzas, and some exotic Asian specialties. If you're looking for traditional American fare, this is probably not the best spot for you, but you know what they say: "When in California, eat like the Californians do," or something like that. Your best bet for the family at the PCH Grill is breakfast, because Minnie Mouse is the star here. She is the "hostess with the mostest" for this fun-filled Disney dining experience that also features a magic act onstage with Mr. Wizard. (Kids get to help perform tricks between bites.) You can order off the menu or cruise the buffet for your favorite breakfast items.

Goofy's Kitchen at the Disneyland Hotel, 1150 Magic Way, Anaheim; (714) 778–6600. Your kids will not want to miss Goofy's, one of the eight restaurants on-site. Open every day—breakfast and dinner. Call for specific hours as they vary seasonally. You can dine with Disney characters (and get your picture taken!), eat Disney Character Meals, try out the all-you-can-eat buffet, and receive a **free** souvenir button. Our kids insist on this "dining experience" every time! $$$

Anaheim Hilton Hotel and Towers, 777 Convention Way, Anaheim; (714) 750–4321. Only 2 blocks from Disneyland, this AAA three-diamond property features 1,576 guest rooms and suites in a colorful, bright motif. The hotel has a heated outdoor pool, four whirlpools, three rooftop garden sundecks, and the Sports and Fitness Center with its indoor pool, health spa, basketball gym, sauna, tanning beds, and massage services. Retail shops, a duty-**free** shop, a beauty salon, eight restaurants and lounges, and foreign currency exchange complete your experience. The Hilton Vacation Station program is specially created for kids up to age twelve. From Memorial Day through Labor Day,

there is a separate check-in desk in the lobby, with trained personnel and a character mascot. Here you will find an impressive lending library of 300 handheld video games and toys from Kenner, Hasbro, and Playskool. At 4:00 P.M. daily, kids (and parents if accompanied by a kid) can take a behind-the-scenes hotel tour, including the massive kitchens and laundry. All Vacation Station activities are gratis for hotel guests. Cafe Oasis, open for breakfast, lunch, and dinner off the main lobby, has an outstanding children's menu that is very affordable. The hotel offers a **free** shuttle bus to Disneyland Resort every thirty minutes and running daily according to park opening/closing times. $$$$

Disneyland Hotel, 1150 Magic Way, Anaheim; (714) 778–6600 or direct to reservations at (714) 956–6400. Just west of Disneyland and connected by the futuristic monorail, this hotel opened at the same time as the park in 1955 and has continued to evolve. It features 990 guest rooms and suites in three high-rise towers surrounding the magical Peter Pan–themed Neverland pool complex (with water slides, bridges, and shallow play areas); a kids' playground; and a sandy beach with rental pedal boats, remote-control tugboats, and dune buggies. There are several restaurants and lounges to choose from, plus four swimming pools, a hot tub, the Team Mickey Fitness Center, gift shops, and an eighty-game video arcade.

This hotel is a destination within itself, and you should plan some time to enjoy all the amenities. Family-friendly features include no charge for children younger than age seventeen staying in same room as parents; **free** roll-aways and porta-cribs, and babysitting referrals to licensed "grandmother types." Value-priced hotel and park package plans are prevalent and include early admission into both parks one and a half hours before the regular opening. Be sure to ask what's available when making reservations. Another great service is the Package Express, which delivers all your park purchases to your hotel room for **free.** $$$$

Disney's Grand Californian Hotel, 1600 South Disneyland Drive, Anaheim; (714) 635–2300. Opened in February 2001, this luxurious 751-room hotel with its striking California Craftsman architectural design is located on the northwest corner of the new Disney's California Adventure. This hotel is the only one to offer direct access straight into the park, a wonderful time-saving feature for your family. More than 160 of the guest rooms feature solid wooden bunk beds—great fun for kids of all ages! From the moment you arrive (and are offered valet parking), you are treated with outstanding hospitality and service. Hotel dining options include 24-hour room service and the excellent Storyteller's Cafe with its tasty breakfast buffet and American cuisine for lunch and dinner daily (and

visits from Disney characters such as Chip'n Dale), plus the stunning Napa Rose Restaurant (with an open exhibition kitchen), Hearthstone Lounge, and White Water Snacks Poolside. You'll appreciate Pinocchio's Workshop, a supervised kids activity center, and the Mickey Mouse–shaped kiddy pool plus two other swimming pools (one with an awesome redwood slide), whirlpools, exercise suite, and Eureka Springs Health Spa. We really like this property and feel the higher room rates are justified given the ease of park accessibility combined with the outstanding amenities and service. $$$$

Disney's Paradise Pier Hotel (formerly Disneyland Pacific Hotel), 1717 Disneyland Drive; (714) 999–0990 or direct to reservations at (714) 956–6400. This fifteen-story, full-service hotel was acquired by Disney in December 1995 and underwent a complete renovation and name change in 2001. It now overlooks the festive Paradise Pier area at Disney's California Adventure. Choose from 502 nicely furnished guest rooms and suites. There are four restaurants and lounges, an outdoor pool and spa deck, a game arcade, convenient indoor/outdoor parking, and gift shops. There is no charge for children younger than age eighteen staying in the same room as parents.

For More Information

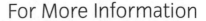

Anaheim/Orange County Visitor and Convention Bureau. 800 West Katella Avenue, 92802; (714) 765–8888 or (888) 598–3200; www.anaheimoc.org.

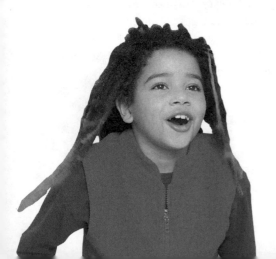

Buena Park

Now it's time to gear up for another round of great family adventure in nearby Buena Park—only fifteen minutes from Anaheim and Disneyland. This area's development began in 1920, when Walter and Cordelia Knott and their three young children arrived and started farming on twenty acres of leased land. The Knotts set up a roadside produce stand on Beach Boulevard to sell their crops, and in 1932 Walter Knott started propagating a cross blend of raspberry, blackberry, and loganberry plants that he named boysenberry. In 1934, to help make ends meet during the Great Depression, Cordelia Knott began serving chicken dinners for 65 cents on her wedding china to passing motorists. Soon Knott's Berry Farm boysenberry fruits, jams, jellies, and pies, along with the Chicken Dinner Restaurant, became so popular that the family decided to build an attraction to keep waiting patrons amused. In 1940 Walter Knott began moving old buildings to the site from various ghost towns. The Calico Mine Ride followed in 1960, and a re-creation of Philadelphia's Independence Hall was constructed in 1966. In 1968 the amusement park area was enclosed, and for the first time a general admission fee was charged. Knott's Berry Farm forms the nucleus for many attractions in this commercial section of Orange County. Plan on spending at least two days here in order to do it all "berry good."

Knott's Berry Farm 🎡 🍴 🛍️

8039 Beach Boulevard at the corner of La Palma Avenue; (714) 220–5200; www.knotts.com. Open daily except Christmas. Summer hours 9:00 A.M. to midnight. In winter the park operates weekdays 10:00 A.M. to 6:00 P.M., Saturday 10:00 A.M. to 10:00 P.M., and Sunday 10:00 A.M. to 7:00 P.M. Extended hours are offered during holiday periods. All admissions after 4:00 P.M. are reduced year-round. Parking across the street and accessed by a special walkway or tram is $7.00 per car. Be absolutely sure to call in advance for current ticket prices and schedules since all are subject to change without notice. $$$$

Knott's Berry Farm was family-owned and -operated until its 1997 purchase by Cedar Fair, L.P. It attracts more than five million guests each year to its entertainment park and marketplace, featuring 165 attractions, rides, live shows, restaurants, and shops. The lushly landscaped 150 acres have plenty of flowers, trees, waterfalls, and shady spots.

Six theme areas include the original Ghost Town, where you can pan for gold and go for a great log ride and take the Ghost Rider, the longest wooden coaster in the West; Camp Snoopy, the official home of the Peanuts gang, including Woodstock's air mail ride; and Fiesta Village, prowling ground for the Jaguar!—a 2,700-foot-long steel roller coaster that winds its way above the park and loops through Montezooma's Revenge (another thrilling coaster with its own 76-foot-high loop). The Boardwalk has a dolphin and sea lion show, Xcelerator, Perilous Plunge, the Hammerhead ride, the Boomerang (ever been on a roller coaster that rolls backward? Definite queasy alert!), Supreme Scream—312 feet of vertical excitement, as well as Sky Cabin, Wipeout, and Kingdom of the Dinosaur. The Mystery Lodge is a magical multisensory show focusing on native North American culture located in the Wild Water Wilderness. Come here at the end of your day if you plan on riding Bigfoot Rapids. Speaking from personal experience, heed the warning signs—you *will* get wet on this ride —most likely drenched! It may feel great on a hot summer day, but squishy shoes and clothing can get mighty uncomfortable mighty fast. "Indian Trails" gives you a chance to dry off and watch Native American arts, crafts, and music.

Knott's Soak City U.S.A.—Orange County

Across the street from Knott's Berry Farm, 8039 Beach Boulevard at La Palma Avenue, adjacent to Knott's Independence Hall, Buena Park; (714) 220–5200. Open daily Memorial Day through Labor Day; open Saturday and Sunday in May, September, and October. $$$$

Opened in summer 2000, this California-beach-theme water park features sixteen separate water rides and attractions, including tube and body waterslides, a wave pool, a lazy river, a family fun house, restaurants, snack bars, a sand beach, a pier, and gift shops.

Ripley's Believe It or Not! Museum

7850 Beach Boulevard, 1 block north of Knott's Berry Farm along the Buena Park entertainment corridor; (714) 522–7045; www.ripleysbuenapark.com. Open Monday through Friday from 11:00 A.M. to 5:00 P.M., Saturday and Sunday from 10:00 A.M. to 6:00 P.M. year-round. $$

Use your parental discretion on the age appropriateness of this attraction. In our opinion, mouse fetus wine, edible maggot jewelry, and a four-eyed man might be a little disconcerting to the very young.

One of the many Ripley's around the country, this 10,000-square-foot structure opened in 1990 with an "Odditorium" featuring a unique collection of the bizarre, the strange, and the beautiful found during the worldwide travels of adventurer Robert Ripley, born on Christmas Day 1893. Some of the exhibits are educational, like the 200 B.C. Venus de Milo statue, Chinese art, and primitive currency.

The Movieland Wax Museum

7711 Beach Boulevard, just down the street from Ripley's; (714) 522–1155; www.movieland waxmuseum.com. Open daily from 9:00 A.M. to 7:00 P.M. Go for the combination ticket with Ripley's for considerable savings. $$$

This is America's first wax museum and one of the world's largest collections (more than 400) of life-size wax images of celebrities from the 1920s until today. If you have seen these stars only on the silver screen or television, you will be able to see them "up close and personal" here. The figures are so realistic you will want to reach out and touch. Don't do it, but take plenty of pictures during your self-guided tour through incredibly detailed sets and originally costumed stars, ranging from Gary Cooper and Bette Davis to Michael Jackson, Whoopi Goldberg, Kevin Costner, and Tom Hanks (as Forrest Gump). The *Star Trek* set is certainly a winner, but young children may want to avoid the Chamber of Horrors, featuring Dracula and Frankenstein as well as Jason and Norman Bates. Since its inauguration in 1962, the museum has been a must-visit on every Southern California tourist's agenda. Put it on yours.

Medieval Times Dinner and Tournament

7662 Beach Boulevard, across the street from Movieland Wax Museum; (714) 521–4740 or (800) 899–6600; www.medievaltimes.com. Open nightly year-round with special Sunday matinees. $$$$

Included is a four-course meal of twentieth-century food (appetizer, vegetable soup, chicken, ribs, baked potato slice, and apple turnover) in medieval style (no modern knife, fork, or spoon to assist you). Make sure you bring plenty of extra cash to buy banners to wave, souvenir programs, and photos taken during dinner. Beer, wine, sodas, and coffee are included in the admission price; however, these prices are subject to change and do not include gratuity for your hardworking serving wenches and serfs. Call the colorful castle for daily show times—advance reservations are *required*. Make sure you arrive at least one hour before your scheduled show time to navigate the parking lot with your chariot and negotiate the check-in line.

This is outstanding family fun that is not to be missed—you and the kids can release all kinds of pent-up vocal energy as you yell for "your" knight in armor during a pageant of excellent horsemanship and tournament games of skill and accuracy. You'll eat in an arena filled with more than 1,100 people, divided into six sections, wearing colored hats, waving streamers, and cheering their favorite knight on to victory over the course of a two-hour eleventh-century show. A pricey outing, but we think you definitely will agree that "your day's not over until you've seen those knights!"

Wild Bill's Wild West Dinner Extravaganza

7600 Beach Boulevard, at the intersection of the Riverside Route 91 Freeway; (714) 522–6414 or (800) 883–1546; www.wildbillscalifornia.com. Show times vary depending on season and run seven nights a week, year-round. Reservations are required. $$$$

This Hollywood-style, family-oriented, two-hour dinner and show experience will have you and the young ones whooping it up. The nonstop action begins the moment you sit down in the 800-seat "barn" at long tables facing an elevated stage. Wild Bill and his sidekick, Miss Annie, serve as master and mistress of ceremonies for the entertainment on stage, which is complete with high-tech lighting and effects and includes singers, cancan girls, roping artists, and Native American dancers. Your servers will provide tableside entertainment as they distribute the hearty family-style menu of soup, salad, fried chicken, ribs, baked potatoes, biscuits, baked beans, corn on the cob, and apple pie topped with vanilla ice cream. The meal includes your choice of soft drinks, beer, or wine. Plenty of audience participation is encouraged during the fun production, including sing-alongs and whooping contests. Wild Bill's is definitely a Southern California version of "how the West was fun."

Where to Eat

Knott's California Marketplace, just outside the main entrance of Knott's Berry Farm, 8039 Beach Boulevard at the corner of La Palma Avenue; (714) 220–5200. This area is filled with shops and restaurants for your family's pleasure, but the best is Mrs. Knott's original Chicken Dinner Restaurant. Hearty American fare is served for breakfast, lunch, and dinner at very reasonable prices. The kids' menu comes complete with crayons and a coloring book. We recommend eating here for lunch (go early or late to avoid crowds). Don't plan on taking any rides anytime near your consumption of that delicious chicken, mashed potatoes, and boysenberry pie. (We speak from experience here. Trust us!) $$

Where to Stay

Radisson Resort Knott's Berry Farm, 7675 Crescent Avenue, adjacent to Knott's Berry Farm; (714) 995–1111; www.radisson .com/buenaparkca. 320 units recently renovated and upgraded with a limited number of "Peanuts" theme rooms with nightly

Snoopy character turndown service. Free Snoopy gift for kids at check-in. Outdoor kiddy pool, adult pool, whirlpool, fitness center, sauna, and steam room. Festive Italian family food at Cucina! Cucina! Cafe. Gift shops. **Free** parking. $$$

For More Information

Buena Park Convention and Visitors Office. 6601 Beach Boulevard, Suite 200, 90261-2904; (714) 562–3560 or (800) 541–3953; fax (714) 562–3569; www .buenapark.com.

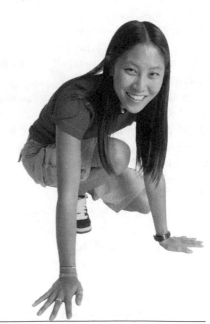

Orange

How would you like to find a slice of the midwestern United States buried in the heart of Orange County? Look no further than the historic city of Orange, sandwiched between Santa Ana and Anaheim, the two largest cities in all of Orange County. Approach the city of Orange by way of eastbound Chapman Avenue, off Interstate 5 or from State Route 57. As you enter downtown, cobblestone, tree-lined thoroughfares take you into the intersection of Chapman and Glassell Streets, where you will discover a circular central plaza. The "Plaza City" boasts a 1-square-mile historic district, where nineteenth-century architecture is preserved and cherished, and the appeal is decidedly homespun and friendly. Check out the living-history lessons presented in the myriad antiques shops scattered around the plaza.

Watson's Drugs and Soda Fountain
116 East Chapman; (714) 633–1050; www.watsondrug.com. $

The best place to soak up the flavor of Orange is on a stool at a joint that has been continuously serving heaping scoops of ice cream, traditional American meals, and remedies at
its Plaza Square location since 1899. Prices for hand-dipped cones start at around $1.00,
and the root beer floats are so frothy you will wonder how you lived this long without one.
Breakfast, lunch, and dinner daily, featuring a kids' menu for those age twelve and
younger, with all items less than $4.00. Go in anytime to see an authentic soda fountain in
action and watch the servers in their period outfits and hairdos play soda jerks.

For More Information

City of Orange Chamber of Commerce.
531 East Chapman Avenue, Suite A,
Orange, 92866; (714) 538–3581 or (800)
938–0073; www.orangechamber.org.

Santa Ana

Orange County's largest city is also the county seat of government and home to the **John
Wayne/Orange County Airport (SNA)** (949–252–5200). Downtown Santa Ana combines
Fiesta Marketplace, a bustling Latino-style pedestrian mall, with a contemporary $50 mil-
lion civic center and about a hundred historic buildings that would make the Spanish
explorer Portola proud of the city he christened in 1796.

Bowers Museum of Cultural Art and Kidseum
2002 North Main Street; (714) 567–3600; www.bowers.org. Open Tuesday through Friday
10:00 A.M. to 4:00 P.M., Saturday and Sunday 10:00 A.M. to 6:00 P.M. Open holidays except
Christmas, Thanksgiving, and New Year's Day. Closed Monday. $$

A significant part of Santa Ana's past is found in its first museum, created in 1936 through
a bequest from Charles and Ada Bowers to preserve the local history of Orange County.
Through gifts and acquisitions, the Bowerses' collections have grown over the years, and
the museum has enlarged its space three times. It is now considered one of the finest cul-
tural arts repositories in the West. The museum specializes in the arts of the Americas,
the Pacific Rim, and Africa, along with its ongoing commitment to chronicle the story of
Orange County. The museum store has unique art treasures, cards, and gifts not readily
available in traditional museum gift shops. Increasing community interaction and family
demand have caused the expansion into an old bank building 2 blocks away.

In December 1994, the 11,000-square-foot Bowers Kidseum opened 2 blocks away at
1802 North Main Street. This amazing center has been competently designed for youth
ages six to twelve as a place where children can learn about other cultures, music, art,
and history through interactive, hands-on exhibits. Hours of operation for the general pub-
lic run Tuesday through Friday from 1:00 to 4:00 P.M. and Saturday and Sunday from 10:00

A.M. to 4:00 P.M. Admission fees are identical and reciprocal with the Bowers Museum. Thematic "explorers' backpacks" covering various cultural differences are just one example of this outstanding opportunity for your kids to actually learn something valuable while vacationing. The Kidseum perfectly bridges the gap between amusement and education.

Centennial Heritage Museum

3101 West Harvard Street; (714) 540–0404. Open Wednesday through Friday from 1:00 to 5:00 P.M. and Saturday and Sunday from 11:00 A.M. to 3:00 P.M. Closed major holidays. $

This historic museum, located in the fully restored, 1898 Victorian Kellogg House, is your family's chance to step back in time to the 1800s. Kids can try on Victorian costumes, wash clothes on a scrub board, play a pump organ, or talk on a hand-cranked telephone. This is a very fun yet informative way to learn early California history.

The Santa Ana Zoo at Prentice Park

1801 East Chestnut Avenue; (714) 835–7484; www.santaanazoo.org. Open daily 10:00 A.M. to 4:00 P.M., extended hours in summer. Closed holidays. $

This charming zoo will calm your kids' animal urges with its 250 species of primates, other mammals, and birds. Refreshments are available in the food court, and vendors around the grounds sell snacks and ice cream. A playground and miniature train rides are available. Call for current programs and times.

Discovery Science Center

2500 North Main Street (at the corner of Interstate 5 and the Santa Ana Freeway); (714) 542–CUBE; www.discoverycube.org. Open daily from 10:00 A.M. to 5:00 P.M. except major holidays. $$$

"The Amusement Park for Your Mind" opened in 1998 in a 59,000-square-foot multistory facility devoted to sparking children's natural curiosity and increasing everyone's understanding of science, math, and technology. More than 120 highly interactive exhibits make you think, search for answers, and participate in the learning process. Eight themed areas include Perception, Dynamic Earth, Quake Zone, Exploration Station, Principles of Flight, Performance, Space, and KidStation (a special area for those younger than age five). Our personal favorites include the Shake Shack to experience an earthquake, lying down on a bed of nails, and dancing on the musical floor. This is a marvelous family activity that you should not miss! Highly recommended.

Irvine and Costa Mesa

The city of Irvine is the largest master-planned community in the United States. It was first developed in 1959 as a site for the University of California-Irvine on an old Spanish land grant. Billboards, overhead power lines, and TV antennas are banned here in an area divided into thirty-eight urban villages featuring a plethora of parks, all connected by greenbelts and bike paths. Shopping centers and services are all conveniently located nearby. The central corridor of high-rise buildings, such as the Irvine Spectrum and Koll Center, provide headquarters for plenty of Fortune 500 firms as well as some family fun.

The adjacent city of Costa Mesa, also home to many corporations as well as a popular residential community, became a player on the Orange County shopping and entertainment scene in 1967 with the opening of the South Coast Plaza Mall, a great place for your family to satisfy those shopping urges.

Irvine Spectrum Center

At the intersection of Interstate 405 (exit Irvine Center Drive) and Interstate 5 (exit Alton), Irvine. Open daily from 11:00 A.M. to 11:00 P.M.; hours can vary during holiday periods and special events. Call (949) 789–9180 for more information or visit www.shopirvinespectrum center.com.

This premier entertainment plaza offers twenty-one IMAX movie cinemas, the NASCAR Silicon Motor Speedway, Sega City, laser light shows, world-class restaurants, nightlife, and specialty shops from around the globe.

Wild Rivers Waterpark (age 3-plus and up)

8770 Irvine Center Drive, Irvine; (949) 768–WILD; www.wildrivers.com. Open daily throughout the summer season from 10:00 A.M. to 8:00 P.M.; call for weekend and winter hours. $$$$

Your high-tech children will definitely want to take advantage of the twenty-acre park with more than forty water rides, including the Edge, the Ledge, and the Abyss, two wave pools, kiddie wading pools, sunbathing areas, a waterslide, log flumes, picnic areas, and a video arcade to complete the family-fun mix.

Palace Park

3405 Michelson Drive, Irvine; (949) 559–8336; www.so-cal.com/palace. Open daily, hours vary according to season and holidays. $$

This indoor/outdoor facility has more than six acres of family entertainment, including miniature golf, batting cages, laser tag, bumper boats, and a state-of-the-art 25,000-square-foot video arcade with the new Galaxian virtual-reality challenge machines, where up to six people compete against the computer. The Palace Playland is specifically created for the younger set, with a large squishy maze.

South Coast Plaza and the Crystal Court

3333 Bristol Street, at the intersection of Interstate 405 and Bristol Street, Costa Mesa; (800) 782–8888 or call the concierge at (949) 435–2034 for a current special event and promotion schedule; www.southcoastplaza.com.

More than one hundred world-renowned stores call this internationally recognized address home, as do restaurants, art galleries, and even a day spa. The kids will clamor to check out the fabulous Disney Store and the Sesame Street Store.

Trinity Broadcasting Network International Headquarters

3150 Bear Street (across Interstate 405 from the South Coast Plaza Mall); (714) 708–5405; www.tbn.org.

This striking, classically inspirational building houses broadcast studios and the popular gift and bookshop of this Christian television network. The Virtual Reality Theater presents **free** motion pictures daily. Call for current titles and show times. All ages are welcome.

Orange County Performing Arts Center

600 Town Center Drive, South Coast Plaza, Costa Mesa; (714) 556–2121 or www.ocpac.org for current events and admission charges.

Opened in 1986, the 3,000-seat Segerstrom Hall is where major symphony concerts, operas, ballets, and Broadway musicals are presented year-round. Children's programs dominate around the Christmas holidays. Call for a schedule of **free** backstage tours.

Orange County Fair and Exposition Center

88 Fair Drive, Costa Mesa; (714) 708–1567 or www.ocfair.com for current activities.

Discover a variety of fun family events, including swap meets, automobile and motorcycle speedway races, and concerts. In July the Orange County Fair takes over, featuring top-name entertainment, livestock, carnival rides, rodeo, foodstuffs, arts, crafts, contests, and demonstrations.

For More Information

Costa Mesa Visitor Bureau. 1631 West Sunflower Avenue, Suite C37, Santa Ana, 92704; (800) 399–5499; www.costamesa-ca.com.

Irvine Chamber of Commerce. 17755 Sky Park East, #101, Irvine, 92614; (949) 660–9112; www.irvinechamber.com.

Huntington Beach

Waterfront action or just plain relaxation will provide a respite from all your inland encounters. Orange County's beaches are part of the defining Southern California experience. Traveling along the Pacific Coast Highway, commonly known as PCH or just the Coast Highway, begin your waterside explorations at Huntington Beach, Orange County's third-largest city (after Santa Ana and Anaheim). It is growing into a thriving resort area with more than 8 miles of uninterrupted shoreline. Between Goldenwest Street and Brookhurst Street along PCH, the Bolsa Chica and Huntington Beaches provide plenty of area for safe swimming, picnicking, and surfing. Beach parking fees are charged and vary according to time and season.

Huntington is one of the surf capitals of Southern California. Your kids will probably know this because of the mega-television coverage afforded the surfing championships and international competitions held here every summer. You can easily spend a day on the beaches of Huntington, just enjoying the beautiful surf, sand, and sea. (Do remember to use your sunscreen liberally. Ask any Huntington Beach surfer dude—sunburn is not cool!) The town's ambitious redevelopment efforts along Main Street, just off PCH, contain postmodern shopping plazas and condos alongside the original turn-of-the-last-century waterfront clapboards, which now house trendy clothing stores, beach shops, and bistros. Strolling the 1,856-foot municipal pier is a favorite pastime. Pier Plaza, on PCH at Main, hosts a farmers' market on Friday and live entertainment.

International Surfing Museum

411 Olive Street; (714) 960–3483; www.surfingmuseum.org. Displays, admission fees, and opening and closing hours change like the tides (well, not really that frequently!), so call for the current schedule and low admission donations, dudes.

An art deco–ish building downtown, home of radical exhibits, artifacts, and memorabilia ranging from vintage surfboards to surf wear and surf films.

Bolsa Chica Ecological Reserve and Interpretive Center

Between Warner Avenue and Goldenwest Street on the Pacific Coast Highway, just opposite the entrance to Bolsa Chica State Beach; (714) 846–1114. Open daily, dawn to dusk. Free.

It is both relaxing and educational to walk through the 300-acre reserve, one of the largest salt marsh preserves in Southern California. The reserve supports such rare migratory waterfowl as avocets, egrets, plovers, and terns. A 1.5-mile walkway with explanatory signs leads the way throughout the ecosystem. **Free** guided public tours are given the first Saturday of each month.

Shipley Nature Center at Huntington Central Park

Goldenwest Street between Slater and Ellis Avenues; (714) 960–8847. Center generally open daily 9:00 A.M. to 5:00 P.M.; park open 5:00 A.M. to 10:00 P.M. Free admission.

For another view of plants and animals, the park is home to hundreds of bird species. For human guests there are picnic areas and playgrounds, plus walking and bicycling trails that wind past ponds, waterways, and woodlands.

Where to Eat and Stay

Dwight's at the Beach, on the Boardwalk, 1 block south of the pier; (714) 536–8083. Open daily; call for seasonal times. Since 1932, serving juicy burgers, hot dogs, ice cream, and famous cheese strips–tortilla strips and cheddar cheese topped with secret hot sauce. $

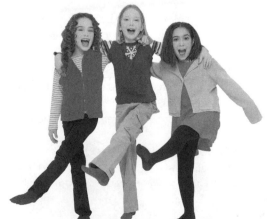

Lazy Dog Café, 16310 Beach Boulevard, at MacDonald Avenue, just south of the 405 Freeway near Huntington Beach in Westminster; (714) 500–1140. www.thelazydogcafe.com. Open daily for lunch and dinner. They're serious about food here, but they don't take themselves too seriously since they offer build-your-own pizzas for kids, a plate of delicious mini chili-cheese dogs, and even a dessert served in a dog bowl. The extensive children's menu, which is broken down into "Puppy Dogs"—ages 0–7 and "Big Dogs"—ages 8–12," also features a special dessert—a cup of string licorice with fruit loops for making your own edible necklace or bracelet. $$

Hyatt Regency Huntington Beach Resort & Spa, 21500 Pacific Coast Highway; (714) 698–1234; fax (714) 845–4636; www.huntingtonbeach.hyatt.com. Garden and ocean views from 517 guest rooms and 57 suites in Andalusian-inspired style. This new luxurious hotel directly across from the beach via a pedestrian walkway features three restaurants (The Californian for fine dining, Pete Mallory's Surf City Sunset Grille, and Mankota's Grill poolside), the Village shopping plaza, and the 20,000-square-foot Pacific Waters Spa. Two Camp Hyatt children's programs are offered daily from 9:00 A.M. to 9:00 P.M. starting at $40 per child. Campers receive a welcome gift upon arrival and a packet describing on-site activities. Kids ages three through seven can become Camp Hyatt Beach Clubbers and make shell necklaces, do beach sand art, and roast s'mores by the fire. The SophistiKids program for youth ages eight through twelve includes cool pool and beach play, koi fish feeding, or surfboard making. Other options include parents and kids shared spa treatments as well as Adventure Hyatt programs such as kayaking, learning to surf, and sportfishing tours. $$$$

For More Information

Huntington Beach Conference and Visitors Bureau. 301 Main Street, Suite 208, 92648; (714) 969–3492 or (800) 729–6232; www.hbvisit.com.

Newport Beach Area

Just south of Huntington Beach along the glittering Pacific lies a city of villages, islands, and private enclaves first incorporated in 1906. The Newport Beach area comprises Balboa, Balboa Island, Lido Isle, Newport Heights, Harbor Island, Bay Shore, Linda Isle, and Corona del Mar. It includes one of the West Coast's most famous yacht harbors, containing approximately 9,000 pleasure craft. In addition, a 6-mile "inland" beach lies along the peninsula between Newport Bay and the ocean. You and your family will discover what many believe to be the trendiest Southern California beach life here.

Balboa Pavilion 🏛 🎣 🍴

400 Main Street, located at the Newport Bay end of Main Street, on the Balboa Peninsula; www.BalboaNewportBeach.com. **Open daily 10:00 A.M. to 10:00 P.M.** Free.

Begin your exploration of the waterfront action at this classic building constructed in 1905 and now listed in the National Register of Historic Places. Here you will discover a marine recreation center offering ferries to quaint Balboa Island and Catalina Island and charter boats for sailing, whale-watching, sightseeing, and sportfishing. The Fun Zone has a carousel, Ferris wheel, and arcade.

Davey's Locker Sportfishing

400 Main Street, Balboa Pavilion, Balboa; (949) 673–1434; www.daveyslocker.com. Open daily; hours vary according to season.

Your headquarters in Newport Beach for harbor excursions, whale-watching, and half-, three-quarter, and full-day fishing excursions for catching yellowfin tuna, bonito, sand bass, and rockfish. Twilight fishing trips are offered in the summer, too. These folks are pros, and they will make you feel very comfortable and safe on the water.

Catalina Passenger Service/Pavilion Paddy Cruises

400 Main Street in the Balboa Pavilion, Balboa; (949) 673–5245; www.catalinainfo.com. Call for sailing times. $$

At the end of the Balboa Peninsula and Pier, do not miss taking a forty-five- or ninety-minute sightseeing cruise aboard the old-fashioned riverboat *Pavilion Paddy*. You will wind your way through the meandering channels of Newport Harbor and see some imposing homes and dazzling yachts of the rich and famous (such as the late John Wayne and Shirley Temple). Tours run mostly year-round. Sunday brunch cruises are also available in season. This is also the dock for *Catalina Flyer* service to Catalina Island offshore. (See sidebar.)

Cruising to Catalina from **Orange County**

The Catalina Passenger Service operates the *Catalina Flyer*, its 500-passenger catamaran vessel, from Balboa Pavilion in Newport Beach. It offers one round-trip seventy-five-minute cruise daily to neighboring Santa Catalina Island, a pristine, unspoiled isle only 26 miles out to sea yet a world away. (See the Greater Los Angeles chapter for Long Beach/San Pedro embarkation choices.) Fares and departure times are subject to change seasonally. Reservations are required. Phone (949) 673–5245 or (800) 830–7744 for current schedules or visit www.catalinainfo.com. $$$$

The Newport Harbor Nautical Museum

151 East Coast Highway, Newport Beach; (949) 673–7863; www.nhnm.org. Call for seasonal hours. Closed Monday. Free admission.

This interesting museum gives a photographic history of the harbor, a fascinating ships-in-a-bottle exhibit, and a display of navigational instruments and model ships housed in the 190-foot *Pride of Newport,* docked near the Back Bay Bridge. Anthony's Riverboat Cafe serves lunch, dinner, and brunch.

Hornblower Cruises and Events

2431 West Pacific Coast Highway, Suite 101, Newport Beach; (949) 646–0155; www.horn blower.com. Cruises on climate-controlled large yachts offered year-round. Evening and Sunday brunch cruise schedules vary according to season and demand for private char-ters. Brunch cruises sail for two hours and include an all-you-can-eat buffet with cham-pagne for adults; children ages four to twelve half-price. Gratuity and cocktails additional. $$$$

Excellent service from nautically attired crew and California cuisine prepared fresh onboard make this an upscale cruising, dining, and sightseeing experience to remember. Recommended for older children; for our families, we like the Sunday brunch cruises best.

Newport Sports Museum

Newport Center Drive, Suite 100; (949) 721–9333; fax (949) 721–0999; www.newport sportsmuseum.org. Open Monday through Friday 9:00 A.M. to 6:00 P.M. and Saturday 10:00 A.M. to 3:00 P.M.. Free admission; donations welcome.

This 6,000-square-foot museum features one of the world's largest collections of sports memorabilia, assembled in fifteen themed rooms containing 10,000 items. Highlights include jerseys from Michael Jordan, Larry Bird, Dr. J, and Wilt Chamberlain; and auto-graphed baseballs from every Cy Young winner. There's even a baseball park with actual seats from places such as Yankee Stadium and Wrigley Field! The collection started in 1953 when John W. Hamilton, at the age of twelve, was given a "Look All-American Foot-ball" by a family friend. Hamilton has been collecting sports memorabilia ever since, with the majority of the items being personally given to him by athletes.

Sherman Library and Gardens

2647 East Pacific Coast Highway, south of Newport Beach in Corona del Mar; (949) 673–2261; www.slgardens.org. Gardens are open daily from 10:30 A.M. to 4:00 P.M. $

This two-acre cultural center has botanical gardens display-ing tropical and subtropical flora in addition to its research library of southwestern history. The touch-and-smell garden is a major wow for your kids; you will enjoy the respite in the tea garden.

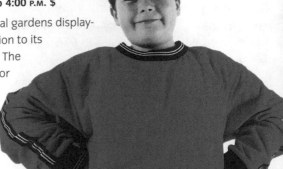

Shopping and More **with an Ocean View**

Luring you away from the Newport Beach and harbor area, but with the ocean firmly in sight, the 600-acre **Newport Center,** just above the Pacific Coast Highway between MacArthur Boulevard and Jamboree Road, is an office, luxury hotel, and entertainment complex built in 1967. It hosts a must-stop shopping center—the trendy **Fashion Island.** Contact (949) 721–2000, the concierge contact number, or www.shopfashionisland.com for schedules of children's activities, fashion shows, and great promotions. Containing more than 200 major chain stores and regional specialty shops, Newport Center is also home to the luxurious AAA five-diamond-rated **Four Seasons Hotel** (949–759–0808; www.fourseasons.com/newportbeach), as well as forty restaurants in the Atrium Court. This is where you and the kids can chill out after a hard day at the beach!

Where to Eat

Hard Rock Cafe Newport Beach, 451 Newport Center Drive (Fashion Island), Newport Beach; (949) 640–8844; www.hardrock.com. Open daily 11:30 A.M. to 11:00 P.M. This is the Orange County version of one of the most famous rock-and-roll restaurants in the world, featuring memorabilia of major rock stars as well as their platinum and gold records. Be sure to make your pilgrimage to at least one of these emporiums for the fun of it! $$$

Tale of the Whale, 400 Main Street, in the Balboa Pavilion, Balboa; (949) 673–4633. Open daily 11:00 A.M. to 11:00 P.M., serving lunch, dinner, and cocktails overlooking the magnificent harbor area. Dressy casual, but a fine children's menu makes this a super spot to dine on the best fresh seafood. Our favorite is cioppino, a fish stew that is a feast. $$

Where to Stay

Hyatt Newporter Resort Hotel, 1107 Jamboree Road, one-half mile from Pacific Coast Highway, Newport Beach; (949) 729–1234 or (800) 233–1234; www.hyattnewporter.com. This 410-room California-casual property has spacious, beautifully landscaped grounds. The value is here for your family, with package plans and special rates. There are three heated pools, a wading pool for the kids, a nine-hole, par-three golf course, plus an exercise room if you're feeling flabby from lying on the beach. Two restaurants serve daily meals. You'll appreciate the shuttle service to nearby shopping and attractions. $$$

The Newport Dunes Waterfront Resort, 1131 Back Bay Drive, just off PCH and Jamboree Boulevard; (949) 729–3863 or (800) 765–7661; www.newportdunes.com. Overnight camping site and a seven-lane boat-launch ramp are open twenty-four hours. This hundred-acre waterfront RV resort provides more than 400 hookups for recreational vehicles and campers, each separated by tropical vine-covered fences. Plus, beachfront cottages that sleep from two to eight people and are equipped with a kitchen make ideal family headquarters. You can rent kayaks, windsurfers, paddleboats, and sailboats here for hours of fun. Call for current prices. $$

For More Information

Newport Beach Conference and Visitors Bureau. 110 Newport Center Drive, Suite 120, 92660; (949) 722–1611 or (800) 94–COAST; www.newportbeach-cvb.com.

Laguna Beach

Unspoiled by time or tide, the dazzling white sands of Laguna Beach, combined with its artist-colony heritage and year-round mild climate, add up to a unique Orange County destination resort worth exploring. All the major beach action along the Pacific Coast Highway can be found here—your kids will "dig" the sand and the playground at Main Beach downtown, while you stroll the art galleries, boutiques, and bistros that line the Pacific Coast Highway.

Festival of Arts and Pageant of the Masters

In Irvine Bowl Park, 650 Laguna Canyon Road, near the ocean. The annual festival is staged in July and August. For a complete program and brochures, call (949) 494–1145 or (800) 487–3378; www.foapom.com. $$$$

The Festival of Arts features 150 of the area's most accomplished artists in a rigorously juried show requiring that all pieces on display or for sale be original, including paintings, sculpture, pastels, drawings, serigraphs, photographs, ceramics, jewelry, etched and stained glass, weaving, handcrafted furniture, musical instruments, model ships, and scrimshaw.

Each summer evening the park's natural amphitheater is the site of the Pageant of the Masters, a world-famous event, where amazingly faithful re-creations of famous artwork are presented on stage by live models. Narrators and a full orchestra make these tableaux vivants (living pictures) an extraordinary dramatic experience, particularly the finale—a stunning live portrayal of Leonardo da Vinci's *Last Supper*. There is so much for your kids to see and do, including participating in hands-on workshops, watching performing artists, listening to music, even viewing the junior art displays of local schoolchildren.

The Sawdust Art Festival Winter Fantasy

935 Laguna Canyon Road; (949) 494–3030 for this year's Winter Fantasy dates and nominal admission fees; www.sawdustartfestival.com. $

This favorite Laguna Beach event is held on four consecutive weekends in November and December in a fragrant eucalyptus grove. Wander three acres of paths containing 150 booths filled with holiday arts and crafts while your kids play in the snow (trucked in daily!). A children's art workshop, food, and entertainment make this a wonderful addition to your wintertime vacation experience in Southern California.

Where to Eat and Stay

Hotel Laguna and Claes Restaurant, 425 South Pacific Coast Highway, Laguna Beach; (949) 494–1151 or (800) 524–2927; www.hotellaguna.com. This historic, sixty-five-room property right on the sand in the absolute center of town was built in 1930. The three-story old girl has undergone several face-lifts over the years but remains a favorite. Don't expect ultramodern furnishings but revel in the California-beach quirky atmosphere. Be sure to request a room on the ocean side, because the street side is way too noisy. Private beach access, complete with your own beach chairs and food/drinks/towel attendant, make this the ultimate place to people-watch while the kids create sand castles. **Free** continental breakfast included. We really enjoy Claes Restaurant and The Terrace for lunch or early dinner (the bar gets a little hectic later on). You can dine overlooking the beach and all the action. $$$

For More Information

Laguna Beach Visitors and Conference Bureau. 252 Broadway (State Route 133), 92651; (949) 497–9229 or (800) 877–1115; www.lagunabeachinfo.org.

Dana Point

At the turn of the nineteenth century, Dana Point (named after Richard Henry Dana, author and mariner) was the only major port between Santa Barbara and San Diego. Now this natural cove has picturesque and modern marinas hosting 2,500 craft. It is famous for its whale-watching cruises from late December through March. The town celebrates its annual Harbor Whale Festival in March with street fairs and plenty of outdoor activities.

Orange County Ocean Institute

24200 Dana Point Harbor Drive; (949) 496–2274. Open daily from 10:00 A.M. to 4:30 P.M.; closed major holidays. Ship tours are Sunday from 10:00 A.M. to 2:30 P.M. Admission fee is voluntary; donations are gladly accepted.

Be sure to investigate this fun place that has outstanding sea-life exhibits, tide-pool tours, and a hands-on aquarium touch tank. While you're there, take a tour of the tall ship *Pilgrim*, a replica of the vessel on which Richard Henry Dana, author of the book *Two Years Before the Mast*, sailed to Southern California in the 1830s. In July and August, musical and dramatic productions with a nautical theme are presented on the *Pilgrim's* deck. Your kids will love the chance to really see sea life in action!

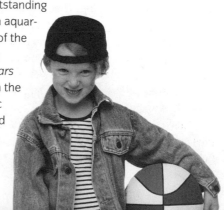

Dana Point Harbor Information Service
P.O. Box 701, Dana Point, 92629; (949) 496–1094; www.danapointharbor.com.

Your best point of contact for waterfront activities and special events, including whale-watching; rentals of Jet Skis, kayaks, canoes, and sailboats; parasailing; and windsurfing.

Where to Stay

Doubletree Guest Suites Doheny Beach, 34402 Pacific Coast Highway, across from Doheny State Beach, next to the Yacht Harbor; (949) 661–1100. This full-service, 196-suite hotel is located along a 10-mile stretch of beautiful white sand beach. All suites have a bedroom and a sitting room (our fave floor plan) with a wet bar, microwave, fridge, two remote control TVs, a VCR, and panoramic views to boot.

If you get bored with the beach (heresy), you can always take a dip in the pool or work out in the fitness center. The restaurant Tresca has a Mediterranean menu, open daily for all three meals and Sunday brunch. $$$

For More Information

Dana Point Chamber of Commerce. 24681 La Plaza #115, Box 12, 92629; (949) 496–1555; www.danapoint-chamber.com.

San Juan Capistrano

The village of San Juan Capistrano is just inland along Interstate 5 north from Dana Point, set in rolling hills between the Santa Ana Mountains and the sea. It has many old adobe buildings, and the 1895 Santa Fe Railroad depot has been lovingly restored and is now an AMTRAK station and restaurant. Since San Juan Capistrano is good enough for thousands of swallows to return to every year, you know you cannot go wrong here, or for that matter anywhere in Orange County—the ultimate family vacation destination.

Mission San Juan Capistrano and Cultural Center
Two blocks west of the junction of State Route 74 and Interstate 5 at 31882 Camino Capistrano; (949) 248–2048; www.missionsjc.com. Open every day except Good Friday, Christmas, and Easter, 8:30 A.M. to 5:00 P.M. $$

This "jewel of the missions" was founded on November 1, 1776, by Father Junipero Serra and is seventh in his famous chain of twenty-one missions along the California coast. On your self-guided walk through history, you will first enter the Serra Chapel, the oldest building still in use in California; then tour the ruins of the Great Stone Church, which was destroyed by an earthquake in 1812; and view the padres' quarters, soldiers' barracks, an Indian cemetery, and the mission kitchen. You can also view the site of an ongoing archaeological dig as well as revel in the majestic gardens. Even the crankiest toddlers seem to unwind here.

Today the mission is famous for the swallows that arrive every March 19 (St. Joseph's Day) and leave on October 23. These remarkably constant birds fly approximately 6,000 miles from Goya, Argentina, to nest and rear their young in San Juan Capistrano. As early

as 1777, a record of their return was first noted in the mission archives, spawning ceremonies and celebrations each year since (not to mention the celebrated song "When the
Swallows Come Back to Capistrano").

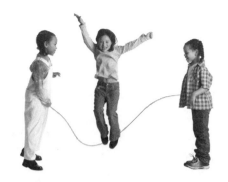

For More Information

**San Juan Capistrano Chamber of
Commerce.** 31871 Camino Capistrano,
Suite 306, 92675; (949) 493–4700;
www.sanjuanchamber.com.

Southern California **CityPass**

The Southern California CityPass debuted in 2003 and is an outstanding
money saver for you and your family. It includes a three-day Disneyland
Resort Park Hopper® Ticket, valid for unlimited admission to both Disneyland park and Disney's California Adventure park for three days; a one-day
visit to Knott's Berry Farm theme park; and ample time to motor down the
coast to stunning San Diego and two world-class parks, SeaWorld and your
choice between the San Diego Zoo or San Diego Zoo's Wild Animal Park. City-
Pass delivers the best of Southern California fun at a savings of more than 30
percent off regular admission fees. Plus, you have fourteen days to take it all
in from the first day you use it! Purchase the Southern California CityPass at
any of the participating attractions or online at www.citypass.com.

the Inland Empire and Beyond

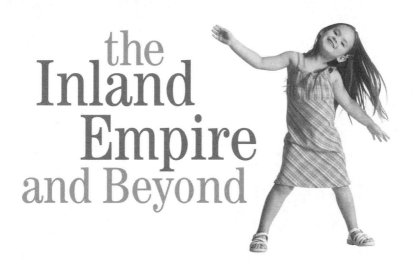

Residents of Greater Los Angeles often think of everything else in California—with the exceptions of San Francisco, San Diego, and a handful of other cities—as "the great outdoors." Indeed, the presence of gold (somewhere) in "them thar hills" aside, what makes California such a gold mine for the nature enthusiast is the wealth of opportunities for outdoor excitement afforded by its vast expanses of wooded mountains, pristine lakes, and other natural areas. As with so many other lifestyle considerations, when it comes to out-of-doors fun, Southern California truly has the edge.

Even those areas with the most striking natural beauty, however, have rich cultural heritages stretching back to the days of the Spanish explorers and Native Americans before them. A wide variety of museums—many geared toward children—sprinkle the scenic splendor of the Southern California wilds. The combination of history, festive special events, and, towering above it all, those glorious mountain peaks makes for an unforgettable family adventure.

When considering which areas to travel to or through, it helps to think like a native Southern Californian: In other words, think big! We tend to take wide-open spaces for granted, but in a state where many counties are bigger than other entire states, can you blame us? We like to drive, and we consider many areas easily within the orbit of Greater L.A. These include, among others, the sizable chunks of San Bernardino and Riverside Counties east of L.A. (a 28,000-square-mile region known as the Inland Empire); vast Kern County north of the city, with its celebrated Kern River; Tulare County, farther north, gateway to Sequoia and Kings Canyon National Parks; and the ski resort of Mammoth, at the southern end of the Sierra Nevada range. The latter areas may be more Central than Southern California, but a true Californian just hops in the car, puts the top down, and goes. Getting there is easy, and with landscapes like these, easily half the fun.

It is California's Inland Empire that furnishes the archetypal images of the Golden State: acre upon acre of lush orange groves guarded by snowcapped mountains in the not-so-far-off distance. To the East Coast eye—that is, one accustomed to cities arranged on neat grids and self-contained countryside speckled with small towns—the Inland Empire can be a bit overwhelming. The valley floor is an immense patchwork of farmlands

THE INLAND EMPIRE AND BEYOND

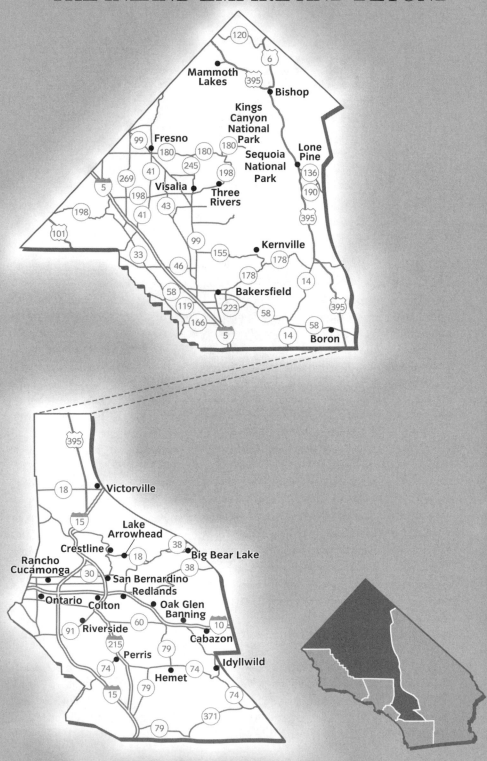

and small cities. It's sometimes hard to tell where one town ends and another begins. Malls, museums, and roadside fruit stands all vie for the motorist's attention. There are more than 660,000 acres of national forest. All this makes for a slightly rough-and-tumble atmosphere, but a relaxed one, too. Though still growing, the palm-studded Inland Empire is a less pressured kind of place than adjacent L.A. County. It's about as far away from stuffy as you can get—and that's *very* Southern California.

If the sight of citrus crops right and left is quintessential Southland, those snowcapped mountaintops house a part of the state perhaps less well-known to the visitor. Mountain vacation spots such as Lake Arrowhead and Big Bear, with its 7,000-foot-high lake, are like old-fashioned New Hampshire lakeside resorts a la California. They offer calm, cool respite from the L.A. basin and surrounding valleys and loads of outdoor activities from the simple to the simply adventurous. But to really appreciate the roominess of the Inland Empire, we recommend that you make stops along the way. Those who value the journey as well as the destination won't be disappointed, and during road trips kids need as much stretch-run-and-have-fun time as itineraries allow.

Ontario

If, like most people, you enter the Inland Empire via Interstate 10, heading east out of Los Angeles, you'll want to make a couple of stops in the Ontario area. With its bustling international airport, Ontario is the hub of this region within a region.

Welcome to the **Ontario International Airport (ONT),** a terrific gateway for families on the grand Southern California tour route! The airport is serviced by all the major carriers. You can start your itinerary from here without the hassle that is LAX. This state-of-the-art $270 million terminal is a major link in Southern California's air transportation network. You can easily rent a van or car from here and head for the hills, mountains, desert, and beyond.

Graber Olive House

315 East Fourth Street, Ontario; (909) 983–1761 or (800) 996–5483; www.graberolive.com. Open Monday through Saturday 9:00 A.M. to 5:30 P.M. and Sunday 9:30 A.M. to 6:00 P.M. Free admission.

This is a fitting place to visit just in case the area's warm Mediterranean-like breezes have put thoughts of—what else?—olive oil in your mind. They've been doing wonderfully delicious things with homegrown olives at Graber House since 1894. An on-site olive processing and packing plant and a museum will enlighten kids and adults alike.

Planes of Fame Air Museum

7000 Merrill Avenue, Chino (just south of Ontario on Highway 60); (909) 597–3722; www.planesoffame.org. Open daily 9:00 A.M. to 5:00 P.M. except Thanksgiving and Christmas. $$

This museum houses a very impressive collection of both vintage World War II airplanes and military aviation memorabilia. It's a vivid reminder of the pivotal role the aviation industry has played in California's history.

Mall **Break!**

If you have visions of a megamall, with everything the kids could ever imagine (more than 200 shops, including Children's Place, Off 5th/Saks Fifth Avenue, plus AMC Theatres, the Improv Comedy Club, and Game Works), you'll be glad to know that the **Ontario Mills,** (1 Mills Circle), Southern California's largest entertainment and outlet mall, is open seven days a week (www.ontariomills.com). At the intersection of Interstate 15 and Interstate 10, Ontario Mills has it all. It's mere minutes from the airport, thirty minutes from Disneyland, and forty minutes from downtown L.A. Start with a noisy lunch at the **Rainforest Cafe** (909–941–7979), where you'll find animated wildlife, environmental education, and a spunky menu with hamburgers, salads, and more. You'll hear the sounds of the rain forest as you dine. **Dave & Busters** is another hit here with state-of-the-art interactive games and simulators, (909) 987–1557. Snackers will like the food court, which is near the Virgin Megastore. Parents will love the smooth-as-silk cheesecake in more flavors than you thought possible at the **Cheesecake Factory.** Dig in!

Where to Eat

Cucina! Cucina! Italian Cafe, 960 North Ontario Mills Drive; (909) 476–2350. Known for its festive atmosphere, Cucina! Cucina! is a popular place in Ontario. Moderate prices and great tasting food. $–$$

New York Grill, 950 North Ontario Mills Drive; (909) 987–1928. Upscale dining and a great Sunday brunch. Special children's menu features hamburgers, hot dogs, and grilled cheese sandwiches. $–$$

Where to Stay

Doubletree Hotel Ontario, 222 North Vineyard; (909) 937–0900 or (800) 222–8733; www.doubletree.com. The Doubletree boasts 484 guest rooms, two restaurants, a pool, and a spa. $$$

Ontario Airport Marriott, 2200 East Holt; (909) 975–5000 or (800) 228–9290; www.marriott.com. This 293-room property is within walking distance of the Ontario Convention Center and restaurants and is close to the Ontario International Airport. Twenty-four-hour **free** airport shuttle. $$

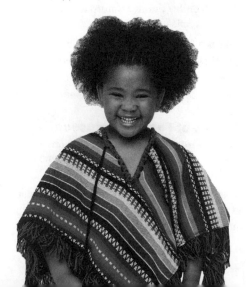

For More Information

Chino Valley Chamber of Commerce. 13150 Seventh Street, 91710; (909) 627–6177; fax (909) 627–4180; www.chinovalley chamber.com.

Ontario Convention and Visitors Bureau. 2000 Convention Center Way, 91764; (909) 937–3000 or (800) 455–5755; fax (909) 937–3080; www.ontariocvb.com.

Rancho Cucamonga

Rancho Cucamonga, northeast of Ontario along historic Route 66, has a name kids love to make fun of. But there's also fun to be had in the town. There's a monument here to Jack Benny (you'll have to explain to the kids who Jack Benny was), as he often mentioned Rancho Cucamonga on radio and television shows. For more civic information, access the chamber of commerce at www.ranchochamber.org.

Where to Eat

Magic Lamp Inn, 8189 Foothill Boulevard; (909) 981–8659. If you want to get more kicks on Route 66 around the dinner hour, visit this legendary, classic 1950s restaurant with its comfortable red banquettes and the look and feel of yesteryear. The menu includes old favorites such as chicken marsala and roast prime rib of steer *au jus*.

Sycamore Inn, 8318 Foothill Boulevard, Bear Gulch; (909) 982–1104; www.the sycamoreinn.com. This historic inn, just across the street from the Magic Lamp, opened in 1848. The children's menu includes the Hot Dogger, Burger Master, Mr. Chicken, and the Big Cheese. Tell your kids this restaurant was in business a long time before McDonald's and Burger King— even before the California burger was invented.

Crestline

All right. You've taken in a bit of culture, a bit of sunshine, and hopefully a bite of something to eat from one of the myriad fast-food establishments along the interstate (**In-N-Out,** 800–786–1000 for locations, makes the best burgers. Try the number three, it's a bargain and includes a burger, fries, and drink.) Now, why not get away from it all, or above it all, as the case may be? There are three main resorts in the mountains framing the northern tier of the Inland Empire: Crestline, Lake Arrowhead, and Big Bear. Choose according to taste: a day for a detour, two or three for a mini-vacation.

On your way to or from Lake Arrowhead, you'll pass through Crestline, a smallish (population 10,000), rather funky, no-nonsense mountain village that lures passersby in for a meal or a lakeside stroll.

No Earplugs **Required**

If you're near Claremont, home of Claremont Colleges, and have an evening free, consider tickets for **Ben Bollinger's Candlelight Pavilion Dinner Theatre** (455 West Foothill Boulevard; www.candlelightpavilion.com), exiting from Interstate 10.

The box office is open Tuesday and Wednesday 11:00 A.M. to 5:00 P.M., Thursday and Friday 11:00 A.M. to 7:00 P.M., and Sunday 10:00 A.M. to 6:00 P.M. Call (909) 626–1254 for performances, times, and cost of tickets.

This is a far cry from a rock concert, so let the kids know in advance. This is where musicals of yesteryear such as *Singin' in the Rain* (based on the MGM film), *The Sound of Music*, and *Ain't Misbehavin'* come alive. Dinner is served a la carte with appetizers, entrees, desserts, and a selection of kid-friendly, nonalcoholic beverages, such as the Melinda May (with coconut cream) and the Show Stopper (a frozen raspberry piña colada and cream concoction).

This is a large theater, which was once a gymnasium. The seating is spacious and comfortable, and the sight lines are excellent, even if you sit in the back at a banquette. It's a perfect way for the family to enjoy live theater and to learn about the marvelous vintage musicals, where you could really hear the words and they meant something, too.

Lake Gregory County Regional Park
24171 Lake Drive, located off Route 18; (909) 338–2233.

The 86-acre Lake Gregory is Crestline's centerpiece, a popular though rarely crowded spot for swimming, shore fishing, and paddle-boarding. Some scenes from Disney's new *Parent Trap* were filmed here as well. From May through September, Friday night in Crestline means Lakeside Family Market Night, a festival of fun that features not only plenty of food and fresh produce but also kids' rides, crafts vendors, and entertainment.

Lake Arrowhead

Summer days find many folks at **Lake Arrowhead Village,** a hundred-year-old resort area named for the arrowhead landmark at the base of the San Bernardino Mountains. No one knows exactly how the 1,115-foot-tall, 396-foot-wide geological imprint got there, but it certainly helps those with a less-than-stellar sense of direction. Virtually every imaginable aquatic activity—swimming, waterskiing, fishing, sailing—is available on the lake, which is ringed by accommodations ranging from camping facilities to deluxe rooms. In the winter this 5,000-plus-foot elevation welcomes snow sports and recreation. A true wonderland only two hours from the beach!

In October 2003, the area suffered from the ravages of the "Old Fire," with 350-plus families directly affected. The flames are gone but not the spirit of hospitality and welcoming community.

The Lake Arrowhead Children's Museum

Lake Arrowhead Village, lower level; (909) 336–3093; fax (909) 336–5815. Open daily. $

Features fun hands-on exhibits, including an ever-popular climbing maze.

Arrowhead Queen

Lake Arrowhead Village waterfront; (909) 336–6992. $$$

A great summertime way to experience the lake. The Louisiana-style paddle-wheel vessel departs hourly.

McKenzie's Waterski School

At the marina; (909) 337–3814.

The longest-running school of its kind in the United States, McKenzie's offers lessons for children of all ages (summertime only).

Snow Valley Mountain Resort

P.O. Box 2337, 35100 Highway 18, Running Springs, 92382; general information: (909) 867–2751, snow report: (800) 680–SNOW. Thirty-five ski trails served by eleven lifts. The longest run is 1.25 miles long.

The seasonal (Thanksgiving to April) Snow Valley Mountain (base elevation 6,800 feet) is located in the heart of the San Bernardino National Forest and operated under a special-use permit with the USDA Forest Service. Resort features include a multitude of food and beverage venues, complete rental operations, a ski and snowboard school, great alpine skiing, and separate snowboarding terrain. Plus, the San Bernardino National Children's Forest provides a means for families with small children to enjoy the wilderness in the off-season.

Where to Eat

Belgian Waffle Works, Lake Arrowhead Village, dockside; (909) 337–5222; fax (909) 337–7862. Open for breakfast, lunch, and dinner. $

Casa Coyote's Grill & Cantina, Lake Arrowhead Village, lower level, Lake Arrowhead; (909) 337–1171; www.casa coyotes.com. This is a full-service family restaurant with southwestern/Mexican favorites. $

Woody's Boat House, Lake Arrowhead Village, lower level; (909) 337–2628; fax (909) 337–9562. Dockside merchants offer another view of the lake, so spend some time exploring this corner of the village. If you are a fan of the Chris Craft boats of the 1950s, stop by for breakfast, lunch, or dinner. Woody's has a salad bar, a separate kids' menu, and fair prices. Beautifully restored Chris Craft boats serve as booths and your platform for viewing the lake. $$

Where to Stay

The Arrowhead Pine Rose Cabins, Highway 189 at Grandview; (909) 337–2341 or (800) 429–PINE; www.lakearrowhead cabins.com. Individuality reigns supreme at this great base camp for sightseeing. It's centrally located between Lake Arrowhead and Lake Gregory. Seventeen cabins (one, two, and three bedrooms) and a five- to seven-bedroom lodge are scattered around five forested acres. No charge for cribs. Children welcome and stay **free** in same cabin as parents. $$

Lake Arrowhead Resort, Lake Arrowhead Village; (909) 336–1511; www.lake arrowheadresort.com. Located on Lake Arrowhead, this 177-room resort has all of the amenities, including its own beach. $$$

For More Information

Lake Arrowhead Communities Chamber of Commerce. P.O. Box 219, 92352; (909) 337–3715; www.lakearrowhead.net.

Lake Arrowhead Village. P.O. Box 640, 28200 Highway 189, Suite F-240, 92352; (909) 337–2533; www.lakearrowhead village.com and www.bluejayvillage.com.

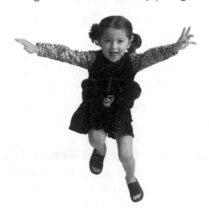

Big Bear Lake

If you follow Highway 18 east from Lake Arrowhead to Big Bear Lake, you'll be cruising along the **Rim of the World Scenic Byway,** with its spectacular vistas of thick forests and the sprawling valley below. It's a fitting entry to the 5-mile-long lake, the perennial favorite of thousands of local residents.

Big Bear is many things to many people. The area includes the city of Big Bear Lake, Fawnskin, Big Bear City, and Moonridge. Some come for the great water sports (23 miles of shoreline), others for the chance to see the stars and meteor showers during the refreshingly cool nights, and others for the hiking opportunities. Hiking trails abound in the area, including a section of the 2,600-mile Pacific Crest Trail that extends from Canada to Mexico. In winter—and often well into spring—Big Bear means top-notch skiing and snowboarding, plus sledding, tubing, and snowball fights. Elevation ranges from 6,750 to 9,000 feet, and the area is dominated by pine and oak forests and rare bald eagles.

Big Bear Discovery Center

San Bernardino National Forest, P.O. Box 66, Fawnskin; (909) 866–3437; fax (909) 866–1781; www.bigbearinfo.com.

Get your family to the marvelous Big Bear Discovery Center before you make any decisions on where to go and what to do. Try one of the tours, such as the Grout Bay Canoe

Tour, Mountain Mining Tour, or Woodland Trail Tour; children are welcome! The USDA Forest Service has made great strides in opening this area to tourists. There is an orientation video, a gift shop, exhibits, an amphitheater, and information on more than fifty activities, from horseback riding, hiking, and backpacking to fishing and bird-watching. Ask about the Children's Forest, a 3,400-acre site on Highway 18 between Running Springs and Big Bear Lake, where kids learn about the preservation of our magnificent wildlands.

Big Bear Queen

500 Paine Road, Big Bear Lake; (909) 866–3218; www.bigbearmarina.com. Seasonal.

Enjoy the water up close during a ninety-minute cruise aboard a paddle wheeler. Dinner cruises available.

Snow Summit

880 Summit Boulevard, P.O. Box 77, Big Bear Lake, 92315; (909) 866–5766; www.snow summit.com. For Snow Summit snow reports, call (909) 866–4621 or (888) SUMMIT–1. $$$$

Here is a paradise for snow seekers, traditional skiers, snowboarders, and families with children. Take it all in from View Haus, where rustic dining will enchant you and the kids with a marvelous mountain view. If there is no natural snow, don't worry, they will make it happen for you! Snow Summit has a drop of 1,175 feet. There is a children's school and a mountaintop family park. Ample **free** parking. During the summer enjoy rides on the scenic sky chair.

Bear Mountain Resort

43101 Goldmine Drive, Big Bear; (909) 585–2519; www.bearmtn.com.

"The Park" at Bear Mountain is the only ski resort in the world devoted almost entirely to free-style snowboarding, with 117 jumps, 57 jibs, and 2 pipes on 195 acres. Bear Mountain boasts a vertical drop of 1,700 feet. Excellent and inexpensive ski instruction centers abound, and plenty of rental companies make downhill and cross-country skiing or snowmobiling easy for those without equipment of their own.

Cruise the Lake with **Captain John**

Pleasure Point Boat Landing is at 603 Landlock Landing Road (Cienega Road off Big Bear Boulevard at Metcalf Bay) in Fawnskin; (909) 866–2455. It is open from 6:00 A.M. daily from May 1 to November 1. Captain John, a real mountain man, casts off daily from the Pleasure Point Marina at noon, 2:00, and 4:00 P.M. for a two-hour cruise around the scenic shoreline of Big Bear Lake. There are also canoes, pedal boats, pontoons, and eight-, ten-, and fifteen-horsepower motorboats at the landing.

Alpine Slide at Magic Mountain

800 Wild Rose Lane, Big Bear Lake; (909) 866–4626. Slide open daily 10:00 A.M. to 4:00 P.M. $$

A Big Bear must. Few can resist the lure of "bobsledding" down the concrete runs. The maximum attainable speed is fast enough to thrill, but not fast enough to frighten. Actually, you control your own pace as you glide down the hillside. There are go-karts and miniature golf, too. In winter, kids can inner-tube down a mountain of snow, then be rope-towed back to the top again.

Moonridge Animal Park

Goldmine Drive, Big Bear Lake; (909) 584–1171; www.moonridgezoo.org. Open year-round 10:00 A.M. to 5:00 P.M. $

Kids will love this zoo, which is a home to many orphaned and injured wild creatures, from ringtail cats, wolves, and foxes to raccoons and cougars. There's even a grizzly bear family in residence.

Solar Observatory

40386 North Shore Lane, Big Bear City; (909) 866–5791. Open July through Labor Day on Saturday only. Free admission; donations welcome.

With more than 300 sunny days annually, Big Bear is an ideal location to study the sun. Check out the rays!

Big Bear **Adventure Passport**

Here's how to get the kids their own Big Bear (the plush, stuffed kind that is). Get yourself a thirty-two-page Adventure Passport (call 800–4–BIG–BEAR). Earn ten Adventure Stamps, including one for lodging, then stop by the visitor center at 630 Bartlett Road in Big Bear and pick up your bear! There are discounts galore with the passport.

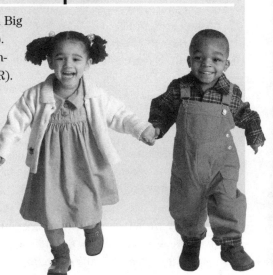

Where to Eat

Mozart's Bistro, 40701 Village Drive, Big Bear; (909) 866–9497. Serving lunch and dinner daily, this great stop has American and German cuisine. Try the salmon! $

Stillwell's (in Northwoods Resort), (909) 866–3121; www.northwoodsresort .com/stillwells.htm. Serving breakfast, lunch, and dinner in a unique, rustic mountain atmosphere. $

Where to Stay

Goldmine Resort, 42268 Moonridge Road, ½ mile east of Big Bear Boulevard, Big Bear Lake; (909) 866–5118; www.big bear-goldmine-lodge.com. Open year-round and only 1 mile to Snow Summit and Bear Mountain. Rustic, old-fashioned accommodations include motel rooms, one- and two-room suites and cabins. Vacation home rentals also offered. Continental breakfast **free.** Large playground,

hot tub, horseshoe pit, and fireplaces; family reunions and weddings welcomed. $$

Northwoods Resort, 40650 Village Drive, Big Bear Lake; Reservations: (800) 866–3121; www.northwoodsresort.com. This 1930s-style, 141-room mountain lodge is great for families. There are even Golden Getaway Grandparents packages that include a full American breakfast plus a box lunch for four to go, mountain bike rental, and a half-day pass at Snow Summit or a two-hour pontoon boat rental. You are right at the village, where there are inviting shops and restaurants, all amid those enchanting whispering pines. $$$

For More Information

Big Bear Lake Resort Association and Visitor Center. 630 Bartlett Road, Big Bear Village, P.O. Box 1936, Big Bear Lake, 92315-1936; (909) 866–6190 or (800) BIG–BEAR; fax (909) 866–5671; www.big bear.com.

Victorville

If you take Interstate 15 a bit north of the San Bernardino Mountains (another section of the Route 66 Heritage Corridor), before you get too far into the Mojave Desert you'll come across the little town of Victorville. In addition to its role as a gateway to the Mojave, it has a few worthwhile stops.

If you're hungry and in a hurry, along the freeway you'll find an In-N-Out (for hamburgers, fries, and lemonade), a Dairy Queen, and Popeye's Chicken. Make sure you have a portable Dust Buster ready to clean up the crumbs in the backseat!

California Route 66 Museum

16825 D Street, take exit D off Interstate 15; (760) 951–0436; fax (760) 951–0509; www .califrt66museum.org. Open Thursday through Monday 10:00 A.M. to 4:00 P.M. **Free.**

Kids may not appreciate the incredible array of memorabilia gathered by Route 66 fans, but this museum will make them wonder and ask questions about what travel was like before freeways. That alone is worth making the stop. From the high desert landmark called Hulaville (once an open-air museum along Route 66 on Victorville's southern fringes built by an eccentric ex-carney) to cute Route 66 fanny packs (for sale), the curiosities displayed here reveal an era of American travel left to the pages of history. Just a refresher, Route 66 debuted in 1926, connecting Chicago to L.A. (Santa Monica).

Check out the historical exhibits, contemporary gallery, research library, and loads of travel info. "Get your kicks" here, on Route 66!

Mojave Narrows Regional Park

18000 Yates Road, off Bear Valley Road; (760) 245–2226; fax (760) 245–7887; www.co.san bernardino.ca.us/parks/mojave.htm.

This picturesque, not-quite-yet-the-desert site spans 840 acres and overlooks the Mojave River. With an 87-unit campground (with 38 full utility pads), year-round fishing, and rowboat rentals, the park is well equipped for families interested in a little communing with nature. Mojave Narrows Regional Park is home to the Huck Finn Jubilee during Father's Day weekend. This festival is loaded with toe-tappin' bluegrass music, a watermelon seed spittin' contest, arts and crafts booths, and a catfish derby.

For More Information

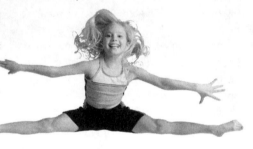

Victorville Chamber of Commerce.
14174 Green Tree Boulevard, 92329; (760) 245–6506; www.vvchamber.com.

Fontana

The city of Fontana is located at the "crossroads" of the Inland Empire at the intersection of Interstates 10 and 15 and State Routes 66 and 30, only ten minutes away from Ontario International Airport. Metrolink rail service makes connections easy to Greater Los Angeles. Your family and the city's population of 139,100 can enjoy easy access to mountains, beaches, twelve regional parks, the desert, and the best-known attraction—the California Speedway just west of downtown. Access www.fontana.org for more information.

California Speedway

9300 Cherry Avenue; (909) 429–5000 or (800) 944–RACE; fax (909) 429-5500; www.california speedway.com.

Known as "America's Ultimate Race Place," California Speedway opened in June 1997 with the Inaugural NASCAR NEXTEL Cup Series California 500. Presented by NAPA, more than 90,000 fans watched Jeff Gordon win the 500-mile race. Since then the speedway has hosted hundreds of NASCAR, IROC AMA Superbike, Grand-Am Cup Series races, IndyCar Series events, CART Champ Car races, and Dayton Indy Lights Series races. The grandstand capacity is 92,000 seats plus there are 63 Terrace Suites overlooking the pit road and 28 luxury Skybox Suites. In addition, more than 1,800 RVs can be accommodated in the infield—a popular choice for families. The speedway is also the home of the quarter-mile NHRA-sanctioned dragstrip—California Dragway. Suffice it to say, if your family loves racing, this is where you need to be! $$$

San Bernardino

On the other side of the mountains, via Interstate 15 to Interstate 215 south, lies sprawling San Bernardino. "San Berdoo," as it's called locally, offers pleasures of a more municipal, but certainly no less stimulating, nature.

Historic Site of the World's First McDonald's Hamburgers
1398 North E Street. Open Monday through Sunday 9:00 A.M. to 5:00 P.M.

In 1948 Dick and Mac McDonald opened their original restaurant on this site on the business district loop of Route 66. There is a display of early McDonald's memorabilia. No food here, though.

Renaissance Pleasure Faire
Glen Helen Regional Park, at the foot of the San Bernardino Mountains where Interstates 15 and 215 meet; (909) 880–0122 or (800) 52–FAIRE; www.renfair.com. Open 9:00 A.M. to 6:00 P.M. on eight weekends plus Memorial Day from beginning of April. $$$

This is indeed a pleasure—a lively re-creation of a sixteenth-century English country fair. This is the largest outdoor theatrical event of its kind. But for the conspicuous absence of fog, you'd swear you were in merry olde England. How often do you get the chance to toast the arrival of Queen Elizabeth I on her royal barge, see knights in shining armor battle one another in a royal joust, and ride an elephant all in the same day?

Then there's the Elizabethan theater, music, and country dance on six stages, old English-style crafts, and historically accurate foodstuffs to partake of (mega-size turkey legs are a perennial favorite). You can also opt to get your palm read by a gypsy, have a fortune teller teach you all about tarot cards, or just pause to chat with a strolling, fully costumed jester. The festive atmosphere at the fair is simply contagious, an unforgettable treat for both youngsters and oldsters.

Glen Helen Regional Park
2555 Glen Helen Parkway; (909) 887–7540; fax (909) 887–1359 for park information and (909) 880–6500 for concert information.

The "jewel in the crown" of the area's regional parks, 1,425-acre Glen Helen comes complete with a half-acre swimming lagoon, a 350-foot waterslide, and a beach. And proof positive that Southern Californians think big, the park also boasts the Glen Helen Hyundai Pavilion (909–88–MUSIC) outdoor concert venue, the largest amphitheater in the United States (total capacity is 65,000).

Route 66 Rendezvous
(800) 867–8366; www.route-66.org.

If you're up for a healthy dose of nostalgic honky-tonk (500,000 were in 2004), check out this four-day affair that kicks off every year in mid-September. Southern Californians have always had a special relationship with their automobiles; what wine is to the French, cars are to us—sacred objects, worthy of adulation. This is clearly in evidence as squeaky-clean vintage Corvettes, Cobras, and Chevys cruise the sunny streets of downtown San Bernardino (some of those streets have replaced the fabled old Route 66). Drag races, an auto sound challenge, and an antique performance parts swap are also on the annual activity roster. Dozens of vendors hawk their wares, which range from antique milk caps and Elvis clocks to new stereo equipment. And to put a little honk into the tonk, celebrities come to life via ongoing Legends in Concert performances. The rendezvous, which is **free** to spectators, is sponsored and produced by the San Bernardino Convention and Visitors Bureau.

National Orange Show
689 South E Street; (909) 888–6788; www.nationalorangeshow.com. Held from Thursday through Monday (Memorial Day weekend). Admission is free.

Here's an event you'll never find in Kansas. Started way back in 1911, the show has been getting juicier ever since. Today it features fireworks, top entertainment, a rodeo, livestock shows, art exhibits, kid-friendly rides, and, of course, a broad range of oranges and orange food products.

Where to Eat

Guadalaharry's, 280 East Hospitality Lane, San Bernardino; (909) 889–8555. Specializing in fajitas, Guadalaharry's is also known for its fried-ice-cream dessert. $–$$

Isabella's, 201 North E Street, #101, San Bernardino; (909) 884–2534. Tasty Italian cuisine in a relaxing atmosphere.

Yamazato of Japan, 289 East Hospitality Lane, San Bernardino; (909) 889–3683. Teppanyaki chefs are very entertaining as they prepare your meal on a grill at your table. It's fun to watch them flip an egg into their hat or a shrimp into their pocket! Delicious teriyaki, tempura, and sushi dishes. $

Where to Stay

Hilton San Bernardino, 285 East Hospitality Lane, San Bernardino; (909) 889–0133 or (800) 445–8667; www.hilton.com. Located off the I–10 at the North Waterman exit. As the street name suggests, this area of San Bernardino is visitor friendly. You'll find an extensive variety of restaurants on Hospitality Lane within walking distance of the hotel, including Guadalaharry's, Yamazato, and others. $$$$

For More Information

San Bernardino Convention and Visitors Bureau. 201 North E Street, Suite 103, 92401; (909) 889–3980; www.san-bernardino.org.

Redlands

Quiet little Redlands, home of the eponymous and highly regarded university, awaits exploration just a few minutes east of San Bernardino on Interstate 10. If you're on the way to, say, Palm Springs and have time for only one detour, make it Redlands. You'll be in excellent company, for in the latter part of the nineteenth century, Midwesterners and East Coasters of certain means began a time-honored tradition of wintering in Southern California, and one of their favorite spots was Redlands. Among the city's attractions are several mansions that bear witness to the Golden State's brief Victorian renaissance.

San Bernardino County Museum

2024 Orange Tree Lane, near the California Street exit from Interstate 10; (909) 307–2669 or (888) BIRD-EGG; www.co.san-bernardino.ca.us/museum/. Open Tuesday through Sunday 9:00 A.M. to 5:00 P.M. $. Children younger than age five admitted free.

This local landmark is easily recognized by its large geodesic dome (actually a seminar room). Here you'll find exhibits on early Californian ranch life and the Native Americans who once lived in these parts. But the real strong suits of the museum are the earth and biological science exhibits, which also happen to be among the most popular with younger children. For starters, there are more than 40,000 birds' eggs, the state's only dinosaur tracks, and a dazzling collection of minerals and gemstones. Kids are captivated by the live insect, reptile, and amphibian displays. Both kids and adults can contemplate the forces that formed the Inland Empire's beautiful mountains by keeping an eye on the always-on seismometer.

Kimberly Crest House and Gardens

1325 Prospect Drive; (909) 792–2111; www.kimberlycrest.org. Open Thursday through Sunday 1:00 to 4:00 P.M. September through July. $

With its commanding views of the San Bernardino Valley, this six-acre estate, purchased in 1905 by J. Alfred Kimberly and his wife, Helen (of Kimberly-Clark fame), features Louis XVI decor on the inside and formal Italian gardens and lush orange groves on the outside. See if you can spot the great southern magnolia, for years the Kimberlys' outdoor Christmas tree. The most impressive of the city's mansions, this French château-style home is off Interstate 10 at the Ford exit. Closed August. Average visit: one hour.

The Frugal Frigate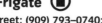

9 North Sixth Street; (909) 793–0740; www.frugalfrigate.com. Open Monday through Friday 10:00 A.M. to 6:00 P.M., Thursday 10:00 A.M. to 8:00 P.M., Saturday 10:00 A.M. to 5:00 P.M., and Sunday noon to 5:00 P.M.

A delightful source for "carefully chosen children's classics," this unique bookstore is located in historic downtown Redlands.

Pizza, Pizza, and **More Pizza**

The Gourmet Pizza Shoppe (120 East State Street; 909–792–3313; www.gourmetpizzas.com) boasts ninety different combinations of pizza, including peanut butter and jelly. Its beverage list features sodas from all over the world, including cream sodas, root beers, black cherry sodas, and six varieties of orange soda! You won't find noisy arcade games or a TV in the dining room. This family-style pizza parlor has seating areas with children's books available for kids to read while they await their favorite pizza.

Pharaoh's Lost Kingdom Theme Park

1101 California Street (I–10 and California); (909) 335–PARK; www.pharaohslost kingdom.com. Open Sunday through Thursday 10:00 A.M. to 11:00 P.M. and Friday and Saturday 10:00 A.M. to midnight. Prices vary. The Sky Coaster costs extra.

An eye-catching eighteen-acre Egyptian-style amusement park with rides, a water park, pyramids, and sphinxes. Some might regard Pharaoh's as yet another Disney imitation (or to others, a monstrosity). Regardless, it's a gauche, comic replication of history plastique. For a moment, when you catch a glimpse of the stately ersatz gold pharaoh, you'll think you've escaped the freeways for Egypt.

At any rate, Pharaoh's is open daily. If your tastes run toward video arcades, the one here is colossal, with the incentive of **free** admission for kids. Once inside, you'll find the tariff rises sharply. We recommend steering the young ones to the rides, the water park, and other activities, such as the King's Pond (bumper boats) and Chariots of Thunder (race cars).

Where to Eat

Doughlectibles, 107 East Citrus Avenue; (909) 798–7321. The bakery has all varieties of fresh pastries and breads. The restaurant serves breakfast, lunch, and dinner. The French toast is worth the calories. Lunch choices include a great patty melt. $

Oscar's Mexican Restaurant, 19 North Fifth Street; (909) 792–8211. Oscar's is an institution in downtown Redlands, serving great Mexican food that is sure to satisfy your appetite. They have great "lite combos" for $6.25. $

For More Information

Redlands Chamber of Commerce. One East Redlands Boulevard, 92373; (909) 793–2546; www.redlandschamber.org.

Riverside

If one views the Inland Empire as a vast stage, its outdoor attractions tend to steal the show. Maybe that's why so few people seem to know much about Riverside, the city built on oranges. Riverside is accessible via Highway 60 or Highway 91, both south of Interstate 10. By 1895 more than 20,000 acres of navel orange trees had made then-sleepy Riverside into the nation's wealthiest city per capita. This distinctly Californian heritage is still evident, thanks to the presence of a handful of old California-style structures: the old **City Hall** (3612 Mission Inn Avenue); restored **1892 Heritage House,** the finest example of Victorian lifestyle in the West; and the city's landmark, the restored **Mission Inn** (3649 Mission Inn Avenue). Originally a twelve-room adobe built in 1875 (a very long time ago by Californian standards), this grand hostelry expanded along with the town.

Riverside Municipal Museum

3580 Mission Inn Avenue; (951) 826–5273; www.riversideca.gov/museum/. Open Monday 9:00 A.M. to 1:00 P.M., Tuesday through Friday 9:00 A.M. to 5:00 P.M. and Saturday and Sunday 1:00 to 5:00 P.M.; admission free.

The area's roots are on display at this museum, with its large collection of Native American artifacts and early citrus industry exhibits.

Jurupa Mountains Cultural Center

7621 Granite Hill Drive; (951) 685–5818; www.jmcc.us. Open Saturday 8:00 A.M. to 4:30 P.M. $

If you missed the San Bernardino County Museum (see the Redlands section in this chapter) and it's Saturday, bring the kids here for an educational guided nature walk. Along with excellent fossil and crystal exhibits, the museum has a cache of moon rocks.

California Citrus State Historic Park

Take Riverside Freeway (Route 91) to Van Buren Boulevard at Dufferin Avenue, look for the big orange; (951) 780–6222; www.parks.ca.gov/?page_id=649.

This California state park was built to celebrate one hundred years of citrus production in Riverside with support from Sunkist growers. Located on the 377 acres are the Varietal Grove, which has a hundred different species of citrus; an outdoor amphitheater where concerts are held on Friday evenings during summer (the last concert is the first Friday in August); and, new in the spring of 2002, a larger visitor center. Many weddings and events are held in the California Craftsman–style building. As you walk around the park, you will encounter interpretive displays and picnic areas.

Botanic Gardens at University of California—Riverside (UCR)

University of California at Riverside; (951) 787–4650; www.gardens.ucr.edu. Open daily from 8:00 A.M. to 5:00 P.M.

These gardens are nestled in the foothills of the Box Springs Mountains in East Riverside and cover forty hilly acres. The gardens boast more than 3,500 plant species from around the world. More than 200 species of birds have been observed in the gardens. From Highway 60/I–215, exit at Martin Luther King Boulevard and turn right. Turn right again at Canyon Crest Avenue and enter the UCR campus. Follow signs to the gardens and park in Lot 13. Admission is **free,** although donations are appreciated.

Rancho Jurupa Park

4600 Crestmore Drive; (951) 684–7032; www.riversidecountyparks.org.

There are thirty-five parks in Riverside County's Regional Park and Open Spaces system. Rancho Jurupa Park is located just outside the city limits of Riverside and provides fishing, biking, hiking, and equestrian trails as well as camping. Don't forget to stop into the Luis Robidoux Nature Center on the park grounds. Only a mile (as the crow flies) from Rancho Jurupa is the Jensen-Alvarado Ranch. This was the first non-adobe building in the Riverside area. Many school groups come to learn how to make homemade ice cream and tortillas (on a potbellied stove!). The Jensen-Alvarado Ranch is located at 4307 Briggs Street in Riverside. Take Freeway 60 west from Riverside, exit at Rubidoux Boulevard, drive south to Tilton Avenue, and head west on Briggs.

Castle Amusement Park

3500 Polk Street; (951) 785–3000; www.castlepark.com. No admission fee; ride tickets and game tokens can be purchased inside the park.

Hold on to your collective hats! This twenty-five-acre park has it all. It was built in 1976 to be the "Ultimate Family Entertainment Park." The three-level castle houses more than 400 state-of-the-art games. The rare Dentzel carousel (built in 1898) is one of the oldest in America and has fifty-two hand-carved, brightly painted animals and two sleighs on highly polished brass poles (one of our family advisers had the family photographed here for a Christmas card). Add to these four world-class, eighteen-hole, championship miniature par-four golf courses surrounded by gorgeous palm trees. The Big Top Restaurant has everything from a salad bar to super sundaes.

Where to Eat

Anchos Southwest Grill and Bar, 10773 Hole Street, Riverside; (909) 352–0240. Take Freeway 91 to La Sierra, head north to Hole, and turn right. Delicious Mexican and southwestern cuisine. Watch the flour tortillas being made and rotating in the warmer. Try the Ribs and Diego Shrimp, which isn't listed on the menu. Wonderful! $

Gram's Mission Barbeque Palace, 3527 Main Street, Riverside; (951) 782–8219.

Gram's reigns supreme in barbecue and Cajun cuisine. $

Mario's Place, 3646 Mission Inn Avenue, Riverside; (951) 684–7755. Some of the most savory Italian dishes available. The Palagi family has made Mario's Place a landmark in Riverside. $$–$$$

Sevilla Restaurant & Club, 3252 Mission Inn Avenue, Riverside; (909) 778–0611. Take Freeway 91 to the Mission Inn Avenue exit. This restaurant specializes in Spanish (not Mexican) food. Entertainment includes flamenco dancers and offers nightlife when the children go to sleep. $$

Where to Stay

The Mission Inn, 3649 Mission Inn Avenue, Riverside; (951) 784–0300; www.missioninn.com. This European-style hotel encompasses an entire city block in downtown Riverside. Come stroll the halls of this great inn, which has hosted several of our nation's presidents. There are 239 elegant rooms and suites, no two alike. The Mission Inn Foundation/Museum offers walking history tours. $. Children younger than age 12 admitted **free.**

For More Information

Greater Riverside Chambers of Commerce. 3985 University Avenue, 92501; (951) 683–7100; fax (909) 683–2670; www.riverside-chamber.com.

Perris

For a taste of the real Riverside County, you have to delve into deep Riverside—in other words, let the country roads be your guide. If you take Interstate 215 south from State Highway 60 (which runs right through Riverside), in about twenty traffic-free minutes you'll come across the little town of Perris. The locals always say there's nothing like Perris in the springtime—a reference to the California golden poppies and other wildflowers that carpet these parts round about April. Even if your visit doesn't happen to coincide with the annual flora show, Mother Nature won't disappoint. Rambling about the Temecula Valley, in which Perris lies at the northern head, is like entering a time warp to old California. Bring your camera.

The Perris area is well known for the outdoor activities afforded by its laid-back country setting. The early morning and late evening stillness, coupled with mild temperatures, spells paradise for aviation buffs. Hot-air balloon, sailplane, hang glider, and even skydiving outfitters abound in the area. It can be quite a spectacle simply to watch these folks in action at the Perris Valley Airport. At ground level, campers, swimmers, boaters, fishers, hikers, and bikers will enjoy a detour to the **Lake Perris State Recreation Area,** 1781 Lake Perris Drive; (951) 657–0676. Visit the YA-I Heki Museum for information on Native American history of the area. It's located at Lake Perris Recreation Area.

Orange Empire Railway Museum

2201 South A Street; (951) 657–2605; www.oerm.org. **Free** admission. Nominal fees for trolley and train rides.

This is the West's biggest railway museum, with electric cars, buildings, and other artifacts. The museum covers sixty acres, so there is plenty of room for a family picnic among streetcars, trains, and municipal buses from yesteryear.

More than 150 historic train cars, locomotives, and streetcars are on display indoors and outside. Are you ready to ride the rails, kids? Each Saturday and Sunday from

11:00 A.M. to 5:00 P.M., vintage streetcars circle the museum property (it takes about seven minutes), and antique Southern Pacific train cars make a ten-minute trip to the Perris Depot and back.

Hemet

If you're heading from the Perris area to Hemet or Idyllwild (more on that next), you could take either Highway 74 east or drive along the **Juan Bautista de Anza National Historic Trail.** This scenic corridor, which skirts Lake Perris, dairy farms, and other quiet farmlands, follows the tracks de Anza made when he explored the region for Spain in 1775.

Ramona Outdoor Play
2400 Ramona Bowl Road; (951) 658–3111 or (800) 645–4465; www.ramonabowl.com. Late April/early May.

Performed by more than 400 of the town's residents, the play is adapted from the 1884 novel *Ramona,* which depicts the romantic spectacle of early California. It has been an annual event since 1923, earning it the designation as the official outdoor play of California. The play runs on weekends from 3:30 to about 6:30 P.M.

Diamond Valley Lake
300 Newport Road, Hemet; (951) 765–2612; www.dvlake.com. Exit I–215 south at Highway 74 east toward Hemet. Head south at State Street to Newport Road. Turn right.

These 4,000 square acres of water storage and recreation land are the great attraction of the Hemet Valley. Inside the visitor center you can see the mastodon exhibit as well as other artifacts retrieved from excavations made as this lake began to fill in 1999.

Highland Springs Resort and **Guest Ranch**

This 900-acre ranch, at 10600 Highland Avenue in Cherry Valley, offers horseback riding, cookouts, hayrides, and barbecues. Once a stagecoach stop for gold panners headed for the Colorado River, this rustic resort has been a good choice for a family vacation since 1884. Palm Springs is 30 miles east, and Idyllwild is 20 miles south. Call (951) 845–1151 or visit www.highland springsresort.com.

Idyllwild

Take Highway 74 east out of Hemet to Highway 243, which leads to the hamlet of Idyllwild. You will be traveling on the **Palms to Pines Scenic Highway,** and as the name indicates, you'll observe desert palm and oak trees giving way to pine and fir forests as the elevation increases. Idyllwild, which looks like a village from the Swiss Alps dropped into the heart of the **San Bernardino National Forest,** makes for one of the most enchanting detours in the Inland Empire, especially in winter. This town, at an altitude of 5,400 feet with zero days of smog, is a mile-high oasis nestled in the San Jacinto Mountains and a favorite choice for a well-balanced family vacation in Southern California. It is devoid of fast-food joints (and their comforts), but the exceptional opportunities for family recreation more than compensate! Check it out by contacting the **Idyllwild Chamber of Commerce** at 54295 Village Center Drive, 92549; (951) 659–3259; fax (909) 659–6216; www.idyll wildchamber.com. Since the town is nestled 5,400 feet up, Idyllwild nights are cool and crisp, even in the summer. Idyllwild is home to fifteen art galleries and more than thirty art events annually. Get ready to tackle the great outdoors by ordering up a savory Belgian waffle first—any time of day—at the **Idyllwild Cafe,** 26600 Highway 243, next to Idyllwild School; (951) 659–2210.

Living Free Animal Sanctuary

54250 Keen Camp Road, at Mountain Center on Highway 74; (951) 659–4684; www.living-free.org. Self-guided tours on Friday, Saturday, and Sunday from 11:00 A.M. to 2:00 P.M. Other days by appointment. Guided tours on Saturday only. Admission free; donations welcome.

This is a most unusual retreat for dogs and cats, a nonprofit animal sanctuary founded by Emily Jo Beard on 180 bucolic acres. The retreat is home to a variety of dogs, plus cats who have found a new life and home in this caring environment. The emphasis is on education, and children will find the dogs "living in harmony" and the cats "contented," enjoying spacious yards, play structures, and shady trees.

Sugarloaf Cafe and Market

70–111 Highway 74 at Mountain Center; (760) 349–9020; sugarloafcafe@aol.com. Open Tuesday through Sunday 8:00 A.M. to 8:00 P.M. $

At this rustic roadhouse, you can order anything from barbecue chicken hot off the rotisserie to sandwiches in a basket. Try one of their homemade soups, the perfect way to start your dining adventures in this majestic region of Southern California. Outside dining on the patio is a nice way to take in the scenery. And the market has a deli and takeout, too.

Idyllwild Arts

P.O. Box 38, 92549 (located at the end of Tollgate Road); (951) 659–2171; www.idyllwildart.org.

Idyllwild Arts offers a family camp in late June and early July. There are separate activities for children, teenagers, and adults, including hiking, wilderness activities, swimming, and just relaxing. Evening activities include concerts, folk dancing, and family talent night.

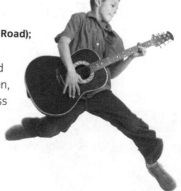

Oak Glen and Yucaipa

Washington State doesn't have a monopoly on apples. Oak Glen, just north of Yucaipa, is the core of the Inland Empire's tranquil apple country, which both tourists and natives are often surprised to find. September through December means apple-picking time at the 900-acre **Los Rios Rancho,** 39610 Oak Glen Road; (909) 795–1005 and **Parrish Pioneer Ranch,** 38561 Oak Glen Road; (909) 797–1753.

In the summer, you can pick raspberries instead—not a bad alternative. The New England atmosphere of Oak Glen is particularly strong in wintertime, when snow often coats the apple orchards. But any time of year, the place is simply charming. Visit www.oak glen.net or call (909) 797–2364 for the latest news on this year's crop and the annual Apple Blossom Festival.

Are you there yet? The town of Oak Glen is like a West Coast version of Sleepy Hollow, with its antiques stores and scent of fresh apple pie wafting out of the windows of little restaurants. The pace is slower up here, and residents seem to like it that way. Not everything's coming up apples, though. At the **Mously Museum of Natural History,** 35308 Panorama Drive; (909) 790–3163, seashells, minerals, and fossils take center stage.

Riley's Farm and Orchard

12253 South Oak Glen Road; (909) 790–2364; www.rileysfarm.com.

"Villagers and country folk" are cordially invited to "come and be one hundred years behind the times." During apple season you can take the kids on a hayride that includes a farm tour, cider pressing, and hot-caramel-dipped apples. Check out their summer tours, dinner events, and "Colonial Farm Life" Adventure Trips.

Where to Eat

Parrish Pioneer Apple Ranch, 38561 Oak Glen Road, Yucaipa; (909) 797–4020; www.parrishranch.com. Home to Apple Dumplin's Restaurant. Stop in for lunch (they have a great selection of sandwiches) and hot apple pie ala mode daily from 9:00 A.M. to 6:00 P.M. $

Dinosaurs, **Fruit, and Shopping**

As you drive along Interstate 10, the kids will make you pull over in **Cabazon** (population 1,400) the instant they see two hulking dinosaurs stalking drivers on the left (exit at Main Street). One's a brontosaurus with a mini-museum and gift shop tucked into his belly. His friend is a not-too-friendly-looking *Tyrannosaurus rex.* Like Pee Wee Herman in *Pee Wee's Big Adventure* (if you haven't seen it, your kids probably have), you can climb up to the dinosaur's jaw to take in the view. These Jurassic monstrosities are California camp at its best. They seem to be made expressly for family vacation fun. You can fill up at the **Wheel Inn** diner (951–849–7012), serving great grub 24/7 since 1964. We love this roadside classic, especially the pies!

There are two more attractions in Cabazon, both easily visible from Interstate 10. The first is **Hadley's Fruit Orchards** (www.hadleyfruitorchards .com), an all-natural dried fruit and produce emporium famous for its deliciously frosty date shakes. The other is **Desert Hills Premium Outlets** and **Cabazon Outlets** (48400 Seminole Road, 951–849–6641; www.cabazonoutlets .com), three rambling outlet complexes. If your kids have been pining for a new pair of Nikes, or you have designs on some off-price Ralph Lauren apparel or home furnishings, you've hit the jackpot. And this isn't even Las Vegas!

Kern County

Unlike many other states, California never quite seems to end. If you thought the sweeping vistas stopped after the San Bernardino Mountains, think again. Just north of them lies Kern County, nestled between the Sierra Nevada and the coastal range. With its 8,073 square miles, Kern is the third-largest county in California and is as large as Massachusetts. It forms the southern tier of the agriculture- and oil-rich Central Valley, the one of *Grapes of Wrath* fame, acre for acre the richest in the world. No matter what time of year you happen to be driving through, you'll see boundless fields of grapes, almonds, carrots, apples, watermelons, tomatoes, and more. The fruits and vegetables grown here are shipped all over the world, but you can sample them first at any of the numerous roadside farmers' markets.

Even if you've never been to Kern County before, you or your kids may feel as though you have, because of the numerous movies that have been filmed here over the years, from *Star Packer* (with John Wayne, 1934) to *Jurassic Park*. This portion of the vast, semi-arid valley is perhaps best known, though, for white-water river rafting on the Kern River. It was the river, in fact, that put the region on the map: Gold was discovered in the riverbed in 1851. There is even more to explore, but basically the area is less tourist intensive than the California that lies farther south. It is, above all, a place to appreciate the great outdoors, slow down a bit, and smell the forest.

Boron

Twenty Mule Team Museum

26962 Twenty Mule Team Road; (760) 762–5810; www.rnrs.com/20muleteam. Open daily 10:00 A.M. to 4:00 P.M. Kids welcome. Free.

If you find yourselves on Highway 58 at the junction of Highway 395 ("Four Corners") and think you're in the middle of nowhere, think again. Another 6 miles and you're here.

Should you have that *Thomas Guide* we recommended in the Greater Los Angeles chapter, you won't get lost. Your kids may not remember the TV series *Death Valley Days* or the product Borax (it used to make our wash sparkle), but here's a good way to refresh your memory. The museum, located in a renovated house from the old Baker Mine campsite, depicts borax mining and early life in Boron. There are plans to add an air and space museum here, so look for an F4D airplane that was retired here. There's also a train station that was brought in from Kramer. Keep your road map handy and your eyes open— there's no telling what you'll find in these parts.

The Borax Visitor Center

14486 Borax Road, off Highway 58 at the Borax Road exit; www.borax.com. Open seven days a week from 9:00 A.M. to 5:00 P.M., excluding major holidays and weather permitting.

Everyone who finds his or her way to this center gets a sample of "TV rock." After watching the seventeen-minute video on the worldwide uses of borax, the kids will understand why there really is a treasure in "them thar hills." And it's borax!

Kernville

Have you been contemplating a **white-water river-rafting adventure** for your family? If so, you're in the right place. From its headwaters at Lake South America in the Sierra Nevada (elevation 11,800 feet), the Kern River falls more than 12,000 feet in 150 miles. That makes it one of the fastest-falling rivers in North America. But the pace of the rapids ranges from wild to mild. According to the International River Classification System, rapids ratings range from Class I—very easy, like a swimming pool with a current—all the way up to Class VI, which is virtually unrunnable. Class I and II rapids are perfectly suitable for most children; older ones who enjoy a good soaking can take on Class III. The important thing to remember is that you don't just drive up to the river and hop in with an inner tube. There are several professional rafting outfitters whose sole purpose is to orchestrate a fun, safe time for everyone who signs up.

Most of these outfitters are based in Kernville, the traditional jumping-off point for rafting trips. If you've never done this kind of thing before, ask them about one-day instruction sessions.

If you happen to be in Kernville in late February (before the rafting season kicks in), enjoy the carnival atmosphere of **Whiskey Flat Days,** when the town travels back in time to the gold-rush days. With a parade, rodeo, whisker and costume contests, and frog races, the event is designed for families in search of a little quality fun time. Call (760) 376–2629 for dates and other information.

Kernville straddles the northern end of **Lake Isabella,** built in 1953 for flood control and as a hydroelectric source and reservoir. It is Southern California's largest freshwater lake. With up to 11,000 surface-acre feet, it also happens to be a prime body of water for Jet Skiing, waterskiing, windsurfing, sailing, and fishing.

The region around the lake is surrounded by the **Sequoia National Forest;** for camping information and details about other outdoor activities, stop by the USDA Forest Service's visitor center off Highway 155, just south of the lake's main dam, 4875 Ponderosa Road; (760) 379–5646.

Sierra South Mountain Sports Outfitters

11300 Kernville Road; (760) 376–3745 or (800) 376–2082; www.sierrasouth.com. Prices vary.

This company offers a wide range of rafting and kayaking excursions, including a two-and-a-half-hour Lickety-Blaster run. On this eminently manageable aquatic jaunt, rafters experience Class II and III rapids. Lake kayaking is an alternative to river rafting for those traveling with kids younger than age twelve, say the folks at Sierra South, because it is more relaxed and there is swimming at Lake Isabella. It's a family paddle adventure at a mellow pace.

Whitewater Voyages

(800) 400–RAFT; www.whitewatervoyages.com. $$$$

Offers Class I and II family trips that accommodate kids as young as age four. Whitewater's guides were stunt doubles for Meryl Streep and Kevin Bacon in *The River Wild.*

Mountain and River Adventures

(760) 376–6553 or (800) 861–6553; fax (760) 376–1267; www.mtnriver.com. $$$$

Offers mountain-biking and rock-climbing rambles in addition to white-water rafting trips—all under expert supervision by guides who know the lay of the land (and water) inside out. New in 2004 was a five-hour docent-led bus excursion to the Giant Sequoia National Monument, including a picnic lunch in the forest.

Kern Valley Turkey Vulture Festival

Contact Kernville Chamber of Commerce; (760) 376–2629 or (800) 350–7390; fax (760) 376–4371; www.valleywild.org/tvfest.htm.

Just when you think you've heard about the most unusual festival imaginable (for instance, the tobacco spitting competition in Calico), along comes this one. Held between September 1 and October 31, depending on when the big birds decide to fly through Kern Valley (during the four-day festival in 2003, some 16,000 birds were tallied), the festival offers such activities as a turkey vulture slide show, workshops on raptor rehabilitation, a bird-banding demonstration, and an official Turkey Vultures Lift-Off. There are turkey vulture T-shirts to buy, designed by John Schmitt, and enough information to satisfy the most rabid bird-watcher (or turkey vulture buff). The festival takes place in Weldon at Audubon's Kern River Preserve.

Where to Eat and Stay

Cheryl's Diner, 11030 Kernville Road. Open from 6:00 A.M. to 9:00 P.M. Breakfast, lunch, and dinner served at family-friendly prices. $

The River View Lodge, P.O. Box 745, Kernville, 93238; (760) 376–6019; www.riverviewlodge.info. This historic eleven-room inn welcomes families and pets. You'll find refrigerators in every room and a picnic area, too. The country-style rooms with two queen-size beds are ideal for families. $$

For More Information

Kern River Valley Chamber of Commerce. P.O. Box 567, 6117 Lake Isabella Boulevard, Lake Isabella, 93240; (760) 379–5236 or (866) KRV4FUN; www.kern valley.com.

Kernville Chamber of Commerce. 11447 Kernville Road, P.O. Box 397, Kernville, 93238-0397; (760) 376–2629; fax (760) 376–4371; www.kernvillechamber .org.

Bakersfield

There are several attractions in and around the pleasant city of Bakersfield, Kern's county seat. Bakersfield has an unexpected culinary surprise: numerous Basque restaurants. One of the largest Basque communities outside the Pyrenees is in Kern County, and no chance to sample their singular cuisine should be missed.

Buck Owens' Crystal Palace

2800 Buck Owens Boulevard; (661) 869–BUCK; (661) 328–7500 for dinner reservations. Call (661) 328–7560 or (808) 855–5005 for show reservations; www.buckowens.com. Daily **free** tours are available.

Opened in 1996, this all-in-one restaurant, museum, and theater is a must-see! Even if the kids are unaware that Buck Owens starred in *Hee Haw,* they'll love the smashingly sensational decor. You'll be amazed by what's above the 50-foot-long bar: the car Elvis never drove, a vintage 1970s Pontiac and yacht, studded with silver dollars! It's mounted at a tilt so you can check out its luxurious interior.

Buck Owens and others perform country favorites evenings, matinees, and weekends. State-of-the-art sound, and lighting and giant screens throughout make this a visual marvel. And we haven't even mentioned the 35-foot mural showing Buck's rise from the cotton fields to Carnegie Hall to entertaining presidents at the White House. Country music has found a home in Bakersfield.

Kern County Museum and Lori Brock Children's Discovery Center

3801 Chester Avenue; (661) 852–5000; www.kcmuseum.org. Open Monday through Friday 8:00 A.M. to 5:00 P.M. and Saturday 10:00 A.M. to 5:00 P.M. $

The museum provides more than a glimpse into the history of Bakersfield and its environs. Kids have room to roam here, for it's a sixteen-acre walk-through site with more than sixty historic and refurbished structures, ranging from the Havilah Courthouse and Jail (1866) and the Calloway Ranch Blacksmith Shop (circa 1880) to an 1898 Southern Pacific locomotive. The Spanish Mission–style main museum building houses permanent and changing exhibitions that chronicle Kern County's history, natural history, and culture. The Lori Brock Children's Discovery Center, with hands-on displays and activities for kids, is also located on the premises.

California Living Museum (CALM)

Just north of Bakersfield, 14000 Alfred Harrell Highway; (661) 872–2256; www.calmzoo.org. Open Tuesday through Sunday 9:00 A.M. to 5:00 P.M. $

Whereas the Kern County Museum focuses on the human history of the area, the natural environment occupies center stage here. This is an ideally situated spot for a family-oriented wildlife experience. The thirteen acres house a botanical garden, petting zoo, and natural history museum. The animal exhibits assemble fauna native to California: coyotes, desert tortoises, shorebirds, and birds of prey, including hawks, raptors, owls, and eagles. The *Mammal Round* exhibit features mountain lions, raccoons, foxes, and bobcats—yes, all native to the Golden State! The Living Museum merits at least a ninety-minute visit.

Tule Elk State Reserve

Twenty-seven miles west of Bakersfield, 4 miles west of Interstate 5, and off the Stockdale Highway, south of Buttonwillow; (661) 764–6881 or (661) 248–6692. Open daily 8:00 A.M. to sunset.

For a slightly wilder look at the wild kingdom, head to this 953-acre site. Tule elks were once as common in California as the antelope of South Africa are today, but they are now a rare species. The State Division of Beaches and Parks keeps a herd of about thirty adult elk at the park, which is equipped with a shaded picnic and viewing area. With the sweeping grassland forming a backdrop, gawking at the elks' regal antlers (which only the males have) is rather like taking a mini-safari. The best times to view the elk are in summer and fall.

Fort Tejon State Historic Park

Interstate 5, 36 miles south of Bakersfield. Exit off Interstate 5, 70 miles northwest of Los Angeles at the top of Grapevine Canyon; (661) 248–6692. Living-history programs held the first Sunday of each month; Civil War reenactments, third Sunday, April through October.

The fort is well worth a few hours' stop, especially for a realistic perspective of the 1850s to 1860s.

Vroom **Vroom**

If you and your kids are feeling the need to see some speed, feel the roar, and taste the dust, Kern County is renowned for its racetracks. Here's where the action is!

Mesa Marin, 11000 Kern Canyon Road, Bakersfield; (661) 366–5711; www.mesamarin.com. A half-mile, high-banked paved oval track and test track. NASCAR California 600, late-model Stock Cars, Modified Stock Cars, Grand American Modified, Craftsman Trucks, and NASCAR Winston West Series 200 held here.

Famoso Raceway, 33559 Famoso Road, McFarland; (661) 399–2210; www.famosoraceway.com. Quarter-mile drag strip featuring the Good Guys Nostalgia March Meet, the NHRA FM series in April, and the NHRA CHRR IX in October.

Willow Springs International Raceway, 3500 75th Street West, Rosamond; (661) 256–2471; www.willowspringsraceway.com. Races held every weekend; five circuits available. Car, motorcycle, kart driving, and racing schools.

Buttonwillow Raceway Park, 24551 Lerdo Highway, Buttonwillow; (661) 764–5333; www.buttonwillowraceway.com. Three-mile road-racing track. Indy cars, sports cars, motorcycles, and go-karts go here.

Where to Eat

A highlight of any meal is the scrumptious Basque salsa, made of chopped tomatoes, yellow and jalapeño chiles, garlic, onions, and salt. Try it at:

Benji's French Basque Restaurant, 4001 Rosedale Highway; (661) 328–0400.

Chalet Basque, 200 Oak Street; (661) 327–2915.

Pyrenees Cafe, 601 Sumner Street; (661) 323–0053. $$

Wool Growers, 620 East Nineteenth Street; (661) 327–9584.

Dewar's Candy and Ice Cream Parlor, 1120 Eye Street, Bakersfield; (661) 322–0933; www.dewarscandy.com. Savor sweet confections and ice cream from the Dewar's family recipes, originating in 1909. $

Noriega Hotel, 525 Sumner Street; (661) 322–8419. One seating at noon and one seating at 7:00 P.M. Our favorite family-style dining spot. Make sure you know how to get there, as first-timers have some trouble. Hungry diners sit at long tables (you may not know who'll be next to you), sharing up to seven courses of hearty Basque food. No set menu. We've tried soup, salad, chicken, ribs, fresh-cut french fries—all excellent. The ambience is, well, plain, but the service is efficient and the fare is robust. Only the most ravenous will have room for dessert. $–$$

Where to Stay

Red Lion Hotel Bakersfield, 2400 Camino Del Rio Court, Bakersfield; (661) 327–0681; fax (661) 637–1822; reservations: (800) RED–LION; www.redlionbakersfield.com. There are 165 rooms and suites, some with Jacuzzis. Prime location at junction of Freeway 99 and Highway 58 (Rosedale Highway exit) for all your family's Kern County adventures. Smokin' Joe's Beach Bar & Woodfired Cuisine restaurant on-site. $$$

For More Information

Greater Bakersfield Chamber of Commerce. 1725 Eye Street, P.O. Box 1947, Bakersfield, 93303; (661) 327–4421; www.bakersfieldchamber.org.

Kern County Board of Trade and Tourist Information Center. Mailing address: P.O. Bin 1312, Bakersfield, 93302; street address: 2101 Oak Street, Bakersfield; (661) 861–2367 or (800) 500–KERN; www.visitkern.com.

Home on **the Ranch**

If your kids spot some elk, they may be disappointed to learn that no, they can't ride or even pet them. However, they can pet and ride horses to their hearts' content at **Rankin Ranch,** minutes north of Bakersfield in Walker's Basin. To get there, take Interstate 5 north to the Lamont–Lake Isabelle exit. The ranch is 38 miles from the exit, past the town of Caliente. Members of the Rankin family have been ranching at their Quarter Circle U since 1863, and they've got the western way of life down pat. This is a working, 31,000-acre, cattle and guest ranch where kids and adults can help out with farm chores and horseback ride at their leisure. Fourteen cozy cabins with no room phones or TV. Family-style meals, horseback riding, swimming, and hiking. Seasonal supervised children's program is first-rate. Call for current rates (which include riding, lodging, and three meals a day) and other information at (661) 867–2511, or visit www.rankinranch.com.

Tulare County

Encompassing 4,863 square miles (slightly larger than Connecticut) in the San Joaquin Valley, Tulare County is nestled between the Sierra Nevada to the east and the Coastal Mountain Range to the west. Tulare County's extensively cultivated and very fertile valley floor is the second-leading producer of agricultural commodities in the United States. The rest of the county is composed of foothills, timbered slopes, and high mountains ranging in elevations from 270 feet to 14,495 feet (the top of Mt. Whitney, the highest point in the continental United States). There are more than 110 mountain peaks in eastern Tulare County, which furnish a backdrop of scenic wonder. Tulare County is home to Sequoia National Park as well as Inyo and Sequoia National Forests–offering an amazing array of dining, lodging, camping, winter sports of all kinds, fishing, boating, backpacking, hunting, hiking, and waterskiing options that attract thousands of visitors annually.

Sequoia National Park and Kings Canyon National Park

Office of the Superintendent, 47050 Generals Highway, Three Rivers; general visitor infor-mation: (559) 565–3341; fax (559) 565–3730; www.nps.gov/seki. The two main entrances, Ash Mountain on Highway 198 and Big Stump on Highway 180, are open daily year-round. Certain areas of the park are open part of the year: The Mineral King area is open late May through October 31 in Sequoia National Park, and the Cedar Grove area in Kings Canyon is open mid-April through mid-November. Crystal Cave, some campgrounds, and several side roads close for the winter. The main park road, the Generals Highway, may close between Lodgepole and Grant Grove during and after storms for plowing. The highest visitation is in July and August. It can be difficult to find a campsite at popular campgrounds on summer Saturdays. Driving times: To Sequoia Park Ash Mountain entrance from Highway 99 at Visalia, take Highway 198 east for approximately one hour. To Kings Canyon Park Big Stump entrance from Highway 99 at Fresno, take Highway 180 east approximately 1¼ hours. Admission per vehicle: $10 for a seven-day pass, $20 for annual vehicle pass. Note: Gasoline is not sold within park boundaries, but it is available at locations near the park boundaries. Be sure to fill up in one of the towns near the park entrances or at one of three locations in the national forest that borders parts of the park.

Tulare County is best known as the home of these parks. Even though it's part of Fresno County, Kings Canyon shares its east-west boundary with Sequoia, and the two parks are generally referred to together. If the wooded retreats of Big Bear and Lake Arrowhead in the Inland Empire are imbued with an "escape from the city" atmosphere, up here you'll really feel a zillion miles away from it all. This is nature at its most unbridled, God's country with a very capital G. With more than 800 miles of marked hiking trails and 1,200-plus campsites and other lodging options, it's no wonder Sequoia and Kings Canyon are a California family favorite for camping and nature trips.

The biggest attractions are trees. Autumn in New England may be prime leaf-peeping time, but the trees of the central Sierra Nevada are marvels to behold anytime of year. This is mainly due to their gargantuan size. Of the thirty-seven largest sequoia trees in the world, twenty giants roost here in Sequoia and Kings Canyon. You'll find the most stupendous grove of sequoias in the Giant Forest, longtime home of the General Sherman Tree. Weighing in at 2.7 million pounds, the 275-foot-tall tree is the largest living thing in the world. At more than 2,300 years, it's also one of the oldest. Each year the venerable Sherman grows enough wood for another 60-foot-tall tree. Imagine the tree-house possibilities! For an easy, rewarding hike the whole family will enjoy, try the 2-mile, two-hour Congress Trail, which begins at the Sherman and circles around the grove.

Kings Canyon is where the General Grant Tree, the earth's third-largest, has its roots. It's also known as the "Nation's Christmas Tree." Annual Noel celebrations are held beneath its considerable and magnificent canopy. Walk along the easy ⅓-mile-long trail, marked with informative signposts, to learn more about trees and the peoples who lived here.

Conservationist John Muir called Kings Canyon a rival to Yosemite, and it's not hard to see why. The depths of the canyon at Cedar Grove, where the Kings River gushes between sheer granite walls, bottom out at 8,000 feet. Both Sequoia and Kings Canyon offer incomparable vistas, hiking trails, camping, and other natural wonders, including more than a hundred caves.

There are several excellent visitor centers throughout the parks that offer **free** information, weather updates, naturalist programs, slide shows, maps, and services. Grant Grove Visitor Center in Kings Canyon (559–565–4307) is open daily. Lodgepole Visitor Center in Sequoia (559–565–4436) is open daily in summer and on weekends only in winter. Cedar Grove Visitor Center is open daily during the summer only.

The new Giant Forest Museum in Sequoia (559–565–4480) is open daily and should not be missed. It is housed in a historic log building in the Giant Forest sequoia grove at 6,500 feet elevation, 16 miles from the Ash Mountain entrance on Highway 198. Wonderful interactive exhibits tell the story of the sequoias of Giant Forest, and what we have learned about how to protect them.

Activities vary according to season, but no matter the time of year, the best way to get into the park is to get out of the car. "Don't leave until you have seen it," advised 1920s park superintendent Col. John R. White, "and this you cannot do from an automobile." In summer, rangers lead walks and talks in the foothills, the sequoia groves, and the high country. Take a tour of the exquisite Crystal Cave. There are rivers to enjoy—carefully—and pack stations offer horseback riding.

Come winter, cross-country skis or snowshoes can be rented to explore the sequoia groves beyond the roads, and there are ranger-guided snowshoe walks. Wolverton is a wonderful free-terrain snow-play area (sometimes even in April). If you prefer warmer activities, trails in the foothills are usually snow-free, and by February they are graced with wildflowers. Check bulletin boards and visitor centers to find what activities are being offered.

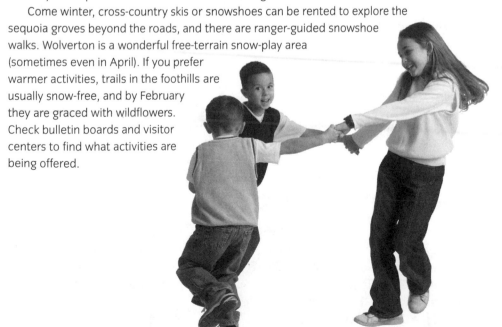

The Biggest **Trees in the World**

Giant Sequoias *(Sequoiadendron giganteum)* grow only on the western slopes of the Sierra Nevada in central California. The groves are scattered across a narrow 260-mile belt, no more than about 15 miles wide at any point in elevations mainly between 5,000 and 7,500 feet. Closely related are the coastal redwoods *(Sequoia sempervirens)* found along the northern California coast. Giant Sequoias are slightly shorter than the coastal redwoods, but they are more massive, and they're considered the largest tree in the world in terms of volume. The largest sequoia and the most massive living organism on the planet is the **General Sherman Tree** in Sequoia National Park.

Where to Eat and Stay

Cedar Grove Lodge, (operated by Sequoia–Kings Canyon Park Services Company); (559) 335–5500; www.sequoia-kingscanyon.com. Open late April through mid-November. Twenty-one motel rooms in Cedar Grove Village, deep in the canyon of Kings Canyon Park. Restaurant, market, gift shop also in building. $$

Grant Grove Village, (operated by Sequoia–Kings Canyon Park Services Company); (559) 335–5500 or (866) JON–MUIR; www.sequoia-kingscanyon.com. Open all year. Here you will find the two-story John Muir Lodge, thirty modern hotel rooms with forest views as well as more than

forty rustic tent and housekeeping cabins, all in the Grant Grove area of Kings Canyon Park, only a half-mile stroll to a sequoia grove. Casual dining on American fare (breakfast, lunch, and dinner daily) at Grant Grove Village Restaurant, next to the visitor center, market/general store, gift shop, and post office. $$$

Montecito–Sequoia Lodge (privately owned and operated by Dr. Virginia Bonds and family for more than fifty years); (559) 565–3388 or (800) 843–8677; www.ms lodge.com. Open year-round. Located on its own Lake Homavalo in Sequoia National Forest, adjacent to Sequoia and Kings Canyon National Parks. This rustic property functions as a weekly Family Vacation

Sequoia and Kings Canyon **Junior Ranger Program**

Kids of any age can participate in this program. Kids ages five through eight earn the Jay Award. Those ages nine through twelve work for the Raven Award, and kids ages thirteen through one hundred and three can earn the Senior Patch. To get started, purchase a Junior Ranger booklet at any visitor center. Follow the instructions and have fun!

Camp in summer and a Cross Country Ski Center in the winter. Thirty-six basic lodge rooms with private baths and thirteen cabins with nearby bathhouses. Reasonable rates vary according to season and include all meals, which are served buffet style in the lodge. On-site summer and children's activities include canoeing, sailing, waterskiing, swimming, horseback riding, tennis, archery, trampoline, riflery, fencing, nature, stream fishing, arts and crafts instruction, theme nights, dances, sing-along campfires, variety shows, water carnivals, fort building, junior gymnastics, and pony rides. $$$

Wuksachi Village & Lodge, (operated by Delaware North Park Services, in Sequoia National Park, 4 miles from the Giant Forest and 23 miles from Sequoia Park entrance); (559) 253–2199 or (888) 252–5757; www.VisitSequoia.com. Open all year. Opened in 1999, the striking log lodge forms the center of the village and houses the full-service dining room (breakfast, lunch, and dinner daily), cocktail lounge, gift shop, and conference rooms, where naturalist-led programs are held (**free** and not to be missed). There are 102 modern rooms housed in three separate log buildings up on the hillside (ask for the Sequoia building for the best views of Mt. Silliman and Silver Peak). The eighteen large family suites have sofa sleepers in alcove sitting areas—ideal for your clan. Reserve early, especially in summer and on weekends. $$$

Mammoth Lakes Area

The Mammoth Lakes area is California's answer to the Alps. Southern Californians have been known to schlep their ski equipment to locales as far off as Chile and Chamonix, but most will agree that some of the best skiing anywhere is found 300 miles north of Los Angeles at **Mammoth Mountain Ski Area** in the heart of the Sierra Nevada. The statistics bespeak world-class thrills: an 11,053-foot summit, a 7,953-foot base, 30 lifts, 150 trails, and 3,500 acres of skiable terrain. The ski season often extends as late as July. Don't let the fact that the U.S. Ski Team trains at Mammoth each spring deter you from coming: Fully 30 percent of the ski runs are rated for beginners. Plus, Mammoth boasts one of the finest ski schools in the country, with family lessons and a children's ski school offered regularly.

Mammoth Mountain went through some big changes during 2003–2004 (its fiftieth anniversary season), but it still retains its spirit of year-round sportsmanship, camaraderie, and friendly hospitality. Throughout the Mammoth Lakes region, not only will your family groove on skiing and snowboarding, but also at cross-country ski centers, on snowmobile rentals, sledding, tobogganing, outdoor ice skating, and snowshoeing. Summer means even more activities to keep the family fit. In the summer, enjoy mountain biking, hiking, jazz and art festivals, swimming, picnicking, fishing, boating, hot springs, and canoeing, kayaking, or riding your Jet Skis and Wave Runners at lakes Topaz, Klondike, Grant, Diaz, Walker, and Crowley. Or check out national monuments—visit Devils Postpile, formed more than 100,000 years ago, or Rainbow Falls, where the San Joaquin River drops more than 100 feet. How about a horseback ride—most of the major canyons in the Eastern

Sierra have pack stations, offering anywhere from a one-hour to full-day or multiday trips. Your family will discover endless choices for accommodations (condos, chalets, hotels, cabins, inns), for dining (from fast food to continental cuisine), and for shopping (from trinkets to fine art), and a shuttle route that connects all the fun year-round!

Mammoth is one of the best choices for a family vacation–summer or winter.

Inyo National Forest
Headquarters, 351 Pacu Lane, Suite 200, Bishop, 93514; (760) 873–2400; www.fs.fed.us/ r5/inyo/.

The name "Inyo" comes from a Native American word meaning "dwelling place of the great spirit." The Inyo National Forest was named after Inyo County, in which much of the forest resides. Here you'll find more than two million acres of clean air, crystal-blue skies, mountain lakes and streams, challenging trails, high mountain peaks, and beautiful views. The Inyo National Forest is home to many natural wonders, including Mt. Whitney, Mono Lake, Mammoth Lakes Basin, and the Ancient Bristlecone Pine Forest, as well as seven congressionally designated wildernesses, comprising more than 650,000 acres of land. Recreational opportunities include camping, picnicking, hiking, backpacking, equestrian use, and off-highway vehicle use. One hundred-plus miles of trails are groomed for multiple-purpose winter use (snowmobiling, skiing, and hiking), and approximately 45 miles of trails are groomed for cross-country skiing and, of course, Mammoth Mountain.

Mammoth Mountain Ski Area
Snowphone: (760) 934–6166 or (888) SNOWRPT; general information: (760) 934–0745 or (800) MAMMOTH; www.mammothmountain.com. Open year-round.

Mammoth Mountain is the leading four-season mountain resort in Southern California, encompassing four day lodges, ten sports shops, nine rental/repair shops, one on-hill snack bar, three food courts/cafeterias, a ski and snowboard school, a race department, lockers, hotel and condominium accommodations, five restaurants, seven bars, child-care area, and game room. Rates for lodging, dining, and attractions are available in a wide range to fit any budget or taste.

Woollywood Children's Ski School
In the Main Lodge, (760) 934–0685, or in the Canyon Lodge, (760) 934–0787; www .mammothmountain.com.

The school is divided into Mammoth Explorers (ages four to six and seven to twelve), the Big Kahuna Snowboard Club (seven to twelve), children's private lessons (four to twelve), the Custom Kid's Camp (seven to twelve), and a three-day ski/snowboard camp. Helmets are required for ages four through twelve.

DJ's Snowmobile Adventures
(760) 935–4480.

Families will enjoy one- and two-hour backcountry self-guided tours or half-hour introductions to snowmobile rides in the flats.

Sledz
(760) 934–7533.

Perfect for kids who love grappling with gigantic inner tubes. Well-matched for kids age three and older. Kids 4 feet and taller can ride the authentic bobsleds with adult supervision.

Children's Fishing Festival (ages 1 to 15)
At Snowcreek Pond every June.

Kids learn how to fish for alpers trout. Best of all, the event is **free** and tackle is provided.

Mammoth Mountain Bike Park (ages 4 and up)
(760) 934–0706 or contact Mammoth Lakes Park and Recreation, (760) 934–8989, ext. 237, for details.

This is a great haven for kids age four and older wanting to learn to ride mountain bikes. Many trails are ideal for younger riders.

Red's Meadow Pack Stations
P.O. Box 395, Mammoth Lakes, 93546; (760) 934–2345 or (800) 292–7758; www.mammoth web.com/redsmeadow/.

If you're in the market for a modern A-frame cabin, these new but rustic cabins are furnished with butane heating, running water, large bathrooms with showers, gas ranges, and refrigerators. From Red's Meadow there are various group riding and hiking trail trips to such places as the John Muir Wilderness, Bishop to Bodie (camping along the old stagecoach route via saddle horse, mule, and wagon), and other off-the-beaten-path tours your family will long remember. These tours begin in late May and end about the first of October. If you're into more comfort, reserve a condominium for the family. Rates are surprisingly reasonable.

Paul Schat's Bakkery
3305 Main Street; (760) 934–6055. $

If the name sounds familiar, you're right. Father Erick has a "bakkery" in Bishop. From delectable caramel-encrusted pecan rolls to scintillating sweet rolls with sweet sliced apples, this place, near the outlets in Mammoth, is an absolute must. Drop by for breakfast or lunch in Cafe Vermeer, where you can order sandwiches on the freshest bread on the planet.

Tamarack Cross-Country Ski Center
Located 2 miles from the town of Mammoth in the Mammoth Lakes Basin on Twin Lakes Road. $$$$

A great bet for families, with its groomed trails that weave through pine forests. It's also home to the Tamarack Lodge and Resort, (800) 237–6879; www.tamaracklodge.com. Ask about mid-week winter ski packages.

Dog Sled Adventures
(760) 934–6270 or (800) MAMMOTH.

Tours (on an honest-to-goodness dogsled) mush off from the Main Lodge at Mammoth Mountain Inn.

Sierra Meadows Ranch
1 Sherwin Creek Road; (760) 934–6161.

You can spend some quality time on one of several theme horse-drawn sleigh rides through Mammoth Meadow (moonlight rides, breakfast rides, etc.) or take a hay or trail ride in summer. The warm months, by the way, are when Mammoth's majesty welcomes back the hiking, fishing, and mountain-biking crowd. Closes Labor Day weekend and opens again Memorial Day weekend.

For More Information

Mammoth Lakes Visitor Bureau. Administrative Office, P.O. Box 48, 437 Old Mammoth Road, Suite Y, Mammoth Lakes, 93546; (760) 934–2717 or (888) GO–MAMMOTH.

Mammoth Lakes Visitor Center/Ranger Station. Highway 203 (at entrance to town); (760) 924–5500 www.visit mammoth.com.

Mammoth Mountain owns Mammoth Mountain Ski Area, June Mountain, Tamarack Lodge and Resort, Mammoth Snowmobile Adventures, Mammoth Mountain Bike Park, and Mammoth Mountain Inn. It also operates Juniper Springs Properties, the Village at Mammoth, and Sierra Star Golf Club in Mammoth Lakes. Visit www.mammothmountain .com or call (800) MAMMOTH.

Manzanar **National Historic Site**

During World War II, Manzanar Relocation Center, just off U.S. Highway 395, 12 miles north of Lone Pine, was one of ten camps where Japanese American citizens and Japanese aliens were interned. Located at the foot of the imposing Sierra Nevada in eastern California's Owens Valley, Manzanar has been identified as the best preserved of these camps. Open all year during daylight hours with free admission.

There is a 3.2-mile-long self-guided auto tour of the camp with a tour description and map available at the camp entrance. A walking tour of the Manzanar Camp takes one to two hours. A self-guiding walking-tour booklet is available at the Interagency Visitor Center in Lone Pine and at the Eastern California Museum in Independence. For more information, call (760) 878–2194 or visit www.nps.gov/manz/.

Lone Pine

How can you not stop in Lone Pine, in southern Inyo County, once you realize you can explore one of the earth's oldest geological formations by car? Among others, these phantasmagoric formations resemble a bullfrog, a polar bear, Hannibal the Cannibal, and an owl. Hundreds of rock sculptures can be imagined in these bizarre hills, and you can drive the route in about half an hour.

You're on historical turf here; this is where Republic Pictures filmed dozens of spaghetti Westerns during the '40s and '50s. Chase scenes from these cowboy flicks, with such stars as Hopalong Cassidy, were immortalized in this stunning landscape. Scenes for *Maverick* (starring Mel Gibson) were shot here. If you see *The Shadow* with Alec Baldwin, you'll recognize the Alabama hills backdrop. Many stars return for the mid-October **Annual Lone Pine Film Festival.** You might just see Virginia Mayo, Rand Brooks, Penny Edwards, Ann Rutherford, or Loren James (Steve McQueen's double for twenty-two years). Of course, the kids may never have heard of these stars. Spending a few hours or a few days here, within view of the majestic Mt. Whitney, is to enter a time warp with California charisma.

You might stop for lunch at the **Totem Café,** 131 South Main Street, or for a burger at the **Mount Whitney Restaurant,** 227 South Main Street.

Overnight accommodations aren't a problem, as so many people stop here to mountaineer for a few days.

Where to Stay

Best Western's Frontier Motel, 1008 Main Street at Highway 395, one-half mile south of Lone Pine; (760) 876–5571, (899) 528–1234, or (800) 428–2627; www.best western.com. Rates include continental breakfast at this 73-room property. Spectacular mountain views from the lawn. $$

For More Information

Lone Pine Chamber of Commerce. 126 South Main Street, 93545; (760) 876–4444, toll free (877) 253–8981; fax (760) 876–9205; www.lonepinechamber.org. The Lone Pine Chamber sponsors such events as the world-class Wild Wild West Marathon, considered to be the seventh-most-challenging marathon in North America; the Early Trout Opener & Derby, which is the earliest trout opener on the eastern side of the Sierra; and the Rod 'N' Cycle Show 'N' Shine Classic Car and Motorcycle Show.

Bishop

Chances are quite good you'll pass through the town of Bishop on your way to or out of the Mammoth Lakes area. You'll see why Bishop calls itself the Mule Capital of the World if you arrive during Memorial Day weekend's **Mule Days** (www.Muledays.org), when the streets are abuzz with mule and chariot races, jumping events, and myriad other equine-related activities. Approximately 40,000 mule lovers gather for what the *Guinness Book of World Records* called (in 1994) the world's longest-running nonmotorized parade. Call (760) 872–4263 for more information.

September in Bishop is a special event in itself thanks to the **Millpond Traditional Music Festival** (760–873–8014 or 800–874–0669) that takes place at Millpond County Park, sponsored by Inyo County and the Inyo Council for the Arts. Featured are top performers of bluegrass, folk, and country music. Families will find this musical weekend ideal for picnics.

Laws Railroad Museum and Historical Site

A bit north of Bishop; (760) 873–5950; www.thesierraweb.com/bishop/laws. **Free;** **donations welcome.**

This eleven-acre indoor/outdoor museum harks back to the rough-and-tumble pioneer days in the Owens Valley. Kids can climb into the cab of locomotive 9 to ring the bell, and explore the compartment cars of the 1883 Slim Princess narrow gauge train, which, says the sign, "began nowhar, ended nowhar, an' stopped all night to think it over." The museum is on the National Register of Historic Places. Check out the bell rack, featuring antique bells from Bishop-area schools; the Original Laws School, refurbished with local artifacts; and a country store with old-time school items and supplies on display.

Erick Schat's Bakkery

763 North Main Street; (760) 873–7156.

This is a local institution. Home since 1938 of the original "sheepherder bread," a hearty country loaf, Schat's also has delicious sweet rolls and scrumptious sandwiches. You'll leave well fortified and ready to tackle another stretch of scenic California.

For More Information

Bishop Area Chamber of Commerce and Visitors Bureau. 690 North Main Street; (760) 873–8504 or (888) 395–3952; www.bishopvisitor.com. Request a copy of the Vacation Planner.

Bishop Creek Recreation Area. 210 South Lake Road, 93514; (760) 873–4484; www.BishopCreekResorts.com.

the Deserts

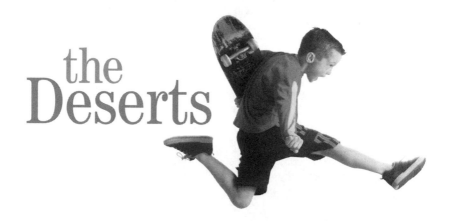

The California deserts conjure up different images for different people. To some they suggest glittering resort cities, brilliant skies, and the verdant greens of impressive Palm Springs golf courses. To others they raise thoughts of a barren, even desolate, landscape of boulders, sand, and cacti lining the freeway from Los Angeles to Las Vegas. To yet others they inspire thoughts of pioneer history, rustic ghost towns, and abandoned gold mines. The advent of tribal Indian casinos has changed tourism throughout Southern California, with five major gaming establishments luring throngs to the desert. It is important to note that Indian casinos do not allow any guests under the age of twenty-one, so they will not be listed in this guidebook. Yet, vast opportunities for family fun endure under the desert sun! Whatever desert-related pictures may come to mind, however, one fact is indisputable: The desert is big. It is immense—stretching from the Mojave Desert and ultra-arid Death Valley National Park in the north to the Colorado Desert area that reaches south to the border of Mexico.

Although the region is strikingly—or starkly—beautiful, much of it is what some might call wasteland or others environmentally pristine. Either way, a good portion is off-limits to nonmilitary personnel. These two attributes certainly make it simpler for families who want to catch the desert's highlights but lack the time (or inclination) to explore every gully or gulch. As a matter of fact, vast tracts of the desert have no highways, and if something akin to a "road" exists, it can be rock-strewn, meandering, sign-less, and dusty, leading you and your clan (best-case scenario) to an old ghost town or some other remnant of long-gone Wild West days, or (worst-case scenario) to nowhere, nowhere at all.

If you are willing to take a modest chance, to be marginally adventuresome in checking out a few of the desert's endless nooks and crannies, you'll find that here, too, the Golden State is indeed a land of contrasts.

As its name suggests, Death Valley—at 282 feet below sea level, the lowest land surface in the Western Hemisphere—is about as dry as a place can get. In sharp contrast, much of Palm Springs and other resort communities of the Coachella Valley, some 150 miles to the south of Death Valley, are as verdant and lush as a tropical oasis—primarily because of irrigation, but partly because of cool mountain streams that have flowed into

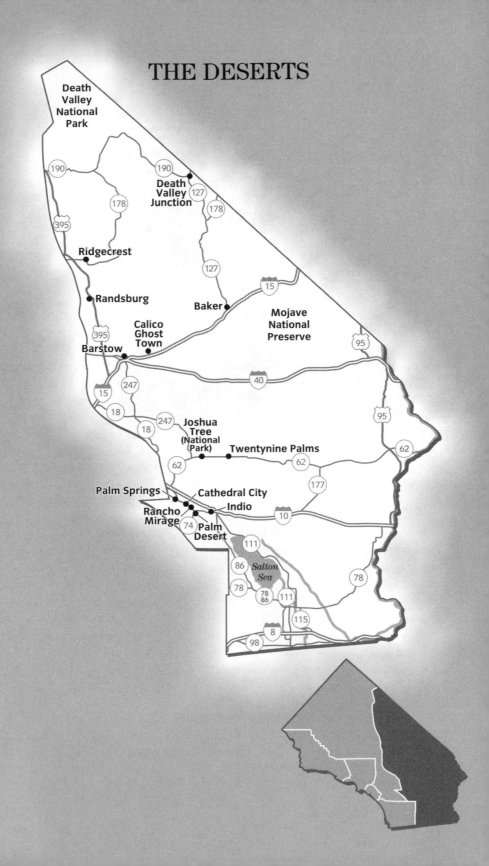

THE DESERTS

Death Valley National Park

Death Valley Junction

Ridgecrest

Randsburg

Baker

Mojave National Preserve

Calico Ghost Town

Barstow

Joshua Tree (National Park)

Twentynine Palms

Palm Springs

Cathedral City

Rancho Mirage

Indio

Palm Desert

Salton Sea

the area for centuries. Even in summer, when 110-plus temperatures expose the desert's true personality, it's still a great time to visit. During the summer months, many Palm Springs–area hotels reduce their rates 50 to 70 percent. And throughout the desert, summer seems to go by a little slower than elsewhere in California. Of course, the sun certainly shines brighter. It's almost as if nature is telling you to enjoy the offerings of the desert at a pace that suits you—and reminding you to bring along the sunscreen!

Palm Springs

Approximately 100 miles east of Los Angeles on Interstate 10 lies the **Coachella Valley,** home to the desert resort communities of Palm Springs, Rancho Mirage, Cathedral City, Palm Desert, Indio, and La Quinta. On the other (north) side of the freeway are the lesser-visited destinations of Desert Hot Springs, Yucca Valley, Morongo, Twentynine Palms, and Joshua Tree. Seen from an airplane window or hot-air balloon, these cities appear as rather artificial patches of green against a flat, arid landscape framed by mountain ridges.

If you drive into the valley from L.A., however, the first thing you'll notice are rows and rows of windmills protruding sentrylike from the hillsides. These are actually working wind turbines that generate electricity for nearly 100,000 homes.

Other desert areas may be more scenic (read: more barren), but the Coachella Valley (local population 243,250, which swells to 500,000 during the peak season from January through April) has the monopoly on recreational attractions and leisure opportunities. Just consider a few valley stats: 600 tennis courts, 16,200 hotel rooms in 130 hotels, and 111 golf courses, meaning more than one golf course per square mile in the desert resort area. Add to these numbers for tennis and golf 30,000 swimming pools, probably a zillion hot tubs (or spas), and 354 days of fun in the sunshine to the recipe, and it's a no-brainer why 3.5 million people visit the area every year. But the valley never seems crowded, even during the peak season, because things are so spread out. To see how vast the desert really is, ride the Palm Springs Aerial Tramway for a "natural high."

World famous as "America's Premier Desert Resort," Palm Springs has ranked high on everybody's Coachella Valley must-visit list since the 1930s, when the small town (current population 43,800) was a favorite playground for California's unofficial royalty—movie stars. Gone but not forgotten are Frank Sinatra and Liberace, who once had estates here. Barry Manilow, Carol Channing, Jack Jones, Suzanne Somers, Howard Keel, and Sidney Sheldon still call the desert home for at least part of the year. It doesn't take a rocket scientist to understand the valley's appeal. Average winter temperatures in the mid-seventies are enough to turn even Los Angelenos green (as in putting green) with envy. And the restaurants and resorts are truly world-class.

The *Coachella Valley Family News* (760–770–6357; www.cvfamilynews.com) is published bimonthly and is **free.** In it you'll find such features as "Now's the Time to Plan a Visit to Joshua Tree National Monument" and "Salton Sea Winter Boat Tours Planned." It's a useful source for desert happenings. Listings include such items as local hikes, museums, various valley attractions, a daily calendar, and information on family-oriented events.

When driving east from L.A. on Interstate 10, you'll know you're near Palm Springs when your kids point out the 150-foot-tall apatosaurus and 55-foot-tall *Tyrannosaurus rex,* the largest in the world. No, they didn't get lost trying to find the outlet mall and Casino Morongo down the road. They are known around these parts as the **Cabazon Dinosaurs,** and they haven't moved in years. Open 365 days a year from 9:00 A.M. to 8:00 P.M. Kids will enjoy dinosaur-related knickknacks at **Dinosaur Delights,** 50800 Seminole Drive, Cabazon; (909) 849–8309.

Windmill Tours

62950 20th Avenue North, Palm Springs; (760) 320–1365 or (877) 449–WIND. Tours between 8:00 A.M. and 4:00 P.M. Wednesday through Saturday. Summer hours may vary. $$$

Look for windmills (you can't miss them; some blades are more than 50 feet long!) and for signs on Interstate 10 at the San Gorgonio Pass, then hold onto your hats because it is very windy out here. There are more than 4,000 windmills "blowin' in the wind," generating pollution-free alternative energy. Experts tell us they provide enough energy to light up all the homes in Palm Springs. There are three 1.5-hour tours (the world's first windmill farm tours). Guests ride in twenty-one-passenger minivans escorted by well-informed guides who enjoy their work and answering kids' questions. This is a terrific and painless way to introduce children to an unusual energy source with enormous future potential.

Whitewater Trout Company

9160 Whitewater Canyon Road, Whitewater. Drive north on Indian Canyon Drive to Interstate 10, west to the Whitewater exit. Continue 5 miles to the Whitewater Canyon exit. (760) 325–5570; www.whitewatertrout.com. It sounds fishy but there are tours, by appointment, at 9:00 A.M. Wednesday through Friday.

Driving on Interstate 10, watch for the Whitewater Trout Company sign; this is the epitome of fishing for the family that loves to fish together! The $3.00 set-up fee includes admission, license, tackle, and bait. Catch any fish? If you do and want to have a fish fry, the cost is $3.28 per pound, live weight. Call in advance for picnic reservations, and they will grill the fish for you for $5.95 per fish.

Moorten Botanical Garden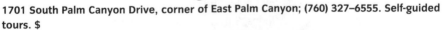

1701 South Palm Canyon Drive, corner of East Palm Canyon; (760) 327–6555. Self-guided tours. $

Kids will learn about the diversity of desert flora at the world's first "cactarium," where 3,000 varieties of cacti flourish in a natural setting. Established in 1938, this unusual botanical garden bristles with cacti in all shapes and sizes. Ask the kids to look for colorful desert flowers because there's "always something in bloom."

Palm Springs International Film Festival

1700 East Tahquitz Canyon Way, Suite 3; (760) 322–2930; fax (760) 322–4087; www.psfilm fest.org.

January 2004 heralded the fifteenth annual film festival, which has become a mecca for buyers seeking films for distribution. The festival also presents an ideal opportunity for families to screen, with the help of an excellent guide, family films. Dennis Pregnolato, executive director, says there is a nice representation of family films, such as *Anton and Anna* (Germany) and *The Great Train Robbery* (United States). Films screened here include comedy, romance, experimental, animation, period pieces, suspense, and thrillers. You're sure to find a few family flicks among the offerings.

Palm Canyon Theatre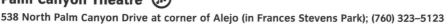

538 North Palm Canyon Drive at corner of Alejo (in Frances Stevens Park); (760) 323–5123 (box office); www.palmcanyontheatre.org. Closed in the summer.

Palm Springs's newest theater group is located in a former elementary school auditorium. Strictly family-type plays such as *Meet Me in St. Louis* and *Brigadoon* make this an ideal choice for a family matinee.

Celebrity Tours

4751 East Palm Canyon Drive, in the Rimrock Shopping Center; (760) 770–2700 (reservations required); www.celebrity-tours.com. Tour A is a narrated one-hour drive including up to forty movie stars' homes. Tour B lasts two and a half hours and adds the Walter Annenberg Estate, country clubs, and the Eisenhower Medical Center. All tours are made in air-conditioned coaches. Pickups at Palm Springs hotels and the tour office. $$

If you've been wondering how to find Elvis's honeymoon hideaway or the place where Liberace entertained, book your family on an air-conditioned coach for a guided tour of the Las Palmas district (also known as the movie colony) and other areas where history was made. Well-rehearsed guides tell all, and you won't want to miss a word of their entertaining narrative. This is far better than a self-guided tour through the quiet neighborhoods of walled villas and winding streets—and it's the only way to get the lowdown on how Hollywood established itself in the desert.

   Edward's Date Shoppe is next door to Celebrity Tours. Before or after your tour, try a deliciously rich date shake. The valley is a world-class date-growing area. Packaged assortments make zippy and inexpensive gifts the shop will ship for you.

Golf Courses

If in L.A., the celebrities are all on the beach in Malibu; in Palm Springs they're probably on the golf course. Although many clubs are private, there are several beautiful courses open to the public. Remember, a licensed driver is required for any golf cart and only two people per cart. Greens fees are substantially reduced at most desert courses in the summer.

Tahquitz Creek Golf Academy. 1885 Golf Club Drive; (760) 328–1005; www.palmer golf.com. Junior and adult clinics can be arranged. After the clinics, children can play at half the adult rate. $$

Desert Dunes Golf Club. 19300 Palm Drive, Desert Hot Springs; (760) 251–5368; www.desertdunesgolfclub.net. $$$$

Cimarron Golf Club. 67–603 30th Avenue, Cathedral City; (760) 770–6060; fax (760) 770–2876; www.cimarrongolf.com. Golfers of all ages will find the thirty-six holes at this club sheer paradise. There is a short and a long course. Inquire about golf clinics and other events. Tee times can be booked up to sixty days in advance. Check bargain twilight and standby fees as well. $$$$

The Golf Resort at Indian Wells. 44–400 Indian Wells Lane, (760) 346–GOLF; www.golf resortindianwells.com. Two Ted Robinson–designed championship courses. Rates range from $45 to $140. Tee times can be made up to seven days in advance.

Desert Willow Golf Resort. 38500 Portola Avenue, Palm Desert; (760) 346–0015; www.desertwillow.com. There is a junior golf program offered on a daily basis. Inquire about summer golf camps. $$$$

Tommy Jacob's Bel Air Greens. 1001 South El Cielo; (760) 322–6062; fax (760) 322–3126. Family-style golf during the season (January through April). Eighteen short holes on a beautiful course for adults and kids (they call it a putt-putt course). This is an all par-three layout. The nine-hole Executive Course is ideal for juniors and adults. New is the ProTour Classic Short Game School, offering lessons. Children age eighteen and younger pay $5.00 for nine holes of golf.

Tahquitz Creek Palm Springs. 1885 Golf Club Drive, Palm Springs; (760) 328–1005 or (800) 743–2211; www.tahquitzcreek.com. Here is the place to enjoy resort golf "without paying for the rest of the resort." The club has two Arnold Palmer–managed courses, Resort and Legend, both rated four star by *Golf Digest* magazine. All-inclusive golf packages feature breakfast, lunch, greens fees, cart, and more.

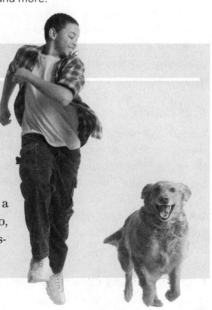

Fab **Family Golf**

If you have a budding Tiger Woods in the family or just want to practice your shot, visit the **College Golf Center of Palm Desert** at the College of the Desert, 73–450 Fred Waring Drive (760) 341–0994, open 9:00 A.M. to 10:00 P.M. A large bucket of balls is $9.00; a medium is $6.00. This is a driving range, and the manager, Dean Mayo, says kids like the junior golf clinics. Professional instruction available.

Agua **Caliente Indians**

The first people to fall under Palm Springs's spell were ancestors of the Agua
Caliente band of Cahuilla (Kaw'-we-ah) Indians, who developed communities
in the palm canyons at the foot of the San Jacinto Mountains. These canyons,
along with other chunks of the Coachella Valley, were deeded in trust to the
Indians in 1876. The Cahuillas control 42 percent of the valley, making them
the wealthiest tribe in North America. Visit www.aguacaliente.org for more
information.

Big Horn Bicycle Rental & Tours
302 North Palm Canyon Drive; (760) 325–3367.

Bike it! Big Horn Bike Adventures has a four-hour 15.5-mile round-trip tour. Visit the Indian
Canyons, bike on Palm Springs's Heritage Trail through the historic Tennis Club District,
and stop to visit Moorten Botanical Garden (see hundreds of cacti, look but don't touch!).
At Palm Canyon there is a hike, then you'll head back to town via the Heritage Trail. You'll
find Burley trailers for infants age ten months and older at Big Horn's Palm Canyon location, along with children's bikes, multiple and single speed. Ask about times and schedules, which change seasonally.

Canyon Jeep Tours' Best of the Best Tours
**15831 La Vida Drive; (760) 320–4600 or (760) 320–1365 for reservations; www.bestofthe
besttours.com. $$$$**

These are awesome adventures in open-air spacious vehicles you'll long remember. All
tours depart from the lobby of the Spa Hotel and Casino in Palm Springs at 100 North
Indian Canyon. The expedition starts at Whitewater Hill (elevation 2,500 feet) and makes
its way through the Cahuilla Canyons of Snow Creek and Chino. Then it's on to the legendary Movie Colony, once a second home to Hollywood stars, including Elvis Presley and
Jack Benny. There is a thirty-minute trek into Andreas Canyon and a drive into Palm
Canyon. Before leaving the Indian Canyons, you'll visit an authentic trading post. It's filled
with Native American souvenirs, maps, dream catchers, cassettes, and exquisite handmade turquoise jewelry. The variety of merchandise crammed into this shop is overwhelming! There is limited parking and a small menu for cold drinks. The most popular
tour, the Bonanza, which lasts from three and a half to four hours, visits the windmills,
canyons, and celebrity homes. Ask about discounts for children age twelve and younger.

Indian Canyons
**Toll-gate entrance, south end of Palm Canyon Drive; (760) 325–3400 or (800) 790–3398;
www.tahquitzcanyon.com. Open fall and winter 8:00 A.M. to 5:00 P.M., spring and summer
8:00 A.M. to 6:00 P.M. $$**

Powwows

While you're in the desert, check with the *Palm Springs' Life Desert Guide* (free and available at most hotels and restaurants) to see if there are any powwows scheduled during your visit. The entire family will find these colorful events a living-history lesson. Adding to the pageantry are the dozens of artisans selling Native American jewelry and arts and crafts. And of course, Indian fry bread is readily available.

The **Morongo Band of Indians** holds an annual powwow adjacent to the Casino Morongo that features gourd dancing, drum contests, exhibitions, and ceremonies that showcase Native American traditions. The costumes, with feathers and fabulous beading, are a sight to behold. Bird songs, a means of aesthetic expression among the Cahuilla people, are preserved and sung at this powwow.

There are other Native American events organized by the **Twentynine Palms Band of Mission Indians,** such as an intertribal powwow.

For more information on powwows, check the *Palm Springs Visitors Guide*, the official publication of Palm Springs Bureau of Tourism (760–778–8415 or 800–347–7746; www.palm-springs.org).

Revenues from admission help fill the tribe's coffers, but this cluster of oases is a priceless natural jewel. With some of the thickest concentrations of palm trees in the world, thanks to the cool mountain streams that flow through them, the site provides a refreshing refuge from the heat of the desert. There are actually four separate canyons, comprising 32,000 acres: Palm, Tahquitz, Murray, and Andreas. All have trails for walking or hiking and well-maintained recreational facilities. The unusual rock formations in Andreas Canyon are the repository of ancient Cahuilla rock art. Tours operate Monday through Thursday 10:00 A.M. to 1:00 P.M. and Friday, Saturday, and Sunday 9:00 A.M., 11:00 A.M., 1:00 P.M., and 3:00 P.M.

Smoketree Stables (ages 7 and up)

2500 Toledo Avenue; (760) 327–1372. Kids ages two to six can ride double with parent or adult. Age seven and older can ride their own horse, led by a guide. Open year-round except July and August, 8:00 A.M. to 4:00 P.M. (when days are longer, hours to 6:00 P.M.) To ride two hours, kids must be age seven or older.

In the same location for fifty years, the stables are next door to Fess Parker's former home (for the young 'uns, he played Davy Crockett). It's Coachella Valley horseback riding at its best.

The Smoke **Tree Ranch**

It's "home on the ranch" Palm Springs's style at the historic Smoke Tree Ranch. Best defined as friendly, casual, and understated, this is one of the most family perfect vacation choices in the Coachella Valley. Enjoying a history as old as Palm Springs, this approximately 400-acre ranch, home to eighty-five "colonists" (the residents, actually), is the desert's best-kept secret. Twenty acres are devoted to fifty-seven comfortable ranch cottages. Activities abound, including tennis at first-rate facilities, hiking, birding, nature trails, swimming pool, hot tub, fitness center, three-hole practice golf course, and, best of all, organized activities for kids at Camp Kawea. Adding to the vintage ambience is an old-fashioned playground.

Ranch guests savor cookouts in the nearby Indian Canyons, marshmallow roasts, cowboy crooners (remember those soothing sounds?), scavenger hunts, and even bonfires. Breakfast rides and cookouts are on the calendar of events, too. The bountiful buffets will keep the family energized, and that's what is needed to explore this pristine desert paradise. The Indian Canyons location reveals a peaceful sanctuary the entire family will find refreshing, reflective of a time when fast food and freeways were not part of our lives. Some more surprises are here: Check out Disney Hall for a collection of Disney memorabilia, since Walt Disney was one of the original colonists.

Rates start at $395 per cottage double occupancy (Full American Plan—all meals and lodging). Children ages five through eleven are $45 each in same cottage as parents. No charge for children younger than age five. Be sure to ask about multiroom cottages and family units. Outstanding venue for family groups and reunions. For additional information and reservations: 1800 South Sunrise Way; (800) 787–3922; fax (760) 327–9490; www.smoketreeranch.net.

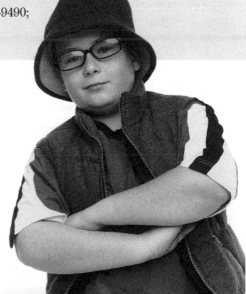

Desert Hills Premium Outlets

48400 Seminole Drive, Cabazon; (909) 849–5018; www.premiumoutlets.com.

It's not a mirage! Just twenty minutes from Palm Springs, this megamall with 130 outlet stores is worth the ride. A stellar collection of the world's leading designers offers savings of 25 to 65 percent (and even more if you're a good shopper).

Kids will love the K*B Toy Outlet, and parents will like the discounted deals at Osh Kosh. Then there is the food court, and strollers are available for a small fee. This is a good place to stop and take a walk, at the very least. Nearby is Hadley's, a bow to old California, with a small cafe serving those legendary date shakes and homemade sandwiches.

Agua Caliente Cultural Museum

219 South Palm Canyon Drive; (760) 323–0151; fax (760) 320–0350; www.accmuseum.org. Open Labor Day through Memorial Day, Wednesday through Saturday 10:00 A.M. to 5:00 P.M. and Sunday noon to 5:00 P.M. Summer hours Friday, Saturday, Sunday 10:00 A.M. to 4:00 P.M. Free.

Artifacts and historical photos from the early Cahuilla era, permanent collections on local history, changing exhibits (example, Cahuilla basketry), plus two shops with jewelry, clothing, music, and assorted Indian arts and crafts from tribes nationwide.

Palm Springs Aerial Tramway

Entrance on the north edge of town, at the end of Tramway Road, off Highway 111; (760) 325–1449 or (888) 515–TRAM; www.pstramway.com. Tram rides depart on the half hour, starting at 10:00 A.M. Monday through Friday, 8:00 A.M. weekends and holidays. Last ride off at 9:45 P.M. There are two new Swiss Rotair revolving tram cars with breath-stopping views. Schedules subject to change without notice. Please call ahead for times and weather conditions. No advance reservations. $$$

If you'd like to know where all those mountain streams come from, take a ride on the spectacular tramway, a thrilling and manageable adventure for the whole family. Two suspended cable cars whisk you from the parched desert floor up nearly 6,000 feet to the top of 10,800-foot Mount San Jacinto (Yah'-sin-toh) in a mere fifteen minutes. Up here there's not a palm tree in sight: This is pine tree country, some forty degrees cooler than the valley below.

From the Mountain Station, which has a gift shop and the Alpine Restaurant, there are breathtaking views of the sprawling valley floor and, off to the left, the unmistakable imprint of the San Andreas Fault. The station is at 8,516 feet.

Mount San Jacinto Wilderness State Park

Behind you at the top of the tramway is the 13,000-acre park, with 54 miles of hiking trails. If it's winter, chances are you'll be able to cross-country ski, too. A Nordic Ski Center, open November 15 through April 15, rents equipment for adults and kids. So you can build a snowman and, back in Palm Springs, take a swim on the same day.

Desert Adventures (ages 6 and up)

(760) 324–JEEP or (800) 440–JEEP; www.red-jeep.com. All two-hour tours leave from the office. Meet at 67-555 East Palm Canyon Drive, Suite E-106. Tours include free hotel pickup service for three- and four-hour tours only. Tours operate year-round.

Now in its sixteenth year, Desert Adventures runs a Mystery Canyon tour, which lasts four and a half hours, covering the area where *Land of the Lost* was filmed. For families, the San Andreas Fault Adventure is the most popular, hands down. For a decidedly more twenty-first-century adventure, and a perfect way for families to explore the desert, consider hopping aboard a red, seven-passenger, four-wheel-drive jeep for one of the tour offerings. The Lost Legends of the Wild West Adventure, Indian Cultural Adventures, and Mystery Canyon jeep adventures are among the tour options. Mary, the owner, says the tours are perfect "for ages six to one hundred and six." Ask about the Night Watch Stargazing Tour.

Covered Wagon Tours

(760) 347–2161; fax (760) 775–7570. Call first for directions, as schedule varies. Tour departs two hours before sunset to a palm oasis and the San Andreas Fault. Reservations required. $$$$

The pioneer-style tour (one hour and forty-five minutes) comes first, then a chuck wagon cookout dinner (barbecued beef, chicken, beans, coleslaw, garlic bread, and apple pie). You'll love the one-man "Singing Cowboy Show."

Palm Canyon **Drive**

For many families, the most enjoyable aspect of Palm Springs is taking a stroll on palm tree–lined Palm Canyon Drive, the historic center of the city. This celebrated stretch of pavement is flanked by a seemingly endless array of cafes, restaurants, boutiques, and theaters.

While you're strolling along Palm Canyon, notice the celebrity stars on the sidewalks. They include such notables as Elvis Presley, Frank Sinatra, Sophia Loren, Leslie Caron, Elizabeth Taylor, Carol Connors (remember the song "Gonna Fly Now" from *Rocky?*), Monty Hall (of *Let's Make a Deal* fame), and Pamela Price, coauthor of this book! Thank local star meister, Gerhard Frenzel, for making this star-studded sidewalk the walk and talk of the town. There seems no end to the Palm Canyon "star placing" ceremonies throughout the year. We've often encountered a ceremony going on in front of one of the stores. Of course, passersby are welcome to watch the festivities. It ain't Hollywood Boulevard, but it's still a kick.

Dollsville Dolls & Bearsville Bears

292 North Palm Canyon, just opposite the Hyatt Hotel; 760–325–2241; www.dollsville.com.

This charming shop is full of teddy bears and an astounding variety of Barbie collectibles. There are literally thousands of dolls and bears to peruse. As much a museum as a shop, it will impress parents and kids of all ages.

The Fabulous Palm Springs Follies (ages 6 and up)

At the Plaza Theatre, 128 South Palm Canyon Drive; (760) 327–0225; www.psfollies.com. Evening and matinee performances beginning in November and running through May. $$$$

A Palm Springs original. Now in its thirteenth season, this three-hour revue has a cast all older than the age of fifty. From Bill Hayes and the Four Lads to Canine Capers, they kick up a storm. This colorful, always humorous vaudeville-style program gives kids a feel for what showbiz used to be all about, despite a few harmlessly off-color jokes now and then.

Villagefest

Palm Canyon Drive, between Baristo and Amado Roads; (760) 320–3781. Open every Thursday 6:00 to 10:00 P.M. except major holidays. Free.

The street fair transforms Palm Springs's main thoroughfare into a lively bazaar with street entertainers, live bands, food booths, 150 arts and crafts vendors, a farmers' market, pony rides, and a Kidzone with inflatable characters. This is your chance to buy anything from a quilted comforter that doubles as a pillow to scrumptious fudge. If you need to park, go early. Villagefest operates rain or shine.

Consignment **Shopping**

Palm Springs is a veritable paradise for consignment-shop fans. Take the kids by the hand when perusing the infinite displays of other people's treasures. Items range from rocking horses to Roy Rogers tin lunch boxes. (Kids, ask your parents if they have any in the attic. They go for at least ten times more than what your parents paid way back when!) A retro place to start your Palm Springs consignment shopping tour of the 1950s through 1970s is **Modern Way,** at 2755 North Palm Canyon Drive (760–320–5455); **Revivals,** one of the best thrift shops in the desert, at 745 North Palm Canyon Drive; and **Panache,** at 725 North Palm Canyon Drive. Fan out from there! And don't rush. This takes time! Ample free parking in the area.

Bus **Around!**

The SunBus will take you to most of the attractions we've tried and tested, from the Desert Museum to the movies, malls, and more. Rides cost $1.00; $3.00 for a day pass for unlimited rides. Contact SunLine Transit for free personalized trip planning and information at (760) 343–3451 or (800) 347–8628; www.sunline.org.

Palm Springs Desert Museum

101 Museum Drive; (760) 325–0189; www.psmuseum.org. Open year-round except Monday and major holidays. Hours are 10:00 A.M. to 5:00 P.M. Tuesday through Saturday, noon to 5:00 P.M. Sunday. Open Thursday until 8:00 P.M., with free admission after 4:00 P.M. $$

The museum specializes in the Coachella Valley environment. It now has 20,000 more square feet with the addition of the new Steve Chase wing. One of its highlights: an anthropology collection of 39,000 artifacts, most representing the Agua Caliente band of Cahuilla Indians. There are also art exhibits. Kids will enjoy the exhibit of once live animals, with dozens of unusual reptiles and insects, plus a sculpture garden. "Jeepers Creepers" was a recent "scary" exhibit. The family programs are exceptional. Nature hikes depart Wednesday and Friday at 9:00 A.M. Five-day camp sessions are held in summer. Geared to first through eighth graders, programs include desert education and hands-on art activities.

Adjacent to the Desert Museum is the Annenberg Theater (760–325–4490) which has weekend concerts, especially during the October through April peak season. The Toor Gallery Café serves sandwiches, salads, and desserts. Hours are 11:00 A.M. to 3:00 P.M. daily.

The Village Green Heritage Center

219–223 South Palm Canyon Drive; (760) 323–8297.

The oldest structure in Palm Springs, dating from 1884, the Village Green is a compact compound of four museums. Desert pioneers are immortalized here. Museums include the McCallum Adobe (houses the Palm Springs Historical Society collection) and Miss Cornelia White's House (built in 1893 from railroad ties!). Next door is Ruddy's General Store Museum, admission 50 cents, where kids will see what a real general store looked like in the 1930s and 1940s—before the behemoth Wal-Marts and Home Depots emerged—complete with soapboxes and soup cans.

Palm Springs Air Museum

745 North Gene Autry Trail; (760) 778–6262; www.palmspringsairmuseum.org. Open year-round 10:00 A.M. to 5:00 P.M., summer hours 10:00 A.M. to 3:00 P.M. $$

While you're on the Gene Autry Trail, visit the Air Museum for a close-up look at propeller-driven aircraft from an era your kids will know only from old movies, documentaries, and (perhaps) their history books. Vintage planes, many colorful and perfectly restored, recall the World War II era. The planes are on display to educate the public about aviation's role in winning the big war. Many guides are wartime vets whose knowledge will amaze you and the kids. The second floor has flight simulators (arrange to use them in advance) and a library. The gift shop carries a treasure trove of aviation gifts, books, and jewelry.

Lucky you if you're in the desert in July, because the Air Museum celebrates Cool Kids Month! with flying model airplane contests and other hands-on activities.

Uprising Outdoor Adventure Center
1500 South Gene Autry Trail; (760) 320–6630 or (888) CLIMB–ON; www.uprising.com.

Anyone can do it! Try rock climbing at this exciting facility. Beginner lessons for age six and older. Shaded, micro-cooled, and open year-round. Family rates are 10 percent off with three or more participants. $$$

Knott's Soak **City Water Park**

1500 South Gene Autry Trail, Palm Springs; (760) 327–0499; www.soakcity usa.com. Museums, movie stars, and "date shakes at Hadley's" aside, here's why kids flock to Palm Springs. The park is an immaculately clean twenty-one-acre fantasy playground where cool water reigns supreme. There is amusement for kids of all ages, from Squirt City and the tranquil Whitewater River inner-tube ride to more than eighteen other waterslides ranging from simple to simply outrageous. The Black Widow slide is a case in point. Those who dare coast in inner tubes along a 54-inch-wide, 450-foot-long slide that at certain points takes riders through total darkness and down a 50-foot drop—yikes! Plus there is stand-up surfing and body boarding. The three-man inner-tube ride is fast and furious!

The most surprising attraction—and arguably the most fun—is California's largest wave-action pool (800,000 gallons), a broad expanse of water that starts out calm but churns away every fifteen minutes to become a sort of Malibu-in-the-desert. Actually, giant fans create the artificial tide, but it feels like the genuine article. If your children are real water bugs, it might be hard to pry them away from this park at day's end.

Open daily mid-March through Labor Day and weekends only through October. $$$. Children younger than age three free.

Where to Eat

Manhattan in the Desert, 2665 East Palm Canyon, Palm Springs; (760) 322–DELI. Open Sunday through Thursday from 7:00 A.M. to 9:00 P.M. and Friday and Saturday until 10:00 P.M. **Free** parking. Opened in October 2004, the desert's newest deli restaurant has as much panache as a Paris bistro. The upbeat, albeit noisy ambience is pure deli-lightful, and there is something on the 12-page menu for everyone including light eaters. There are marvelous soups from cold borscht to sweet and sour cabbage, and a terrific home-style chicken soup (with choice of rice, noodles or matzo ball). Try Super Combo Number 12—brisket, pastrami, and jack cheese served on an onion roll with lettuce and tomato. The "Just for Kids" menu (age ten and under) features a $5.95 lunch special with a choice of tuna, egg salad, or grilled cheese sandwich or hamburger, hot dog, or chicken strips; french fries or applesauce; milk or fountain drink; and a yummy sprinkle cookie. With fair prices and friendly service, this Manhattan-style deli is worth a visit.

Ruby's Diner, 155A South Palm Canyon Drive; (760) 416–0138; www.rubys.com. One of a chain (also in Rancho Mirage). Breakfast, lunch, and dinner daily with very reasonable prices and fast service. Re-creates the diner era of the 1950s with deluxe malts, shakes, blue-ribbon burgers, fries, and breakfast served until 11:30 A.M. Dee-lish! $

Simba's Ribhouse, 190 North Sunrise Way; (760) 778–7630; fax (760) 322–1985. Closed July through October. Closed Monday. You'll find Simba in the kitchen cooking up her homemade specialties. Dinner means southern fried chicken, tender sliced turkey, corn bread, mashed potatoes, macaroni and cheese, and a lavish salad and fruit bar. Then there could just be chicken enchiladas, seafood pasta, yams, and catfish—all are Simba's pride and joy! $

Top of the Tram Restaurant, (760) 325–1391. The closest you'll come to being in Switzerland without leaving Palm Springs. Cafeteria-style lunch served from 11:00 A.M. Winter specialties include prime rib; summer brings barbecue beef, pork ribs, or chicken and vegetarian lasagna and roasted turkey. Kids will love the world's largest rotating tram car as it silently speeds to the 13,000-acre San Jacinto State Park, taking you from the palms to the pines. Upon arriving, view the film *Building on a Dream,* which explains how this daunting tram ride came about. This aerie is also the gateway to 54 miles of hiking trails. For camping information, call (909) 659–2067. Remember, no pets allowed in this sky-high paradise. $$

Tyler's, 149 South Indian Canyon Drive; (760) 325–2990. Open Monday through Saturday 11:00 A.M. to 4:00 P.M. Lunch only. This tiny hamburger haven was once a bus station and then an A & W root beer stand. It reopened as Tyler's, serving, as far as this coauthor is concerned, the best hamburgers in town. The half-pound burger is $4.50 and worth every cent.

Kids will like the sliders, three mini hamburgers that can be decorated with hot sauce, pickles, grilled onions, and ketchup. The menu is small, but the essentials are there, from chili dogs and egg salad sandwiches to homemade potato salad and coleslaw. Before noon every bar stool along the counter is taken with serious foodies. The root beer floats ($2.50) are divine, and the fresh lemonade ($1.50) is like grandma used to make.

During winter, Diana, the proprietor, prepares soups you dream about, from red pepper to fresh mushroom. On Friday, ask for the clam chowder. There is a small patio in the back, but it's advisable to arrive early because this landmark beacon of comfort food, par excellence, fills up fast. You might try the take-out service if there is a long wait. And be sure to tell Diana, a whirlwind, that Pam sent you.

Where to Stay

Casa Cody, A Country Bed & Breakfast Inn, 175 South Cahuilla Road; (760) 320–9346 or (800) 231–2639; www.casa cody.com. Historic and charming, this twenty-three-room inn reflects all that made this desert destination resort a living legend. Founded in the 1920s by Harriet Cody, cousin of Buffalo Bill, accommodations are in early California–style adobe bungalows framed by bougainvillea and citrus-filled courtyards. The 1910 adobe, recently restored, was the getaway of Lawrence Tibbett, the bon vivant Metropolitan baritone turned movie star, and his good friend Charlie Chaplin. Children and pets always welcome here.

Desert Hotel Reservations, (800) 896–7334; www.deserthotelreservations .com. Local agency in business since 1988, providing personal service. One of the largest sources of hotel accommodations in the Palm Springs area. You pay no fee and get the rooms and rates you want. Highly recommended. $$$$

Palm Springs Riviera Resort, 1600 North Indian Canyon Drive; (760) 327–8311 or (800) 444–8311; fax (760) 325–8572; www.psriviera.com. On acres of classic desert gardens, eight low-rise buildings house 476 spacious, newly remodeled rooms and suites (many connecting). Kids seventeen and younger stay **free** in parents' room. Choose from three swimming pools including a small kiddie pool, east family pool, and the largest pool in Palm Springs. (Newcomer singer Destiny's Child was discovered here. Elvis and Sinatra frequented in their day as well.) Eighteen-hole putting course, basketball court, and sand volleyball court are **free** for guests. Nine tennis courts, lessons, and rentals at an additional charge. Kids' menu featured in The Grill, poolside, and Starbucks Espresso Café. $$$

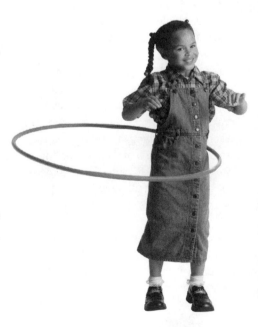

Cathedral City and Rancho Mirage

The desert communities of Cathedral City and Rancho Mirage are small in population (42,000 and 14,965, respectively) but are host to many golf courses and resort communities, even more than in Palm Springs proper. Again, don't make the mistake of thinking all those emerald green courses are for members only. Many are open to the public and/or have reciprocal arrangements with specific hotels. Rancho Mirage is known as the "Realm of the Desert Big Horn" and covers almost 25 square miles.

Cathedral **City**

Once a sleepy, nondescript community on the way to somewhere else, Cathedral City now offers many reasons to stop and spend a day. Ever imagined visiting Yankee Stadium, Fenway Park, and Wrigley Field all in one day? It's possible at the thirty-acre **Big League Dreams Sports Park,** 33–770 Date Palm Drive; (760) 324–1133 or (760) 324–5600; fax (760) 770–6541; www.bigleaguedreams.com. Sports enthusiasts will go for the batting cage stations and sand volleyball courts. This is the nation's first amateur sports facility of its kind and merits at least a two-hour visit. There's a "Tot Lot" for the younger set.

And while you're in the neighborhood, try **Applebee's Neighborhood Grill & Bar,** 32400 Date Palm Drive; (760) 324–6911. Just a minute's drive from the Sports Park, this family-style restaurant has a kids' menu with all entrees under $3.99. All kids' meals come with a choice of soft drink, HiC fruit punch, or milk. The restaurant has a fascinating photograph exhibit of local history including Amelia Earhart's visit to Indio, plus memorabilia from local teams and sporting events.

The big news in Cathedral City is the big screen. "Learning at the Edge of your Seat" is what kids love at the **Desert IMAX theater;** the screen is 50 by 70 feet—that's six stories high! Show times are subject to change, so call the information line first at (760) 324–7333; www.desertimax.com. Free parking at the Cathedral City Civic Center. The theater is on the corner at 68–510 East Palm Canyon Drive at Cathedral Canyon Boulevard.

Children's Discovery Museum of the Desert

71–701 Gerald Ford Drive, Rancho Mirage; (760) 321–0602; www.cdmod.org. Open 10:00 A.M. to 5:00 P.M. Tuesday through Saturday, noon to 5:00 P.M. Sunday. $$

This 8,000-square-foot facility with more than fifty hands-on exhibits encourages kids to touch, explore, and discover. Youngsters can paint a Volkswagen Beetle, dig for Cahuilla Indian treasures, or make a pretend pizza in the Pizza Place. An ideal museum for children and parents who enjoy experiencing hands-on activities. Upstairs there are trunks and suitcases, costumes, and hats. Kids can dress up; this is a good photo opportunity!

Boomer's Family Fun Center

67–700 East Palm Canyon Drive, Cathedral City; (760) 321–9893. Open 365 days a year; Monday through Thursday 11:00 A.M. to 10:00 P.M. (extended hours during the summer and on holidays), Friday 11:00 A.M. to midnight, Saturday 10:00 A.M. to midnight, and Sunday 10:00 A.M. to 10:00 P.M. Admission **free,** but inside fun is pay-as-you-play, with varying ticket prices for combinations. $$$

For some decidedly nonprofessional-level golf action, take the tykes to the home of three fun eighteen-hole miniature golf courses. There are also bumper boats, go-karts, batting cages, a 10,000-square-foot games pavilion, 200 video and sports games, and a rock wall.

The River

71–800 Highway 111, corner of Bob Hope, Rancho Mirage; (760) 779–5664.

For dining, strolling, movies, book browsing, or a scoop of ice cream, this desert mirage is the place to visit. For the best family dining in this 200,000-square-foot complex, check out The Yard House, Johnny Rocket's, Ben & Jerry's, and the newly opened Cheese Cake Factory.

Finding **the Fault**

You've heard about it on the radio, you've seen it on television and probably the Internet—the infamous **San Andreas Fault.** Now there is a four-hour Earth in Motion tour designed by Jurassic Expeditions, taking visitors by bus to the world's most famous earthquake fault. This is "edu"-tainment and soft adventure at their best. The motor-coach tour is produced and directed by Charles Watson, creator of "Seismo-Watch," a column read by millions weekly. The big Cardiff bus leaves from various pick-up points. Call (760) 862–5540 for reservations; www.jurassicexpeditions.com.

Where to Stay

Westin Mission Hills Resort, the corner of Dinah Shore and Bob Hope Drive; (760) 328–5955 or (800) 544–0287; www.westin .com. The Cactus Kids Club program designed for children ages four to twelve offers a good mix of arts, crafts, nature walks, games, and swimming. Hours are daily 8:00 A.M. to noon and 1:00 to 5:00 P.M. There are rental bikes and in all guest rooms, the Sony Playstation. Kids love the 60-foot, S-curved waterslide, basketball, softball, and bicycle rentals. Then there are two golf courses and tennis courts. Inquire about the Summer Magic Getaway Package.

For More Information

Palm Springs Bureau of Tourism. 777 North Palm Canyon Drive, Suite 201, 92262; (760) 778–8415; fax (760) 323–3021; www.palm-springs.org. Open Monday through Friday from 8:30 A.M. to 5:00 P.M. Publishes the *Palm Springs Visitors Guide,* which highlights the wide variety of dining, attractions, shopping, art galleries, events, and lodging establish-ments in the city. This guide is updated twice a year to reflect the latest information for many of the listed establishments.

Palm Springs Chamber of Commerce. 190 West Amado Road, 92262; (760) 325–1577; www.pschamber.org.

Palm Springs Desert Resorts Convention and Visitors Authority. (760) 770–9000 or (800) 41–RELAX; fax (760) 770–9001; www.palmspringsusa.com. Open 8:30 A.M. to 5:30 P.M. Monday through Friday. Ask for an updated vacation planner. The bureau has the latest information on all the desert resort communities: Palm Springs, Cathedral City, Rancho Mirage, Palm Desert, La Quinta, Indian Wells, Indio, and Desert Hot Springs.

Palm Springs Visitor Information and Reservation Center (operated by the Palm Springs Bureau of Tourism). 2901 North Palm Canyon Drive, 92262; (760) 778–8418 or (800) 347–7746. Open daily 9:00 A.M. to 5:00 P.M. for one-stop lodging and information services.

Palm Desert

In recent years Palm Desert, "where the sun shines a little brighter," has been something of a boomtown, with shopping and dining opportunities to rival—some would say surpass—those of Palm Springs. Palm Desert helps make the Coachella Valley the "golf capital of the world," not only on account of the many courses it boasts, but because golf carts are legal transportation on several city streets. There's even a **Golf Cart Parade** every November, in which a hundred carts decorated as floats parade along El Paseo, the "Rodeo Drive of the Desert."

Palm Desert is home to one of the most interesting street fairs in Southern California. Look for the College of the Desert Street Fair, 435 Monterey Avenue in Palm Desert— there's plenty of **free** parking. Kids will love wandering through the farmers' market and checking out the endless vendors selling original art, jewelry, T-shirts, designer eyeglass frames, and faux designer purses. You name it . . . it's for sale here somewhere. Open Saturday and Sunday year-round. Don't miss it! And now, we will go from simple to "simply elegant" shopping, from the street fair to El Paseo.

The undisputed style center of the desert is a few blocks away on **El Paseo,** a 7-block drive between Highway 74 and Portola Avenue.

While strolling on El Paseo, stop at the **Daily Grill,** 73–061 El Paseo (on the corner); (760) 779–9911; www.dailygrill.com; open 11:00 A.M. to 10:00 P.M. Monday through Saturday and 10:00 A.M. (for brunch) to 10:00 P.M. Sunday. There's something for everyone, from a delicious cobb salad to a hearty serving of meat loaf and mashed potatoes. The children's menu has the usual—hamburgers, grilled cheese, and chicken fingers. Wash it down with a giant glass of fresh lemonade. At the **Gardens on El Paseo** (between San Pablo and Larkspur), sample a taste of the Caribbean at **Tommy Bahamas,** 73595 El Paseo (upstairs); (760) 836–0188. The conch fritters are truly a taste from the islands. Downstairs is a boutique with shirts in wild designs—chic but expensive.

If the adults want to slip away for a few hours, there is **Sullivans Steakhouse,** 73505 El Paseo, also on the upper level with a delightful eight-ounce petite filet mignon for $22.99. The meal includes the best lettuce wedge (with diced tomatoes) in the desert. Reservations are essential. Call (760) 341–3560. If you take the kids, my advice is to go early, around 6:00 P.M. The noise level is a challenge even for kids!

Tri-A-Bike 🚲
44841 San Pablo Avenue; (760) 340–2840.

Tri-A-Bike is the oldest bike rental company west of the Mississippi. You'll find mountain and road experts here able to answer your questions about exploring the desert terrain. Tri-A-Bike rents assorted bikes (including mountain, road, tandem, and kids') for rates starting at $19.00 a day (based on twenty-four hours) and $9.00 (and up) an hour for mountain or road bikes (be sure to ask about special family packages). Kids' (age four and older) bikes rent for $4.00 an hour, $16.00 daily. Kids too young to ride? Tri-A-Bike has a trailer to pull the little ones. Along with that comes **free** delivery and pickup of bicycles

Path of the **Big Horn**

Kids, be on the lookout for a posse of creatively decorated bighorn sheep wandering around the Coachella Valley. This is actually a public art project exhibiting more than one hundred painted, life-size sculptures of these legendary sheep—all placed in locations around the desert for public viewing. Celebrities (Cher, Chevy Chase, Phyllis Diller, and Stephanie Powers) decorated many of these sheep sculptures. This is an on-going project to learn about taking responsibility for the environment. Visit www.pathofthe bighorn.com.

Santa Rosa and San Jacinto Mountains
National Monument

Be sure to visit the **Santa Rosa Mountains National Scenic Area Visitor Center,** 51–500 Highway 784 (3.25 miles south on Highway 111 at the base of the mountain). The **Friends of the Desert Mountains Bookstore** at the visitor center (760–862–9084), stocks hiking and nature guides, giving you a fuller picture of what to expect in this rugged corner of Southern California. This area is under the stewardship of the Bureau of Land Management (760–862–9984). Open Friday through Monday 9:00 A.M. to 4:00 P.M. (except federal holidays). Walk along the Native Plant Garden Interpretive Trail and try the interactive exhibits dealing with natural and cultural resources of the Coachella Valley and surrounding mountain before you embark on exploring this area.

(depending on rental agreement and area), a lock, a helmet, and a map of the Coachella Valley Bikeway. This segmented route stretches from Desert Hot Springs all the way to the Salton Sea. The 4-mile-long Morning Side Loop passes by the Morningside and Springs Country Clubs.

Living Desert Zoo and Gardens

47–900 Portola Avenue; (760) 346–5694; www.livingdesert.org. Open daily year-round. $$

This 1,200-acre preserve lets parents and kids have a close-up look at everything from a desert cactus to a bobcat. Common desert inhabitants roam freely in addition to the world's smallest fox, bighorn sheep, gazelles, tortoises, and zebras. Although much of the desert fauna is nocturnal (cooler temperatures bring out the animals), you will surely encounter some of it, especially if you take a hike on one of the several trails on the premises. The family will enjoy the live animal shows daily in the outdoor Tennity Amphitheater. One favorite: the Critter Close-Up, a daily event that permits kids to see small desert animals. The newest exhibit is Gecko Gulch Play Land. At the Village Watutu, kids can get up close with camels, hyenas, birds, and a petting kraal. Stop for a cool drink at the Thorn Tree Grill and peruse the souvenirs at the Kumba Kumba Market.

Westfield Shopping Town

72–840 Highway 111; (760) 341–7979; www.westfield.com.

The largest mall in the Coachella Valley. The fully air-conditioned shopping center has more than one hundred stores and eateries, including a Resort Ten, for the latest films, and Charlotte Russe, an upscale young people's store. Look for family-friendly specialty shops such as the Disney Store.

McCallum Theatre 🎵

Bob Hope Cultural Center, 73000 Fred Waring Drive; (760) 340–ARTS; www.mccallum theatre.com.

For the culturally inclined, the popular McCallum features theatrical, dance, classical, and celebrity events such as Broadway on Ice and the Emmet Kelly Jr. Circus.

Sky Watcher Star Gazing Tours

73-091 Country Club Drive, Suite A 42; (760) 831–0231; www.sky-watcher.com.

If the kids insist upon staying up late at night, consider Sky Watcher Tours as the solution. A sky guide leads a tour of the heavens using high-powered telescopes and sky binoculars. It's mythology mixed with astronomy and a stellar story kids will enjoy.

Lake **Cahuilla**

Riverside County Park, 58075 Jefferson Street, La Quinta, offers day use, a swimming pool ($1.00 daily), camping, and fishing. A fishing license isn't required but fish stocking fees are charged. The sunsets on Lake Cahuilla are gorgeous, and there is plenty of space for kids to run around. A perfect break if you want to pause from driving and just relax. Lake Cahuilla now has genuine camel rides January through Memorial Day!

Where to Eat

Bananaz Grill, 72–291 Highway 111; (760) 776–4333. American-California casual dining for lunch and dinner. Located on "restaurant row." Easy to find and easy on your pocketbook. $$

Cosmos Italian Kitchen, 73–155 Highway 111; (760) 674–3431; www.cosmos.com. For reasonable prices and homemade Italian standbys, from spaghetti and meatballs to pizza, this is the best choice. Large booths and tables are served by a friendly waitstaff. The desert is rife with expensive pasta places, but why outspend yourself for lunch or dinner when you can dine on hearty portions at half the prices charged by nearby restaurants. Mama Mia! Try Cosmos' and you'll see what we mean when that giant pepperoni, mushroom, and tomato pizza hits your table. Children's menu with no entree costing more than $4.00.

Where to Stay

Desert Springs, A JW Marriott Resort & Spa, 74855 Country Club Drive; (760) 341–2211 or (800) 331–3112; www .marriott.com. Among the many lodging options available in the Palm Desert area, this one stands out above the rest. As you enter this immense resort, you will be surrounded by the sounds of water flowing and birds calling. Marriott's preferred mode of transport? Gondolas, Venetian style. While some find this a bit Disneyland-esque, people still flock here for the dramatic ambience of this 884-room mega-resort. A full-service spa, shopping colonnade, and two eighteen-hole golf courses mean there is something to please every member of the family.

This sprawling resort is home to the Kid's Klub, where kids can spend quality time pursuing their own recreational activities while Mom and Dad are on the golf course or in the spa. Designed for ages four to twelve (kids younger than age four require a babysitter, available through the concierge), the program operates seven days a week and features arts and crafts, putt-putt golf, boat rides, animal tours, lunch, and films such as *James and the Giant Peach*. Non-resort guests can also use the facility. Night Parties take place on holiday weekends between 6:30 and 10:00 P.M. The charge is $60 per child. There are different themes, such as a cooking party where kids make their own pizzas and desserts and a beach party, with sandcastle building and limbo contests, and play group games such as beach volleyball. Kids are served hot dogs, hamburgers, and fries. $$$$

La Quinta Resort & Club, 49499 Eisenhower Drive; (760) 564–4111 or (800) 598–3828; www.laquintaresort.com. La Quinta is the ideal resort for families, with something for everyone. Parents can enjoy golf, a full-service spa, and spacious casitas and grounds. Children will like Camp La Quinta from 9:00 A.M. to 3:00 P.M. seven days a week. Programs include nature walks, arts and crafts, and miniature golf. Evening programs are from 6:00 to 10:00 P.M. Friday and Saturday only, and the charge is $35 per program per child. Up to two children stay **free** in a casita with parents. $$$$

The Renaissance Esmeralda Resort and Spa. 44400 Indian Wells Lane, Indian Wells; (760) 773–4444 or (800) 228–9290; www.renaissancehotels.com. At the Esmeralda, there is all a family could ask for, including a "sand" beach, three swimming pools, lots of space to spread out, and family-friendly rates. Up to five guests are allowed in each spacious room. Here is the place to kick back and relax; Dad can try the links and Mom can indulge in the stunning new Spa Esmeralda. Or, if there's a babysitter on hand, parents can have a "couples" treatment in one of the private suites. Farmaesthetics fine herbal skincare preparations and June Jacobs products are used here.

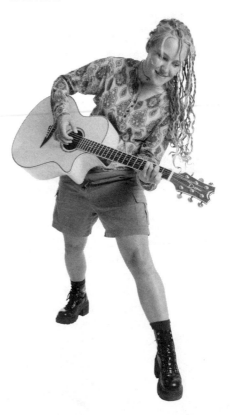

Ace, Deuce, **Forty Love**

The **Indian Wells Tennis Garden** is a $75 million state-of-the-art facility that opened in March 2000 and is the home of the premier ATP Masters Series event, the Pacific Life Open. Including the second-largest tennis stadium in the world, with 16,100 seats, the Indian Wells Tennis Garden operates a full-service tennis club that features eleven sunken championship courts, six practice and clinic courts, and two clay courts. Year-round programs include adult and junior clinics, tournaments, and lessons. USTA and collegiate events are also hosted. Families who love tennis must check out this facility. In addition to world-class tennis, the venue has hosted the world's best entertainers, such as the Boston Pops, Mariachi USA, and Luciano Pavarotti, as well as other festivals and special events, such as the Indian Wells Art Festival each spring. For more information, schedules and times, contact the office at 78–200 Miles Avenue (between Highway 111 and Fred Waring Drive), Indian Wells; (760) 200–8200; www.iwtg.net.

Indio

The first city in the Coachella Valley, Indio—also known as the Date Capital of the Desert—was founded in 1930. Fully 95 percent of the dates grown in the United States are cultivated in and around Indio.

This is truly the "city of festivals," beginning with the **National Date Festival,** which was founded here more than fifty years ago. Indio looks rather plain until you drive by the fairgrounds and glimpse the exotic entrance, which comes alive each February for the National Date Festival. The multicolored plaster domes, reminiscent of a scene from *Arabian Nights,* are sure to make your kids wonder if they have just seen Disneyland. But there's more on this stretch of highway!

Empire Polo Club and Equestrian Park

81–800 Avenue 51 (at Monroe); (760) 342–2762. Open 9:00 A.M. to 5:00 P.M. Monday through Friday. For a polo schedule call (760) 342–2223; www.empirepoloevents.org.

Indio is paradise for polo lovers. If you want to see polo in action, plan to have breakfast or lunch at the Empire Polo Club's Polo Grille Restaurant. This former horse shelter turned restaurant is open seven days a week from 7:00 A.M. to 9:00 P.M. Off the beaten path at Avenue 51 and Monroe, the setting is peaceful and a far cry from the weekend crowds and traffic. There is a great children's menu with burgers, hot dogs, and mac and cheese.

The park covers 175 acres of landscaped grounds, including five world-class polo fields, a picturesque rose garden, and the tropical Medjhool Lake (named for the delectable dates that grow on the Indio date farms).

Riverside County Fair and National Date Festival

Riverside County Fairground, 46–350 Arabia Street, Indio; (800) 811–FAIR; www.datefest .org. $$

For ten days each February, Indio celebrates its principal crop—the tasty, versatile date. The festival is held in conjunction with the annual Riverside County Fair. The festive ambience attracts families for rides, food, games, local entertainment, and camel rides. Don't miss the Arabian Nights Musical Pageant each evening.

Oasis Date Gardens

59–111 Highway 111, Thermal; (760) 399–5665; www.oasisdategardens.com. Open 8:00 A.M. to 5:30 P.M. daily.

This is a 250-acre working date farm, where you can take a guided tour of the groves, have a picnic in a palm garden, or simply partake of the offerings at the Country Store. There are always **free** samples available (ask for a **free** date shake). If you like dried fruits and nuts, this is the place to stock up.

Salton Sea

If you're heading south from Indio, explore the 35-mile-long Salton Sea, the largest body of water entirely in California and saltier than the ocean. A haven for bird life, it is part of the vast (36,527-acre) **Salton Sea National Wildlife Refuge and Imperial Wildlife Area** (760–393–3052). In the **Salton Sea State Recreation Area,** boating and saltwater fishing are the order of the day. Several campsites and nature trails are located around the "sea" shores.

Ship of the **Desert**

None other than a Palm Springs camel can take you on a desert tour. Operating seasonally in March through June and October and November, weather permitting, this expedition departs from the Oasis Date Gardens, 59–111 Highway 111, in Thermal (about 45 minutes from Palm Springs). Children must be six years old and ride on the same camel as the adult. A one-hour ride is $75. Call (760) 399–5665 or (909) 926–1194 for information, or visit www.movie landanimals.com. Have a nutritious and delicious date shake while you're waiting for the camel to pick you up!

Joshua Tree National Park and Chiriaco Summit

Joshua Tree National Park, 74485 National Park Drive (park headquarters), Twentynine Palms, 92277-3597; visitor information line (760) 367–5500; fax (760) 367–6392; www.nps.gov/jotr. Open year-round. Each season adds its personality to the desert's character. Three entrances to the park—Oasis Visitor Center, open all year 8:00 A.M. to 5:00 P.M.; Cottonwood Visitor Center, open all year 8:00 A.M. to 4:00 P.M.; and Black Rock Nature Center, open October through May, Saturday through Thursday 8:00 A.M. to 4:00 P.M. and Friday noon to 8:00 P.M.

The Joshua Tree National Park charges a $10 fee per car entering the park and allows unlimited entry and exits for seven days. Persons with a Joshua Tree National Park card or a Golden Eagle Pass can enter the park without paying the fee. The JTNP card is $25 per year and is only valid at this park. The Golden Eagle Pass is $50 per year and is valid at all U.S. national parks.

Joshua Tree National Park lies 140 miles east of Los Angeles and less than an hour north of Palm Springs. You can approach it from the west via Interstate 10 and Highway 62 (Twentynine Palms Highway). The north entrances to the park are located at Joshua Tree Village and the city of Twentynine Palms. The south entrance at Cottonwood Spring, which lies 25 miles east of Indio, can be approached from the east or west, also via Interstate 10. Motels, stores, restaurants, and auto services are located in the nearby towns of Yucca Valley, Joshua Tree Village, and Twentynine Palms.

Visitor centers and wayside exhibits, providing opportunities to acquaint you with park resources, are located along main roads leading into and through the park. Park rangers are here to help you have an enjoyable, safe visit. Detailed information on

Gublers **Orchids**

If anyone in the family is fascinated by orchids, by all means stop by **Gublers Orchids,** 2200 Belfield Boulevard, Landers, 92285; (760) 364–2282, fax (760) 364–2285; www.gublers.com. You'll find it "off the map" when traveling on Highway 62 toward Joshua Tree National Park. This state-of-the-art orchid farm is in the middle of nowhere, it seems. However, once you see the gorgeous display of orchids, marvel at the climate-controlled greenhouses and the solar greenhouses, and peruse the bromeliads, ferns, and yes, even carnivorous plants, you'll be glad you went out of your way. Free tours Monday through Saturday 10:00 A.M. to 4:00 P.M. Closed Sunday and major holidays.

Joshua Tree **Park Center**

Visit Park Center, 6554 Park Boulevard, Joshua Tree (take Interstate 10 to Highway 62, turn right at Park Boulevard in Joshua Tree) at the west entrance to the national park. Open 9:00 A.M. to 5:00 P.M. Sunday through Thursday and 8:00 A.M. to 8:00 P.M. Friday and Saturday. The Park Center is forty-five minutes from Palm Springs, two and a half hours from Los Angeles and San Diego. Stop here to purchase maps, books, souvenirs, handcrafted gifts, and fine art. You can also visit a sculpture garden. The cafe opens at 6:00 A.M. and sells freshly prepared sandwiches and pastries. This privately owned business is dedicated to helping your family enjoy Joshua Tree National Park. Call (760) 366–3488 or visit www.joshuatreeparkcenter.com.

weather, road conditions, backcountry use, campgrounds, and regulations may be obtained at visitor centers and entrance stations. Walks, hikes, and campfire talks are conducted chiefly in the spring and fall; information is posted on campground bulletin boards, at ranger stations, and at visitor centers. Ranger-conducted activities can increase your enjoyment and understanding of the park.

There are nine campgrounds with tables, fireplaces, and toilets. You must bring your own water and firewood. Several picnic areas for day use are available. Ask about the Junior Ranger Program.

Even if your kids have never been to Joshua Tree National Park before, they will probably recognize the short, bristly, and oddly contorted trees that thrive here from the cover of the popular U2 album *The Joshua Tree*. It was actually Mormon settlers who named the trees. They thought their thick branches, which protrude toward the sky, resembled the biblical Joshua praying.

Less than an hour's drive north of the Coachella Valley, and worth at least a half-day detour, Joshua Tree is where the southern Colorado Desert (elevation less than 3,000 feet) meets the vast expanse of the Mojave (high desert). The park, formerly a national monument, covers 794,000 acres and in some places affords unobstructed views of more than 50 miles. The highlight for many kids will be scrambling about the lower portions of giant quartz-monzonite boulders and monoliths in the Mojave Desert portion of the park.

Try to schedule your visit to Joshua Tree around a sunset. The photographic opportunities here are unparalleled, especially when the shadows dance on the colossal rock formations and the cholla cacti and Joshuas seem to glow in the fading sunlight. The whole place has the feel of a rather eerie lunar landscape, a boundless place in which to take time out and wonder. It's not a geographical experience anyone in your family will soon forget.

Music in **Joshua Tree**

The California high desert is known for nurturing budding talent—such as groundbreaker Gram Parsons, folk-rock-guru Donovan, and English blues legend Eric Burdon. Irish rockers U2 found inspiration here in the 1980s (remember their hit album *Joshua Tree?*).

The annual **Chuckwalla Fest: Two Days of Music and Art in the High Desert** is held every spring in Joshua Tree on the grounds of Mentalphysics. More than fifty locally based bands and performing and visual artists will converge to support arts education in the Morongo Basin. High Desert Living Arts Center (HDLAC) produces the event as its largest fund-raiser. The all-weekend, all-ages event is accessible at only $5.00 per entry. Besides the great music on two stages, the festival features "Camp Chuckwalla" for the younger participants, complete with bouncing castle and **free** arts and crafts activities during the day. Arts fair and a variety of food and other vendors will round out the event. The event was held May 1–May 2, 2004. For current information, visit www.chuckwallafest.com.

The privately owned Joshua Tree Lake Campground (located 9 miles from the park entrance) is soul central for the emerging **Joshua Tree Music Festival.** On-site are two performance stages featuring world music, funk, soul, jazz, and blues, plus a world market, tasty food village, and kidzville—eco-education with Joshua Tree Tortoise Rescue, stargazing, arts and crafts, open mike, storytelling, face painting, juggling, playground, volleyball, bubbles, puppets, and nature walks and talks. Families are encouraged to camp for the entire three-day event. There are hot showers, tent sites, picnic tables, barbeque pits, a lake for fishing, and ample parking. One adult three-day music and camping pass is $75. Children age ten and younger are admitted **free!** In 2004 the festival was held May 7 through May 9. For current information, visit www.joshuatreemusicfestival.com.

General Patton Memorial Museum

#2 Chiriaco Road, Chiriaco Summit; (760) 227–3483; www.ca.blm.gov/needles/patton.html. Open daily 9:30 A.M. to 4:30 P.M. Children younger than age twelve admitted free. $

Thirty miles east of Indio and 70 miles from the Arizona state line on Interstate 10 is a museum not to be missed. Exit at Chiriaco Summit and look for the American flag. You are at what was once the entrance to Camp Young, the famous Desert Training Center. This is the site chosen by Maj. Gen. George Smith Patton Jr. in March 1942 as a training center for desert warfare. Nearly one million American servicemen and -women trained here. Patton commanded the camps for four months, departing in August 1942 to lead Operation Torch, the allied assault on German-held North Africa. The camp closed on April 30, 1944. The museum has an excellent twenty-six-minute video, plus exhibits. Many of the artifacts were donated by servicemen and -women. There are armored tanks on display, along with memorials and a small outdoor chapel.

Next to the General Patton Memorial Museum is the Chiriaco Summit Travel Center, (760) 227–3227, owned by the Chiriaco family. There is a U.S. Post Office here and a service station, as well as a Fosters Freeze fast food and the largest minimart in Riverside County. Enjoy the gift shop with antiques. Plus, there's a selection of fresh fruits, nuts, and desert dates.

The General Patton Museum was established through the tireless efforts of Margit Chiriaco Rusche and the Bureau of Land Management. Margit recalls seeing the tanks from her front yard as a five-year-old, when the Desert Training Center was in full swing. Be sure to have breakfast, lunch, or dinner at the charming coffee shop, where comfortable booths have looked out on the desert since 1933. Margit bakes the best chocolate cake, slathered with chocolate frosting and walnuts, for miles! On the menu is the DTC (Desert Training Center) burger, made with Spam (kids, ask your grandparents about that!). There are also corn dogs with chips and lots of sandwiches kids will enjoy. The Traveler's Special breakfast costs $4.50, and that includes two each of pancakes, eggs, sausage patties, and bacon. It's worth driving out to Chiriaco Summit for this breakfast bargain! On the weekend, enjoy the *carne asada* and on Wednesday don't miss Grandma Ruth's pot roast—a family recipe.

Twentynine Palms

Located between Interstates 15 and 10 on State Highway 62, 57 miles east of Palm Springs and incorporated in 1987, the city of Twentynine Palms encompasses 53.75 square miles (larger than the city of San Francisco) and has grown from a population of 11,000 to more than 28,000 today. Twentynine Palms hosts the headquarters offices of Joshua Tree National Park as well as the **Marine Corps Air Ground Combat Center** (www.29palms.usmc.mil). Since the 1950s the Combat Center has grown from a few buildings, a glider runway, and about 120 Marines to more than 19,000 Marines, sailors, family members, and civilian workers, the largest and fastest-growing base in the Marine Corps.

Twentynine Palms has pristine air, beautiful natural surroundings, and a small-town family lifestyle your family will enjoy visiting. Highlights include Oasis of Murals (www.oasisofmurals.com) and the Old Schoolhouse Museum. The most-well-known special event is the annual celebration **Pioneer Days,** held during the month of October, with the excitement of outhouse races, a carnival, a parade, dances, contests, chili cook-offs, and lots more fun stuff. Dig out your Stetson, your boots, and your bandana and come on along!

Where to Eat and Stay

Rattler Fine Foods, 62705 Twentynine Palms Highway, Joshua Tree; (760) 366–1898. Here's where children of all ages will find a delightful menu of organic sandwiches, such as the Integration (that's a desert oddity) and the Lily and J.D. Special (organic peanut butter and raspberry jam on thick-sliced honey white bread). The owner and her busy helpers are on hand to pack up a lunch box for hungry families to take for desert exploration at Joshua Tree National Park. One of three park entrances is around the corner off to the right at Park Road.

Oasis of Eden Inn and Suites, 56377 Twenty Nine Palms Highway, Yucca Valley, Eden; (800) 606–6686; www.oasisof eden.com. If you've had a dream about spending a night in a Grecian, Roman, safari, or Oriental suite, make a reservation at the one and only Oasis of Eden Inn and Suites, where high desert hospitality means a full or studio kitchenette with adjoining rooms (perfect for a family), deluxe complimentary continental breakfast, free in-room movies, including HBO and Disney, and a marvelous large heated pool, surrounded by a colorful, hand-painted mural. This is a one-of-a-kind hideaway with a personality.

Spin and Margie's Desert Hideaway, Joshua Tree, off Route 62, and ten minutes from Joshua Tree National Park; (760) 366–9124; www.deserthideaway.com. This adorable little property has a fun Southwest feel. With only four suites with kitchens, there is definitely a "get away from the hustle and bustle of city life" feeling here. There are videos in the rooms for the children when they are through discovering the desert for the day. $$$

The Twenty Nine Palms Inn, 73950 Inn Road, Twentynine Palms; (760) 367–3505; www.29palmsinn.com. Founded in 1928, this is another high desert discovery. Its cozy restaurant serves lunch and dinner. Yes, you are slightly off the beaten path, but the high desert air is invigorating and kids will find the spacious grounds perfect for exploring. Guests spending the night enjoy a complimentary continental breakfast. Brunch is served on Sunday from 9:00 A.M. to 2:00 P.M. Desert cottages are roomy and ideal for a family; the decor is authentic with vintage furnishings. You may want to linger an extra day.

But you're almost at the entrance of Joshua Tree National Park, an 850-square-mile plant and wildlife sanctuary, worth another full day of exploration.

For More Information

California Welcome Center–Yucca Valley. 56711 Twentynine Palms Highway (Route 62), Yucca Valley, 92284; (760) 365–5464; info.yuccavalley@visitcwc.com. Located 22 miles off Interstate 10 on Highway 62. Open daily for complete area information, lodging referrals, and public Internet access.

City of Twentynine Palms/Visitors Bureau. 6136 Adobe Road, P.O. Box 995, 92277; (760) 367–6799; fax (760) 367–4890; www.ci.twentynine-palms.ca.us.

Indio Chamber of Commerce. 82–503 Highway 111, 92201; (760) 347–0676 or (800) 44–INDIO; fax (760) 347–6069; www.indiochamber.org.

Joshua Tree Chamber of Commerce. 61325 Twentynine Palms Highway #F, P.O. Box 600, Joshua Tree, 92252; (619) 366–3723; www.joshuatreechamber.org.

Twentynine Palms Chamber of Commerce. 6455-A Mesquite Avenue, 92277; (760) 367–3445; fax: (760) 367–3366; www.29palmschamber.com.

Yucca Valley Chamber of Commerce. 56300 Twentynine Palms Highway, Suite D, Yucca Valley, 92284; (619) 365–6223; www.yuccavalley.org .

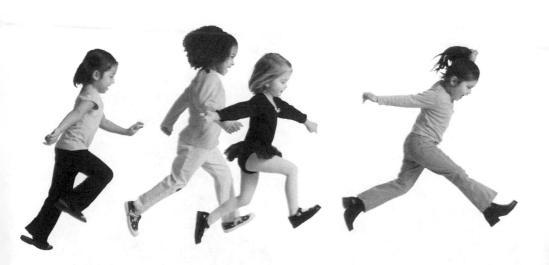

Magical **Mystery Tour**

En route to Joshua Tree National Park, if you've exited from Interstate 10 to Highway 62, you'll be on a stretch of highway that takes you through some fascinating scenery and worthwhile places to stop. This is a two- to three-hour trip in itself, especially if you stop for lunch and visit a few museums and art galleries along the route.

The high desert sweeps the vast area straddling San Bernardino and Riverside Counties. You know you've arrived when the temperature dips about ten degrees from that of the stunning sun-dappled mountains of the ritzier side of Interstate 10, that being Palm Springs. Families head for the high desert when they want to explore a portion of the 800,000-acre Joshua Tree National Park.

Along the way you'll pass Morongo Valley and Yucca Valley prior to arriving at Joshua Tree. The Yucca Valley lies at the gateway to the Mojave Desert's Morongo Basin.

At the Community Center Complex, 57116 Twentynine Palms Highway, you'll find the **Hi-Desert Nature Museum** (open Tuesday through Sunday 10:00 A.M. to 5:00 P.M., **free.**) This is a family-oriented facility related to the high desert's unique natural and historical environments. The museum shop has nature theme gifts and children's science gifts (open 10:00 A.M. to 5:00 P.M. Tuesday through Sunday). Kids can interact with resident snakes and insects or spend some time on arts and crafts.

Twentynine Palms is home to the Marine Corps Air Ground Combat Center. While this immense military base, rivaling the size of the state of Rhode Island, is not open to the public, it is the site on occasion of military events on the parade ground, such as the Battle Color Ceremony presented by the Marine Corps.

While in the area, make it a point to stop at **Pappy & Harriet's Palace** (760–365–5956; www.pappyandharriets.com) on Pioneertown Road ("eatin', drinkin', and sleepin' in an old western town" says their ad). They serve up great food and entertainment Monday through Wednesday from noon to 8:00 P.M. and Thursday through Sunday from 11:00 A.M. to 2:00 A.M. This is a far cry from any chain restaurant. The ambience is authentic; Old West, rustic, and noisy. Local characters looking like vintage cowboys are often sitting around. There's so much going on here with dinners and western entertainment that a monthly schedule is published.

Pioneertown (www.pioneertown.com), 4 miles out of the Yucca Valley, was founded by Gene Autry, Roy Rogers, and Dick Curtis in 1946 and was used as a filming location. The kids may not remember the film **Gunfight at the OK Corral,** but a few parents and grandparents might. This was filmed here along with many other stories of the Old West. This area is truly a time warp, but it's the real McCoy.

Several hiking trails start here, such as the 2-mile Water Canyon Trail and the Pipes Canyon Trail, where you can see the original "pipes," or springs, that attracted the first settlers.

As you enter the town of Twentynine Palms along the **Twentynine Palms Highway** (it's the alternative route to Arizona, the Colorado River, and Las Vegas, by the way), look for the magnificent historical murals painted on the sides of eleven buildings throughout the town. They depict Indians, miners, homesteaders, and ranchers. One mural kids might find interesting is found on the south wall at 6308 Adobe Road, *Jack Cones the Flying Constable.*

Bet you never thought there was so much to see and do along the way. Like an experienced travel writer once said, "Value the journey as well as the destination."

Mojave National Preserve

The Mojave National Preserve is open-year round. The preserve is easily reached via Interstate 15 or Interstate 40 east of Barstow and west of Needles, California, and Las Vegas, Nevada. Six freeway exits provide visitor access. Road conditions vary from paved, two-lane highways to rugged four-wheel-drive roads; see map for major routes. Maps showing all dirt roads are available at park information centers. The Baker Desert Information Center is open from 9:00 A.M. to 5:00 P.M. daily; 72157 Baker Boulevard, P.O. Box 241, Baker, 92309; (760) 733–4040; e-mail: MOJA Baker Interp@nps.gov. Hole-in-the-Wall Ranger Station is open on Friday, Saturday, and Sunday from 9:00 A.M. to 4:00 P.M.; (760) 928–2572. The Office of the Superintendent, Mojave National Preserve, is located at 222 East Main Street, Suite 202, Barstow, 92311; headquarters (760) 255–8800; www.nps.gov/moja/.

Many visitors to Southern California are surprised to learn how extensive the state's desert lands really are. Unless you consider yourself to be a true desert rat, you may want to make only a detour to the Mojave National Preserve, a 14,000-square-mile tract—twice the size of New Jersey. Some of the most prominent natural features in the preserve are the **Kelso Dunes,** situated in the southern section. Rising to 600 feet, the dunes are the third highest in the United States. Shifting sands on the steep side of the dunes create a unique rumbling sound that has given these mobile mounds the alias "the singing dunes." The dunes are ringed by high mountain ranges, and the overall effect is one of a great, stark beauty. A red-tailed hawk soaring above may be the only reminder that this is Southern California, not Mars.

Providence Mountains State Recreation Area

P.O. Box 1, Essex; (760) 928–2586; www.calparksmojave.com/providence/ or www.parks.ca.gov. In the northern portion of the preserve.

Some three dozen ancient volcanic cinder cones are scattered throughout the area. Bighorn sheep are often sighted near the visitor center, which is close by the limestone Mitchell Caverns. Park rangers lead visitors on ninety-minute tours of the caves. The star attraction of this area, however, is the Cima Dome, a geological formation created by volcanic action that rises 1,500 feet above the desert floor and measures 10 miles in diameter. Covered with the largest Joshua tree forest in the world, the dome is best viewed from Mid Hills, several miles away. Several designated state scenic roads, including the Kelso-Cima Road, Essex Road, and Lanfair-Ivanpah Road, crisscross the preserve. This is California's most remote state park, 56 miles from Needles via Interstate 40 and 116 miles east of Barstow.

For More Information

California Desert Information Center. 831 Barstow Road, Barstow, 92311; (760) 255–8760; www.caohwy.com/c/caldesic .htm. Open 9:00 A.M. to 5:00 P.M. daily except holidays. The center provides maps and other information about the Mojave National Preserve and other scenic desert drives.

Barstow Area Chamber of Commerce and Visitors Bureau. 409 East Fredricks Street, P.O. Box 698, Barstow, 92311; (760) 256–8617 or (888) 4–BARSTOW; www.barstowchamber.com.

Barstow Area

The western portions of the Mojave, though as desolate as the lands to the east, offer a very different kind of experience. Barstow, once a railroad crossroads and transportation center, lies halfway between L.A. and Las Vegas at the junctions of Interstates 15 and 40. Right in the center of the Mojave, it's the traditional base from which to explore Calico Ghost Town, Rainbow Basin, and Mitchell Caverns.

California Welcome Center at Tanger Outlets

The state of California has eleven official welcome centers placed strategically throughout the state. The Barstow Center is located at 2796 Tanger Way, Suite 106; (760) 253–4782;

e-mail: info.barstow@visitcwc.com. Located off Interstate 15, exit Lenwood Road. Follow the "traveling bear" signs to the Tanger Outlet Center (one hundred stores filled with discount merchandise). California welcome centers provide information on all twelve regions. Other welcome centers are located in Rohnert Park, Pier 39 in San Francisco, Carlsbad, Santa Ana, and the Shasta-Cascade region, to name a few. Check out www.visitcwc.com for locations of all welcome centers.

Bun Boy

1890 West Main Street, Barstow; (760) 256–9118. $–$$

One of the main attractions in Barstow itself is stopping for lunch at a more-than-fast-food-but-less-than-a-restaurant kind of eatery, where all Southern Californians seem to have had a burger at some point in their lives. It's the kind of place you might imagine Jack Kerouac pulling into for a quick bite before waxing beatific about the experience.

There is another Bun Boy in Baker, off Interstate 15 North (72155 Baker Boulevard; 760–733–4660), and here you will find the world's highest (134 feet) thermometer—and probably some of California's hottest weather as well! Nevertheless, families will enjoy giant-size servings of homemade peach, strawberry, and apple pie. Both Bun Boys open at 6:00 A.M. and close at 10:00 P.M.

Rainbow Basin and Owl Canyon

Once you've filled your gas tank (and your tummy tank), it's time to leave civilization behind again. You won't miss the sounds of the city one bit as you head north on Fort Irwin Road, out of Barstow, and enter the realm of Rainbow Basin (760–252–6000; www.ca.blm.gov/barstow), a national natural landmark, where the colors of the rainbow decorate gorge walls housing an inestimable quantity of fossilized remains that are ten- to thirty-million years old.

And may the force be with you as you drive through the rock-strewn, otherworldly landscape of Owl Canyon, where the movie *Star Wars* was filmed. If your kids don't know R2D2 from C3PO, this would be the place to fill them in.

The Bureau of Land Management (BLM) field office in Barstow administers Owl Canyon; (760) 252–6091; general location: 8 miles north of downtown Barstow, off Irwin Road. The canyon is open year-round and **free,** although there is a fee for primitive camping sites. Activities to enjoy include bird-watching, camping, hiking or backpacking, picnicking, rock hounding or gold panning, scenic driving, and wildlife and wildflower viewing.

Calico Ghost Town

Located minutes off Interstate 15, east of Barstow, 36600 Ghost Town Road, Yermo; (760) 254–2122 or (800) TO–CALICO; www.calicotown.com. Open daily 7:00 A.M. to dusk (shops, playhouse, and railroad hours 9:00 A.M. to 5:00 P.M.).

A not-to-be-missed item on your Mojave Desert itinerary, the ghost town—the most celebrated of many such once-booming settlements that pepper the Mojave—contains remnants of the flourishing mining culture of more than a century ago. As you approach, keep a lookout for small cavelike openings in the mountains above the town. These once were the entrances to the miners' homes. In the town's heyday in the 1880s, some 4,000 people called this dusty outpost home. Before you begin to feel too sorry for them, remember they made fortunes from silver mines that yielded $65 million worth of rich ore. One interesting nugget of information: The town was prosperous enough to keep twenty-two saloons in business.

In 1896 the price of silver plummeted, as did the town's fortunes. In the bat of an eye-lash, Calico went from boom to bust. Today the restored mining town lives on after a fashion as part of the San Bernardino County Regional Park. A stop in Calico is about as close to time travel as you'll ever get. Some of the town's original buildings, such as Lil's Saloon, Lucy Lane's House, and the General Store, have been restored so well that western-theme movies continue to be filmed here.

But Calico is more than atmospheric building facades. You can actually enter Lil's or the Top of Hill Cafe and Ice Cream Parlor for some modern-day refreshment. There are twenty-three shops along Main Street—the only street—a favorite being the 1880s-style candy store. You and the kids also might hop aboard a narrow-gauge train for a ride to the silver mine areas north of town.

At Maggie's Mine, the very adventurous can get an inside look at the miner's work-place, the 30-mile network of tunnels and mine shafts beneath Calico, by taking a guided tour. Maybe you'll even spot a wedge of silver. But if you're like us, you'll stay above-ground and pan for gold, boo the villain at the town playhouse, or dress up like an 1890 pioneer and have your portrait taken. This is one ghost town that is very much alive!

Festivals in Calico take place throughout the year. Palm Sunday weekend, for example, is Calico Hullabaloo time, when "horseshoe pitchin', stew cookin', and tobacco spittin' " are the order of the day. But you can take a walking tour with "Lefty," the town historian, or listen to Sheriff "Lonesome George" spin a yarn throughout the year.

Peggy Sue's 🍴 🎞️ 🔒

Interstate 15 at Ghost Town Road exit, Yermo, 8 miles east of Barstow; (760) 254–3370. Open daily for breakfast, lunch, and dinner.

Soda fountain, ice-cream parlor, pizza parlor, burgers, steaks, homemade chili and soups, old-fashioned candy, 1950s music, a 1950s-style dime store, TV and movie memorabilia, curios, and souvenir shop. The kids will appreciate the game arcade plus a park featuring cool lagoons and sparkling waterfalls surrounded by shady weeping willow trees.

Ridgecrest

While Barstow is the crossroads of the Mojave Desert as a whole, little Ridgecrest, a town of some 30,000 about 70 miles to the northwest, is the best base camp for branching out to explore the natural wonders and attractions of Mojave's northwestern portions.

Ridgecrest is the hub high desert community for visiting the natural attractions of **Mount Whitney** and **Death Valley,** a two-hour drive away. For further information, contact the **Ridgecrest Area Convention and Visitor's Bureau,** 100 West California Avenue; (760) 375–8282 or (800) 847–4830; fax (760) 371–1654; www.visitdeserts.com.

You've seen Ridgecrest in dozens of movies, television shows, and videos. More than 500 television commercials have been filmed here since 1990. Think back to *Star Trek V, Flight of the Intruder, ET,* and *Dinosaur,* which was filmed on location at the Trona Pinnacles. Jawbone Canyon has seen the likes of *Wayne's World II, Desert Blue,* and *Woman Undone.* And Olancha Sand Dunes hosted *Star Trek V.*

Head east out of Ridgecrest on Highway 178 and take in the panorama of the **Panamint Mountains,** which frame Death Valley. About 20 miles up the road, the **Trona Pinnacles** pierce the clear desert sky. The pinnacles, more than 500 in number, are composed of tufa (a porous rock formed as a deposit from springs and streams) and reach heights of 150 feet.

Maturango Museum

100 East Las Flores Avenue, at China Lake Boulevard; (760) 375–6900; fax (760) 375–0479; www.maturango.org. Open 10:00 A.M. to 5:00 P.M. Monday through Sunday. **Free** admission to visitor centers. $

The museum was established in 1962 to tell the story of the northern Mojave Desert. There are exhibits showcasing animals, birds, paleontology, and Native American displays. The hands-on Discovery Area appeals to children of all ages. The museum is also home to the Death Valley Tourist Center and the Northern Mojave Visitor Center.

BLM Wild Horse and Burro Corrals

(760) 384–5765 or (800) 951–8720; www.wildhorseandburro.blm.gov.

Three miles east of Ridgecrest, off Highway 178, a right turn just as the road reaches the top side of the rise brings you to the Bureau of Land Management's Wild Horse and Burro Corrals. This is where the animals are held, fed, and prepared for adoptions locally and throughout the country. It is open Monday through Friday 7:00 A.M. to 4:00 P.M. Closed in July.

U.S. Naval Museum of Armament and Technology at China Lake

East end of Blandy Road in the old Officer's Club building; (760) 939–3530; www.chinalakemuseum.org. Open 10:00 A.M. to 4:00 P.M. Monday through Friday. Guest passes allowing entrance to NAWS China Lake must be obtained in advance to visit the museum.

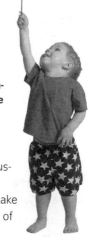

China Lake has been a research, development, and test site since 1943 and covers more than a million acres in Southern California's Mojave Desert. The museum focus is on technical advances in the defense industry made at China Lake. Soon to come: the refurbishment of an FA–18 Hornet aircraft, the first of twenty prototypes manufactured for China Lake in the late 1970s. Kids can see missiles, free-fall weapons, and a variety of other intimidating weapons of war such as a Tomahawk submarine, a Shrike, and a Maverick. More benign is the Lunar Soft Landing Vehicle. Kids should find the actual Sidewinder missile to be especially awesome.

On quite a different note, the Naval Air Weapons Station (NAWS) China Lake houses the largest cache of ancient Native American rock art in North America. Little Petroglyph Canyon, the only site open for public tours, is about 1.2 miles long, with walls 20 to 40 feet high. Elevation is about 5,000 feet. The road to the site is steep and mostly paved, with only the last 7 miles being dirt. The canyon floor is a sand and rocky wash bottom. Visitors have to negotiate over and around a variety of rocks and boulders to enter the canyon. From there, the walk is moderate.

The round-trip from the NAWS main gate is about 90 miles. To arrange for a tour, call the Corporate Communications/Public Affairs Office (PAO) at least two months in advance at (760) 939–1683. The PAO representative will explain how to coordinate your tour and how to get assistance in securing NAWS-approved guides, mandated post–9/11. Questions regarding the petroglyphs may be directed to NAVAIR, Naval Air Warfare Center Weapons Division, Code 750000D, 1 Administration Circle, China Lake, 93555-6100; www.nawcwd.navy.mil/.

Where to Eat and Stay

Texas Cattle Company, 1429 North Chinalake Boulevard, Ridgecrest; (760) 446–6602; fax (760) 446–2378; www.texascattlecompany.com. This family-oriented restaurant is adorned with a train that runs around the ceiling and a toy chest ready for waiting children. $$

The Heritage Inn & Suites, 1050 North Norma Street; (760) 446–6543 or (800) 843–0693. The hotel offers 170 comfortable guest rooms and features complimentary American breakfast for guests. Film crews stay here often, as do many military personnel from nearby China Lake Naval Air Weapons Center.

Randsburg Area

Twenty-two miles south of Ridgecrest, off Highway 395, is the home of the living ghost town of Randsburg (population 80). While not as well known as Calico Ghost Town, Randsburg shared much the same fate as its desert neighbor. Today, visitors can stop for a snack, browse among antiques stores, and take a peek at the bullet slug still lodged in one of the local bars. When you turn off Highway 395 at the sign to Randsburg, the first building you will see is the old jail to your left. Park your car and browse among the vintage structures. This area is desolate but photogenic and has been used as a location for movies and television productions.

Desert Tortoise Natural Area 🛅 🛅 🛅
South of Randsburg; (760) 384–5400; www.ca.blm.gov/ridgecrest.

You've come this far, so don't miss the Desert Tortoise Natural Area (DTNA), just southwest of Randsburg. This 40-square-mile chunk of land has been reserved for the protection and preservation of the largest known population of the shy desert tortoise, an endangered species. There is an information kiosk and self-guided interpretative trails. If you want to see this desert reptile (California's official reptile) at its most active, make your **free** visit in April or September.

Red Rock Canyon State Park

Red Rock Canyon State Park Headquarters; (661) 942–0662; www.calparksmojave .com/redrocks/. Open year-round.

This beautiful, scenic wonder of California was established as a state park in 1968, located where the southernmost tip of the Sierra Nevada converge with the El Paso Range. After wet winters the park's floral displays are amazing. Wildlife includes roadrunners, hawks, lizards, mice, and squirrels. The colorful rock formations in the park served as landmarks during the early 1870s for 20-mule-team freight wagons slogging through the desert.

Just south of Red Rock Canyon State Park, stop by the Jawbone Canyon Visitor's Center on Highway 14, site of the annual Moose Anderson Days spring festival. For more information, contact Friends of Jawbone Canyon, P.O. Box 1902, Cantil, 93519; (760) 373–1146; www.jawbone.info.

Red Rock Canyon State Park is a favorite site for filmmakers, and the beginning scene of *Jurassic Park* was filmed here. There is a self-guided nature trail offering a good introduction to indigenous plants, animals, and awe-inspiring vistas. If you'd like to see more breathtaking desert-scapes, cross over to Highway 14, which skirts red-, pink-, orange-, and white-colored canyons that seem to change color as the light shifts.

Death Valley

It's awesome to imagine that twenty-seven acres of "empty" California desert comprise what we now know as Death Valley. The region is one of 265 areas worldwide recognized and preserved by the Man and the Biosphere organization. This one, the **Mojave and Colorado Desert Biosphere Reserve,** is the ideal place to share with your children the importance of environmental protection.

Before you enter the dazzling desolation of Death Valley, consider making a stop in **Darwin Falls,** a little bit off Highway 178 before the valley. The whole family can manage the half-mile hike to the oasis of lower Darwin Falls. The upper falls aren't far behind. Your memories of green will serve you well as you head into Death Valley, the lowest point in the United States and reportedly the hottest place on earth. Average summertime highs are 115 degrees, and with scarcely a tree in sight, there isn't much shade to cool off in. If you happen to come here between June and September, remember to take it easy and drink water frequently—dehydration is dangerous and can happen faster than you think.

But don't let the heat deter you from visiting. Or the intimidating name, for that matter. With a rich mining heritage dating from 1849 and modern tourist facilities, Death Valley can actually be a very lively place. Geological wonders have, however, always been at center stage. You can see the famous ones in a day or so, but savor the barren beauty slowly.

Artist's Palette Drive is a famous byway that winds through pastel-colored hills laced with minerals. Early morning is the best time to take photographs from **Zabriskie Point,** which overlooks ancient lake beds. By contrast, **Golden Canyon** is at its best in the afternoon. In between, you could investigate the bizarre salt formations of the **Devil's Golf Course** and get an elevated perspective from 5,474 feet up at **Dante's View,** where the Panamint Mountains and snowcapped Mount Whitney will be visible.

Death Valley National Park

The hottest, driest, lowest place in the Western Hemisphere. Open year-round. Office of the Superintendent, P.O. Box 579, Death Valley, 92328; (760) 786–3200; www.nps.gov/deva/. Furnace Creek Visitor Center and Borax Museum, open year-round 8:00 A.M. to 5:00 P.M.; Stovepipe Wells Ranger Station, open all year, seasonal hours.

California Highway 190, the Badwater Road, the Scotty's Castle Road, and paved roads to Dante's View and Wildrose provide access to the major scenic viewpoints and historic points of interest within the park. More than 350 miles of unpaved and four-wheel-drive roads provide access to wilderness hiking, camping, and historical sites. All vehicles must be licensed and "street legal." Admission fees are by permit, $10 per car for seven days. Death Valley Annual Pass for $20 per passholder/vehicle.

Amargosa Opera House and Hotel (ages 5 and up)

(760) 852–4441; www.amargosaoperahouse.com. Doors open 7:45 P.M.; show starts 8:15 P.M. Saturday only during October, December, and January through mid-May; Saturday and Monday during November, February, March, and April. $$

Plan your trip so that you can visit this site in the ghost town of Death Valley Junction, near the junction of State Routes 127 and 190. Performances star Marta Becket, who plays all of the characters. Murals depict gypsies, revelers, clerics, and Spanish royalty. Eccentric, yes, but charmingly unusual. The fourteen-room hotel is a rustic, historic hoot. No phones or TV mar this quirky outpost.

Scotty's Castle

(760) 786–2392; www.nps.gov/deva/Scottys/Scottys_main.htm. Daily guided, living-history tours of Scotty's Castle main house interior are conducted 365 days a year, 7 days a week. The first tour begins at 9:00 A.M., and the last begins at 5:00 P.M. Castle grounds close at 6:00 P.M. Tours last approximately fifty minutes and are given at least once every hour. Limited to nineteen people per tour, the guided tour is the only way to get inside the main house. Tour tickets are sold on a first-come, first-served basis. $$

Located in the northern part of the valley in an area known as Grapevine Canyon, this Spanish Moorish–style mansion was the creation of Walter Scott (and some of his desert friends), who built his home in the 1920s at the cost of $200 million. The building took ten years to complete, but you can see it inside and out in considerably less time. Save your visit here for the second day of your Death Valley tour. Near the castle is the Ubehebe Crater and the Sahara-scale sand dunes.

Where to Eat and Stay

Furnace Creek Inn and Ranch Resort, Highway 190, Box 1, Death Valley, 92328; (760) 786–2345; fax (760) 786–2514; www.furnacecreekresort.com. This privately owned property operated by Xanterra is actually one resort with two hotels: the historic 1927 luxurious, 66-room Furnace Creek Inn (open only mid-October to mid-May) and the more family-friendly 224-room Furnace Creek Ranch, circa 1933, recently renovated and open year-round. Choose the ranch for you and the kids and the inn for a couple's private romantic getaway. Wandering around the western-theme ranch grounds, you'll feel like you've been transported back to the 1800s but with all the twenty-first-century amenities: air-conditioning, TV, telephones, a spring-fed swimming pool, tennis courts, and a children's playground. Ride a horse, take a hike, or challenge your kids to a game of horseshoes. Visit the general store for a quick snack and some great gifts. Check out the antique stagecoaches, mining tools, and the steam locomotive at the Borax Museum. Visit the eighteen-hole Furnace Creek Golf Course, the world's lowest golf course at 214 feet below sea level. For year-round casual, American-style dining, choose from the Wrangler Steakhouse and Buffet, the 49'er Café, and the Corkscrew Saloon.

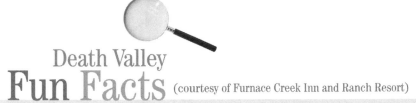

Death Valley
Fun Facts (courtesy of Furnace Creek Inn and Ranch Resort)

- The hottest recorded temperature in Death Valley was 134 degrees (Fahrenheit) in 1913.
- The average rainfall in Death Valley is 1.8 inches per year.
- Death Valley was named a national monument on February 11, 1933, by Pres. Herbert Hoover.
- Death Valley became a national park on October 31, 1994, by an act of Congress.
- The average humidity in Death Valley ranges from zero to 5 percent.
- Death Valley has more than 900 species of plants, 6 types of fish, 5 amphibians, 36 reptiles, and 51 mammals native to the region.
- There are 346 species of birds that migrate through or reside in Death Valley.
- *Death Valley Days* ran as a radio show from 1930–1944 and as a television series from 1952–1968.

San Diego County

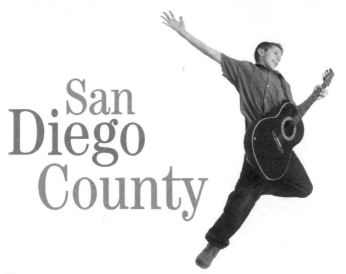

What does summer vacation mean to your family? How about one with plenty of outdoor recreation—boating, hiking, biking, picnicking, swimming, golfing, baseball, surfing, or sunbathing on miles of beach? Does it include excursions to great parks full of wildlife and sea life, exciting museums with hands-on displays of fun things from outer space to automobiles, old sights with new twists, all surrounded by the Pacific Ocean, mountains, and desert and capped by a clear blue sky with mega-sunshine? The year-round answer is San Diego County, Southern California's endless summer vacation destination, encompassing metropolitan San Diego, the coastal areas of North County including Oceanside, and to the east, the mountains and desert of the Back Country, featuring Julian and Anza-Borrego.

San Diego County's location at the extreme southwest corner of the contiguous United States not only helps explain its temperate climate (an average year-round temperature of seventy degrees) but also its friendly spirit. In this geographically varied, 4,205-square-mile region, you can head west out to sea, south into Mexico, east into forested mountains that receive more rain and snow than Seattle and deserts that are hotter and drier than Phoenix, and north into 70 miles of sandy, palm-lined beaches that rival Florida. You will find country kitchens and apple farms, cosmopolitan bistros and burger joints, craft shops and giant retail malls, high-rises and bungalows, dirt roads and ten-lane freeways—inhabited by 2.9 million culturally and ethnically diverse people. Their sheer numbers make San Diego America's seventh most populous area and the Golden State's second-biggest metropolis, after Los Angeles.

Kudos! San Diego came out a big winner ranked second (to Honolulu) in the 2004 *Travel and Leisure* survey of favorite U.S. cities; and ranked in the Family-Friendly 2001 Travel Awards, published in the April 2001 issue of *FamilyFun* magazine. For the second consecutive year, San Diego was named the "coolest city" in the southwestern United States, and the magazine gave San Diego's beaches and the San Diego Zoo highest scores. Plus, the San Diego Zoo and SeaWorld San Diego were both listed among the top twelve nationwide favorite attractions.

SAN DIEGO COUNTY

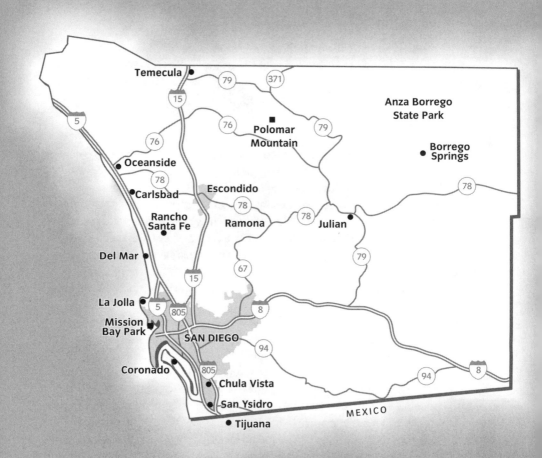

Temecula
79
371
15
Anza Borrego
State Park
5
76
Polomar
76
Mountain
79
Borrego
Springs
Oceanside
78
Escondido
78
Carlsbad
Rancho
Santa Fe
Ramona
78
78
Julian
Del Mar
67
79
15
La Jolla
5
805
Mission
8
Bay Park
SAN DIEGO
Coronado
94
805
8
Chula Vista
94
San Ysidro
MEXICO
Tijuana

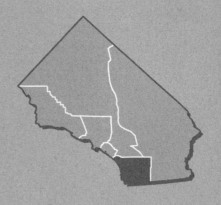

Metropolitan San Diego

Touring the greater San Diego area is best accomplished by automobile. Your choices of activities and attractions are incredibly diverse. Many families start in the Mission Bay area at SeaWorld and are entertained by the penguins, sharks, and killer whales. Or you might begin at the world-famous San Diego Zoo with its exotic and rare species of animals and plants. Or the San Diego Wild Animal Park may beckon, where the animals roam **free** and really wild. Balboa Park's museums, art galleries, and theaters provide you with some fantastic cultural attractions. If outdoor recreation is your family's favorite, there are hundreds of beaches, parks, sailing, and fishing options. We like to begin at the beginning by visiting the Old Town State Historic Park and Presidio district, then touring the first California missions, downtown's restored Gaslamp Quarter, or Point Loma's Cabrillo National Monument, which commemorates the first European to set sight on San Diego Bay. But no matter how you divide and conquer it, you will find incredibly fun things to see, do, and taste throughout metropolitan San Diego.

Cabrillo National Monument

1800 Cabrillo Memorial Drive, State Route 209, off Interstate 5; (619) 557–5450. Open 9:00 A.M. to 5:15 P.M. daily, possibly extended in summer. $$

Cruising the Pacific Coast north of Mexico in 1542, explorer Juan Rodriguez Cabrillo first landed at Point Loma, a 400-foot-high peninsula separating San Diego Bay from the ocean. He claimed it (and everything else in sight) for Spain. Today you can marvel at the same view Cabrillo had of the southernmost tip of this narrow finger of land. On Point Loma's plateaulike surface are two military reservations, a cemetery, and informative attractions for young and old alike. You can get your bearings at the visitor center, tour the monument's small museum, and take in a **free** film or a ranger-sponsored program in the auditorium. Then let the kids climb Old Point Loma Lighthouse, with its breathtaking panorama of the city meeting the sea. This is a superb spot for winter whale-watching.

Old Town San Diego State Historic Park and Presidio Park

Located in a 6-block area bounded by Wallace, Juan, Twiggs, and Congress Streets, sandwiched between Interstates 5 and 8; (619) 220–5422. Open daily 10:00 A.M. to 5:00 P.M. Free admission. Free guided walking tours depart the Robinson–Rose House daily at 2:00 P.M. All buildings are closed New Year's Day, Thanksgiving, and Christmas.

In 1769, a mere 167 years after Cabrillo arrived, Gaspar de Portola established the first Presidio Royal (military fort) while Father Junipero Serra founded the first in a string of twenty-one California missions. Since both the fort and the mission were built in San Diego, they earned the city the moniker "birthplace of California." This is, of course, California-ish hyperbole, because for centuries before de Portola or Serra, Native Americans—quite successfully, in fact—had prospered from the area's fertile lands and bountiful seas.

The fort and mission were located originally in what today is called Old Town. The cluster of adobe buildings at the base of Presidio Hill has swollen over time into a fascinating complex of historic landmarks, museums, art galleries, shops, and ethnic restaurants. These include the Black Hawk Smith & Stable, the Colorado House/Wells Fargo Museum, the Courthouse, the Johnson House, La Casa de Estudillo, the Machado-Stewart Adobe, the Mason Street School, the Plaza, the Robinson–Rose Building, the San Diego Union Newspaper Museum, Seeley Stables, and the Whaley House. Our best advice is just to go, park, walk, and enjoy this family-friendly district.

Junipero Serra Museum

2727 Presidio Drive, in Presidio Park; (619) 297–3258; www.sandiegohistory.com. Open Tuesday through Saturday from 10:00 A.M. to 4:30 P.M. and Sunday from noon to 4:30 P.M.; closed major holidays. $$

This museum stands above the sites of the eighteenth-century presidio and Father Junipero Serra's first mission in Alta, California. It's a great place to learn about San Diego's early Spanish and Mexican periods. Exhibits include artifacts from archaeological excavations at the site.

Who Was **Alonzo Horton?**

For some years after California won statehood in 1850, San Diego remained a relatively quiet community with a Spanish and Mexican flavor. That changed dramatically when Alonzo E. Horton arrived in town from San Francisco in 1867. Buying up some 960 acres of waterfront land, he began the process of developing what was to become today's downtown area. The **Gaslamp Quarter,** bounded by Broadway, Fourth, and Sixth Streets and Harbor Drive, is the historic 16-block quarter where Horton made his first land purchase and where his legacy lives on. A twenty-year restoration and cleanup campaign to return the Gaslamp Quarter to its gay 1890s splendor has paid off: The area sparkles with period streetlamps, old-time trolley stops, and, of more recent vintage, trendy restaurants, hotels, offices, artists' studios, and nightspots. For complete information including walking tours and audiotapes, contact the **Gaslamp Quarter/Historical Society Museum,** 410 Island Avenue; (619) 233–4692; www.gqhf.com. Open Monday through Friday 10:00 A.M. to 2:00 P.M., Saturday 10:00 A.M. to 4:00 P.M., and Sunday noon to 4:00 P.M.

Mission Basilica San Diego de Alcala

10818 San Diego Mission Road (east on Interstate 8, exit Mission Gorge Road north to Twain Avenue, then drive west to San Diego Mission Road); (619) 281–8449; www.mission sandiego.com. Open 9:00 A.M. to 4:45 P.M. daily except Thanksgiving and Christmas. $

Father Serra's first mission, relocated east to its present location in 1774, was burned down by Indians the following year. Rebuilt in 1781, the fully restored mission remains an active parish. Behind the chapel is a small museum containing robes, relics, and original records in Serra's own handwriting.

Horton Plaza

Between Broadway, First, and Fourth Avenues and G Street, downtown; (800) 214–7467; www.hortonplaza.shoppingtown.com. Open Monday through Saturday 10:00 A.M. to 9:00 P.M. and Sunday 11:00 A.M. to 7:00 P.M. Hours adjusted seasonally and during holiday periods. Three hours of free parking with any purchase.

Named after Alonzo Horton, but opened in 1985, this five-story, lavishly decorated and landscaped open-air mall houses more than 150 shops and restaurants, fourteen movie theaters, and two live performance stages. Parking is available at an adjacent garage. Kids will love the festive atmosphere and food courts.

Old Town Trolley Tours/Historic Tours of America

(619) 298–8687; www.historictours.com/sandiego/. Every thirty minutes, daily, beginning at 9:00 A.M. $$$$

Two-hour narrated tours of most of the key San Diego sites are available on propane-powered vehicles. You can exit and reboard anytime during the day at any of the ten fun stops (such as Balboa Park, Horton Plaza, Gaslamp Quarter, Seaport Village, Embarcadero, Old Town, and Coronado) along the route. This is a wonderful way for the entire family to become acquainted with the city without the hassles of driving and parking your own car. Also available is "Boat on Wheels," a hydra-amphibious land and sea tour, plus the new "Ghosts and Gravestones" tour. Highly recommended.

San Diego Trolley System and the Transit Store

102 Broadway, near Horton Plaza; (619) 233–3004 or (619) 685–4900. Runs daily 5:00 A.M. to 1:00 A.M. every fifteen minutes. One-way fares start at $1.25; day-tripper passes (unlimited use of all types of public transit) are $5.00 per day.

An electric trolley run by the Metropolitan Transit System. The North-South Line runs from downtown San Diego to the Mexican border at San Ysidro; the East-West Line runs along the bay and includes Seaport Village, the Gaslamp Quarter, downtown, and El Cajon.

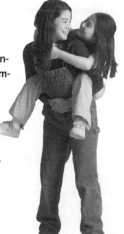

San Diego **Art & Soul**

This is an unprecedented cooperative partnership formed between the San Diego Convention and Visitors Bureau, the City of San Diego Commission for Arts and Culture, and hundreds of organizations and businesses to promote the rich cultural diversity of the area. For an updated daily list of events, links to hundreds of art, music, and cultural Web sites, and a **free** color brochure, access www.sandiegoartandsoul.com or call (619) 533–3050.

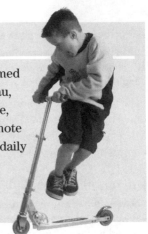

Firehouse Museum

1572 Columbia Street; (619) 232–3473; www.sdfirehousemuseum.org. Open 10:00 A.M. to 4:00 P.M. Thursday through Sunday; closed major holidays. All firefighters **free.** $

Admire antique fire equipment and helmets from around the world in San Diego's oldest firehouse.

Museum of Contemporary Art–San Diego

1001 Kettner Boulevard at Broadway; (619) 234–1001; www.mcasd.org. Open Thursday through Tuesday 11:00 A.M. to 5:00 P.M. (**Free** to all the first Tuesday of every month.) $

In the spectacular thirty-four-story America Plaza, the museum features four galleries on two levels with permanent and changing exhibits of modern paintings, sculpture, and designs. The all-glass exterior gives dramatic views of the San Diego Trolley Station, Amtrak Depot, and the skyline. Call for current exhibitions.

San Diego Aircraft Carrier Museum/USS *Midway*

Navy Pier, 910 North Harbor Drive; (619) 544–9600; fax (619) 238–1200; www.midway.org. Open daily 10:00 A.M. to 5:00 P.M. except on holidays. Admission: $13.00 adults, $10.00 seniors (age 62-plus, military ID, college ID), $7.00 youth (6 to 17 years of age); **free** to children younger than age six and active-duty servicemen and -women in uniform.

Opened in June 2004, the museum is located aboard the USS *Midway,* permanently docked at Navy Pier in San Diego Bay. Marvel at a floating "city at sea" and share in an odyssey that began in 1945 when the USS *Midway* was commissioned as the largest ship in the world. Audio guide provided. More than thirty-five exhibits and displays. You have access to the mess deck, berthing spaces, hangar deck, and flight deck. The museum includes flight simulators, a gift shop, and a cafe.

San Diego Children's Museum/Museo de los Ninos de San Diego
(ages 2–12)

200 West Island Avenue on the corner of Front Street (just a block from the Convention Center); (619) 233–5437 (visitors' line) or (619) 233–8792 (administrative offices);

www.sdchildrensmuseum.org. **Open Tuesday through Saturday 10:00 A.M. to 5:00 P.M.; closed Monday except during holidays. $$**

This facility has dozens of interactive, hands-on exhibits that spark the imagination in you and your kids. Kids can play basketball in Virtual Hoops, a virtual reality–based contest, or paint on the Curious Canvas, even go on stage at the Improv Theatre.

Maritime Museum of San Diego

1492 North Harbor Drive; (619) 234–9153; www.sdmaritime.org. Open daily 9:00 A.M. to 8:00 P.M. $$

The museum will really get your family in a seafaring mood. You can explore three ships: the square-rigged *Star of India,* launched in 1863 and the oldest merchant vessel afloat; the ferry boat *Berkeley,* circa 1898; and the *Medea,* a steam-powered luxury yacht built in 1904.

Seaport Village

West Harbor Drive and Kettner Boulevard; (619) 235–4014; www.seaportvillage.com. Open daily 10:00 A.M. to 9:00 P.M.

Encompassing fourteen acres, this village looks like a transplanted New England fishing town, complete with a carousel, lighthouse, and clock tower along with almost one hundred shops, theme eateries, and restaurants. The Loof Carousel, circa 1890, is worth a whirl. You could easily spend most of the day here wandering the waterfront and enjoying a harbor cruise.

Balboa Park

Just northeast of the downtown business district; (619) 239–0512 for general information; www.balboapark.org.

In 1868 some farsighted city leaders set aside 1,200 acres of barren pueblo land for a city park. Now that land contains the world-famous San Diego Zoo and thirteen museums (the largest concentration outside the Smithsonian in Washington, D.C.). The best way to see the rest of Balboa Park's attractions is on foot. Park at the Plaza de Panama lot (by Laurel Street near the Cabrillo Bridge crossing) or take the **free** tram from the Inspiration Point parking lot (the tram has eleven stops through the park).

Passport to Balboa Park Is a **Great Value**

There are so many incredible things to see and do in Balboa Park, it would probably take you a week to do it all! The **Passport to Balboa Park** is designed with that in mind. Experience up to twelve Balboa Park museums for $21 (a $56 value). This Passport to Balboa is valid for seven days. Obtain yours at any of the museums or the Balboa Park Visitor Center House of Hospitality at 1549 El Prado. Call (619) 239–0512 for more information.

San Diego **by the Sea**

The **Embarcadero,** located at the west end of Broadway, is the thoroughfare forming the heart of downtown San Diego's waterfront action. It's home to the **Broadway Pier,** with berths for cruise ships and freighters, a debarkation platform, U.S. Customs offices, and a cool observation deck. Definitely plan on taking the kids on one of the San Diego Bay excursion cruises to view all the action around Harbor Island, Shelter Island, Point Loma, and Coronado Island. Dinner cruises and whale-watching trips also depart here. Here are some options.

The Original San Diego Harbor Excursions. 1050 North Harbor Drive; (619) 234–4111 or (800) 442–7847. $$$. Dinner cruises also available. Scheduled departures vary seasonally. Generally they are daily between 10:00 A.M. and 5:30 P.M. Sights you will enjoy include the Navy fleet and the stunning Coronado Bay Bridge.

Orion Sailing Charters. 1380 Harbor Island Drive; (619) 574–7504. $$$$. Guided sailing and whale-watching cruises.

San Diego–Coronado Ferry. 1050 North Harbor Drive; (619) 234–4111; www.harborexcursion.com. Operates daily beginning at 9:00 A.M.; last trip 9:00 P.M. $. Every hour on the hour departs San Diego and takes you to Ferry Landing Marketplace in Coronado. Reservations not necessary. This is a super way to do Coronado for the day!

Hornblower Cruises and Events–San Diego. 1066 North Harbor Drive; (619) 686–8715; www.hornblower.com. $$$. Reservations required for one- or two-hour cruises, brunch, and dinner/dancing excursions aboard these deluxe vessels.

San Diego Zoo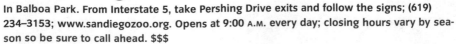

In Balboa Park. From Interstate 5, take Pershing Drive exits and follow the signs; (619) 234–3153; www.sandiegozoo.org. Opens at 9:00 A.M. every day; closing hours vary by season so be sure to call ahead. $$$

Let the zoo be your San Diego headquarters for at least two days of family adventure. The Spanish Colonial buildings here were built originally along El Prado (the Promenade) for the 1915 Panama-California Exposition. Part of the exposition was a modest menagerie, which a certain Dr. Harry Wegeforth took over, expanded, and turned into what is now one of the world's rarest collections. The zoo's size is formidable: more than 4,000 animals, more than 900 species, and 100-plus magnificently landscaped acres with 6,500 exotic plants.

Animals are "on display" outdoors year-round. Viewing is enhanced by many exhibition areas having no bars. Areas include Gorilla Tropics (with incredibly humanlike primates), the Tiger River section, a tropical rain habitat, the Sun Bear Forest, a Southeast Asian jungle, a Hippo Beach (with underwater viewing to see how graceful a swimmer this huge land mammal can be), and the largest koala exhibit outside of Australia. (Get ready for new stuffed teddy bear requests after this particular show!)

The Children's Zoo is user-friendly, with more chances for your kids to pet animals than you can wave a carrot at, plus an incubator for baby chicks and an animal nursery. The Skyfari tram is a great way to see the zoo by air. Our recommendation for "doing the zoo" is the Deluxe Tour, which includes admission to the big zoo, a 45-minute double-decker bus tour (marvelous view), the Children's Zoo, and a Skyfari aerial tramway ride.

Reuben H. Fleet Space Theatre and Science Museum

In Balboa Park, 1875 El Prado; (619) 238–1233; www.rhfleet.org. Open daily 9:30 A.M.; closing times vary. $$

This awe-inspiring facility features a planetarium, hands-on exhibits, and the incredible OMNIMAX, which features new IMAX films. From birds to the Wright brothers to jets, you and the kids will thrill to the history and magical science of flight. Don't miss this!

San Diego Hall of Champions Sports Museum

In Balboa Park; (619) 234–2544; www.sandiegosports.org. Open daily 10:00 A.M. to 4:30 P.M.; closed major holidays. $

Offers a fascinating peek into local sports history via photographs, memorabilia, video tapes, and audiotapes.

San Diego Aerospace Museum & International Aerospace Hall of Fame

In Balboa Park, in the Ford Building; (619) 234–8291; www.aerospacemuseum.org. Open daily 10:00 A.M. to 4:30 P.M.; closed major holidays. Admission is free to all on fourth Tuesday of every month. $$

Check out the replica of Lindbergh's *Spirit of St. Louis* and an A-12 Blackbird. The hall of fame honors heroes of aviation and space flight.

San Diego Model Railroad Museum

In Balboa Park in the Casa de Balboa Building; (619) 696–0199; www.sdmodelrailroadm .com. Open Tuesday through Friday and some holidays 11:00 A.M. to 4:00 P.M., Saturday and Sunday 11:00 A.M. to 5:00 P.M. Admission is free to all on first Tuesday of the month. $

Four scale-model railroad layouts detail the geography and development of the railroad industry in Southern California. Your kids will love the hands-on model railroad.

San Diego Museum of Art

In the center of Balboa Park; (619) 232–7931; www.sdmart.org. Open Tuesday through Sunday 10:00 A.M. to 4:30 P.M.; closed major holidays. $$

The lovely facility has a permanent collection of Italian Renaissance works, Spanish baroque Old Masters, and American, Asian, and Native American art and culture.

San Diego Museum of Photographic Art

1649 El Prado, in Balboa Park; (619) 239–5262; www.mopa.org. Open daily 10:00 A.M. to 5:00 P.M. Admission is **free** on second Tuesday of every month. $$

Devoted exclusively to the photographic arts. Year-round changing exhibitions display everything from fine-art photography to images from around the world.

San Diego Museum of Man

In Balboa Park, the group of buildings around the California Quadrangle; 1350 El Prado; (619) 239–2001; www.museumofman.org. Open daily 10:00 A.M. to 4:30 P.M.; closed major holidays. Admission is **free** on third Tuesday of the month. $$

These multifaceted exhibit halls explore the origins of humankind and feature the cultures of American Indians, ancient Egypt, Mexico, and Latin America. Special features on folk art, textiles, and early man.

San Diego Natural History Museum

East end of Balboa Park; (619) 232–3821; www.sdnhm.org. Open daily 9:30 A.M. to 5:30 P.M.; hours may be extended seasonally. Admission is **free** on first Tuesday of the month. $$

Houses both permanent and changing exhibits and displays detailing the plants, animals, and geology of San Diego County as well as Baja California. Be sure to call for current displays.

Timken Museum of Art

1500 El Prado, in Balboa Park; (619) 239–5548; www.timkenmuseum.org. Open Tuesday through Saturday 10:00 A.M. to 4:30 P.M. and Sunday 1:30 to 4:30 P.M.; closed major holidays. **Free** admission and tours.

This charming gallery contains Old Masters, eighteenth- and nineteenth-century American paintings, and Russian icons.

Botanical and Floral Gardens, Botanical Building

In Balboa Park; (619) 235–1100. Gardens are open year-round. Building is open 10:00 A.M. to 4:00 P.M. daily except Thursday. **Free.**

Revitalize yourself and give the kids some fresh air by heading into Balboa Park's magnificent display of botanical wonders. Included are more than 7,600 trees, 67 kinds of palms, 2,200 rosebushes, plus desert cacti, lilies, ferns, orchids, bamboo, and other oxygen-rich flora. Tour the building (an old Santa Fe railroad station) for explanations of what you've just encountered.

Other Things to See and Do
in Balboa Park

Museums, galleries, and gardens are not the only things going on in Balboa Park for your family. The forty-eight-passenger **Miniature Railroad** will take you and yours into a bygone era. The **Carousel** will set you spinning. The **Starlight Bowl,** where the San Diego Civic Light Opera Association presents delightful musicals, is a sure hit, so call (619) 544–7827 for current schedules. The **Spreckels Organ Pavilion** has free concerts on weekends. The pavilion houses the world's biggest outdoor pipe organ; call (619) 235–1100 for program information. The **Morley Field Sports Complex,** in the northeastern section of the park, can satisfy just about every recreational need your family can dream of (no matter how complex), with a tennis club, two golf courses, a swimming pool, a kiddy pool, some bocce courts, a fitness center, a playground, an archery range, a couple of baseball diamonds, assorted picnic areas, two recreation centers, and a zippy eighteen-hole Frisbee golf course.

Qualcomm Stadium
9449 Friars Road, in Mission Valley; home to the National Football League's San Diego Chargers (619–280–2121 for schedules); www.chargers.com.

This venue, formerly known as Jack Murphy Stadium, was the site of the Super Bowl in 1998 and 2003, and hosts many other events during the year.

PETCO Ballpark
Located downtown, within walking distance to hotels, shopping, and the waterfront; (888) MY–PADRES; www.padres.com.

Major League Baseball's San Diego Padres inaugurated the new PETCO Ballpark in spring 2004. The 46,000-seat facility has spacious concourses, garden terraces, and state-of-the-art services and amenities.

Mission Bay Park
2688 East Mission Bay Drive, just minutes west from Mission Valley; (619) 276–8200 (phone for visitor center). Open 9:00 A.M. to dusk daily. Free.

The park is on a former mudflat transformed into a 4,600-acre aquatic playground by creative dredging, filling, and landscaping. You can easily worship outdoor recreation at its finest here: swimming, power boating, fishing, sailing, volleyball, softball, horseshoes, bicycling, roller-skating, kite flying, Frisbee tossing, and jogging—framed by 27 miles of beaches on Mission Bay and 17 miles of Pacific Ocean frontage. Spread throughout Mission Bay are great resort hotels and campgrounds. The *Bahia Belle* is an old-time sternwheeler that plies the bay between the Bahia and Catamaran Hotels most evenings during the summer and weekends in the winter.

SeaWorld San Diego

1720 South Shores Road, on Mission Bay; (619) 226–3901 or (800) SEA–WORLD; www.sea world.com. Open daily 10:00 A.M., earlier in the summer; closing hours change daily and seasonally. Be sure to call for current times. Parking is $7.00 per car. $$$$

For kids, this is probably the number one reason to visit San Diego. Opened in 1964, this celebrated 189-acre marine amusement park features trained killer whales, ponderous sea lions, playful otters, and lovable dolphins. You can take in five different shows and more than twenty educational exhibits, including the Penguin and Shark Encounters, containing the world's largest collection of these species. New in May 2004, the park welcomed Journey to Atlantis, probably the most exciting attraction in the park's forty-year history: a multimillion-dollar project featuring a wet and wild thrill ride with a 60-foot plunge into a lake, and a new, 130,000-gallon Commerson's dolphin habitat. Also opened in May 2004, Caribbean Realm just south of Dolphin Stadium includes the new Calypso Bay Smokehouse restaurant and Pineapple Pete's Island Eats plus two retail stores—Splish Splash, a children's water gear and clothing store, and Caribbean Breeze gifts.

How about Forbidden Reef, an underwater cave with eels and bat rays, and the not-to-be-missed whale and dolphin Petting Pool? Of course, you've got to see Baby Shamu, only the sixth killer whale to be born in a zoo in a fantastic performance alongside other killer whales (www.shamu.com). You and the kids will scream with laughter at the crazy antics of Clyde and Seamore, the infamous sea lion duo. Try out the new family adventure land, Shamu's Happy Harbor, where you get to crawl, climb, jump, and definitely get wet in a

Diversity **Dining**

From ethnic takeout to historic hangouts to oceanfront glimmer, San Diego chefs use the region's freshest ingredients to create hearty and intriguing dishes. The county's estimated 6,400 restaurants offer everything from new taste sensations to traditional favorites and are attracting some of the nation's top culinary talents. You can sample the tastes of Thailand one evening and Mexico the next, and snack on such local favorites as fish tacos and smoothies in between. Best bet? Ask your hotel's front desk for nearby favorite dining spots or contact the San Diego Convention and Visitors Bureau for its list of restaurant members (more than 250 choices). Contact www.sandiego.org.

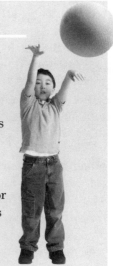

dozen or so play areas. In 1999 Shipwreck Rapids opened as the park's first adventure water ride—a wet and wild experience for sure! Shipwreck Reef Cafe will handle any castaway's appetite (the best dining among twenty or so food options). The Sky Tower and the Aerial Tram ($2.25 each or $3.50 for both) are great ways to see the park.

Belmont Park (icons)

3146 Mission Boulevard, Mission Bay; (619) 491–2988; www.giantdipper.com. Open every day, but hours vary with the season. Free admission to amusement park, but you pay as you go for your choice of rides and games.

Fun, fun, and more fun. Take a ride on the Giant Dipper, a completely restored and rowdy 2,600-foot-long wooden roller coaster, first put into service in 1925 (current cost is $4.00). Then take another dip in The Plunge, the world's largest indoor swimming pool. Pirate's Cove is an indoor playground designed for children ages two to twelve, accompanied by parents. The arcades and Virtual Reality Zone will send everyone for another loop.

SeaWorld **Special Programs**

For some unforgettable experiences, check out these special programs. You can share a meal with an orca family in Dine with Shamu—a scrumptious all-you-can-eat buffet with SeaWorld's biggest star. You will eat at a reserved table alongside the killer whale habitat in an area restricted to trainers and animal-care specialists. Buffet breakfast or dinner includes a special just-for-kids menu.

For an amazing hour and $10.00 for adults, $8.00 for kids, take a public behind-the-scenes tour that brings you to areas you will not find on the SeaWorld map. Many of the tours are interactive, and each is a unique aquatic adventure! Offered daily, this one-hour tour gives you a glimpse at animal care, training, and rehabilitation. Group size is limited to twenty-five plus the educator/guide so you really get the "insider's view."

The Public Animal Spotlight Tour is a two-hour interactive tour with a chance to touch and feed bottlenose dolphins, feed moray eels and sea turtles, and touch sharks. This tour is offered Wednesday through Sunday year-round for an additional $35 per adult/$31 per child that is well worth the time and money.

Other specialized tours include Saving-a-Species Tour, Wild Arctic Experience, and Penguin Experience. Private tours can also be arranged as well as Trainer for a Day, Sleepovers, and group day-camper programs. All are highly recommended as wonderful ways to enhance your family's up-close nature experience.

Hotel Circle Drive and **Mission Valley**

Mission Valley is a suburban area of metro San Diego that is bisected by Interstates 8 (east-west) and 805 (north-south). **Fashion Valley Center** and **Mission Valley Center** are megamalls in this district that can provide you and your family with plenty of dining and entertainment options. They are conveniently located next to a big concentration of accommodations at Hotel Circle Drive, where you will find an abundant selection of family-friendly properties, such as the Comfort Inn & Suites at Hotel Circle (619–881–6800); Ramada Plaza Hotel (619–291–6500); Doubletree Club Hotel (619–291–8790); and Red Lion Hanalei (619–277–1101).

Where to Stay

Omni Hotel San Diego, 675 L Street, San Diego; (619) 231–6664; www.omni hotels.com. Opened in March 2004, this thirty-two-story luxury hotel with 511 rooms and suites is connected via sky bridge to the new PETCO Ballpark, home of Major League Baseball's San Diego Padres. With an excellent location in the heart of the historic Gaslamp Quarter and across the street from the recently renovated Convention Center, the hotel is a superb headquarters for enjoying the city's top sites and attractions only minutes away. The San Diego Trolley stops in front and the train station is 6 blocks away, so staying car-free is an option, too. (Moreover, the hotel is only eight minutes/4 miles from San Diego International Airport.) All accommodations have a choice of views of San Diego Bay, PETCO Ballpark, or the city; are very attractively furnished with outstanding twenty-first-century amenities (and windows that open, unique for a high-rise, so you can catch the fresh ocean breezes). For dining, the hotel offers McCormick & Schmick's Restaurant which serves forty varieties of fresh seafood, pastas, and salads in a casually elegant atmosphere; open for breakfast, lunch, and dinner. Morsel's espresso bar and gift shop has an assortment of delicious desserts and treats. The Terrace Grill offers great barbecue food and poolside beverage service with a view of the bay. Be sure to ask about ballpark packages and other family discount specials—you will score a lodging home run for sure at this property. $$$$

Shelter Pointe Hotel, on Shelter Island, 1551 Shelter Island Drive, San Diego; (619) 221–8000 or (800) 566–2524; www.shelter pointe.com. Located on thirteen acres of spectacular beachfront property, only five minutes from San Diego International Airport, this hotel features 206 guest rooms and suites—all with bay- and marina-view balconies or patios. There are two heated pools and spas, a fitness club, a sand beach with volleyball, bicycle and boat rentals, and a 524-slip marina. American Grille and Bar serves breakfast, lunch, and dinner daily. You'll love the location for the water vistas, as well as easy accessibility to everything you want to see in San Diego. Other highlights are outstanding value packages, plus a $3 million renovation completed in January 2002. $$$

Sommerset Suites Hotel, 606 West Washington Street, San Diego (just west of State Route 163, near Balboa Park and San Diego Zoo); (619) 692–5200 or (800) 962–9665; www.sommersetsuites.com. Eighty one-bedroom suites with fully equipped kitchens. Complimentary continental breakfast and evening refreshments. Outdoor pool, spa, barbecue area. Very family-friendly environment; call for special rates and packages. $$$

Town & Country Resort Hotel, 500 Hotel Circle North, in Mission Valley, San Diego; (619) 291–7131 or (800) 77–ATLAS; www.towncountry.com. This thirty-two-acre resort has 1,000 rooms and suites of every motif and configuration to suit your family's particular needs. There are four swimming pools and spas, nine restaurants and lounges, an eighteen-hole golf course, tennis courts, and a shopping village. Best of all, kids stay **free,** and there

are innumerable package plans that include tickets to nearby SeaWorld and the zoo. A venerable choice for your San Diego headquarters. $$$

For More Information

San Diego Convention and Visitors Bureau. 401 B Street, Suite 1400, San Diego, 92101-4237; (619) 232–3101; www.sandiego.org.

San Diego International Visitor Information Center. 1040½ West Broadway, on the Embarcadero, corner of Harbor Drive and West Broadway; (619) 236–1212. Open 8:30 A.M. to 5:00 P.M. Monday through Saturday year-round. In the summer, open on Sunday from 11:00 A.M. to 5:00 P.M. Experienced, multilingual staff members are super helpful to all visitors, especially foreign travelers.

Chula Vista

Located in the southern tip of San Diego County, the suburb of Chula Vista offers an interesting variety of visitor attractions, all less than twenty minutes from downtown and twenty minutes to the Mexican border.

ARCO/U.S. Olympic Training Center

Eight miles east of Interstate 805 at Telegraph Canyon Road and Wuente Road, 2800 Olympic Parkway; (619) 656–1500; www.usolympicteam.com. Free hourly tours are available daily from 10:00 A.M. to 3:00 P.M.; holidays excluded, varies seasonally.

This is the nation's first warm-weather, year-round, multi-sport Olympic training complex, which complements the U. S. Olympic Committee's other training centers at Colorado Springs, Colorado, and Lake Placid, New York. The 150-acre training site includes a fifty-lane archery range and support building; a six-bay boathouse and a 2,000-meter course for canoeing, kayaking, and rowing; a cycling course and support building; a synthetic surface field hockey pitch and support building; four regulation grass fields and support buildings for soccer; a four-court complex and support building for tennis; a 400-meter track and support building; and a separate, dedicated five-acre throwing area for field events. In the Copley Visitors Center, a short film captures the dedication and emotion involved with the Olympic movement. After the film, you'll be taken on a narrated tour of the 150-acre campus. Inspiring!

Knott's Soak City U.S.A.—San Diego ⊗ 🍴 🚫 🏛

2052 Entertainment Center (next to the Coors Amphitheater); (619) 661–7373; www.knotts.com/soakcity/sd. Open daily Memorial through Labor Day; Saturday and Sunday only during May, September, and October. Hours of operation vary; be sure to call ahead on your preferred day to splash. $$$$

Thirty-two waterlogged acres packed with twenty-two of the most intense water rides imaginable and appointed with a 1950s San Diego surf theme. Body slides, tube slides, wave pools, beaches, and a kiddy play zone will supply your youth with a water wonderland filled with surprises. Food and snacks available on the premises.

For More Information

Chula Vista Chamber of Commerce. 233 Fourth Avenue, 91910; (619) 420–6603; www.chulavistachamber.org.

Coronado

The beaches of Coronado (translated as Crown City) lie between San Diego Bay and the Pacific. Many people call this an "island," but it is actually a peninsula connected to the mainland on the south by a long, narrow sandbar, the Silver Strand. However, you will want to enter this picturesque city, immensely popular for its boating, swimming, golf, tennis, and sunbathing, by way of the dramatic San Diego–Coronado Bay Bridge. This 2-mile expanse of graceful splendor dates from 1969. The **Ferry Landing Marketplace** has plenty of shopping and dining options to handle your family's needs if you come over by ferry (another pretty option, especially if you just plan on spending the day).

Bikes & Beyond 🚲

1201 First Street at the Ferry Landing Marketplace; (619) 435–7180; www.hollandsbicycles.com. Rates vary; call for current hours and schedules.

Your family's source for rental bicycles, skates, and surreys in Coronado. A super way to explore Crown City.

Where to Stay

Hotel Del Coronado, 1500 Orange Avenue, Coronado; (619) 435–6611 or (800) 468–3533; www.hoteldel.com. "The Del," as the hotel is known here, has attracted the rich and famous, including thirteen U.S. presidents, since its opening in 1888. The turrets, tall cupolas, hand-carved wooden pillars, and Victorian fili-grees of this stunning, magnificently restored 691-room national historic land-mark resort have served as the backdrop for many movies and films. So much his-tory has unfolded within the Del's walls that a cassette walking tour has been made available. For example, at its open-ing more than a century ago, it was the largest structure outside New York City to be electrically lighted, and the installation was supervised by Thomas Edison himself!

Today the Del offers a wide variety of accommodations to suit any family's taste and pays close attention to the needs of children, with special programs, babysit-ting services, and children's menus. Choose from the formal main dining room, two restaurants, and a twenty-four-hour deli. The Del's beach provides great swim-ming and sunbathing, plus rental boats, windsurfers, and paddleboats. Just watch out for some of the smaller, original rooms, and you'll be in grand shape at this venera-ble place. World-renowned and definitely worth a visit! $$$$

Loews Coronado Bay Resort, 4000 Coronado Bay Road, Coronado; (619) 424–4000 or (800) 815–6397; www.loews hotels.com. Located on a private, fifteen-acre peninsula named Crown Island, sur-rounded by water and astonishing views of the downtown San Diego skyline and marina. Five guest-room towers feature 438 very deluxe guest rooms with minibars and fax machines. There are three outdoor pools, whirlpools, and decks, five tennis courts, an exercise club, and a private eighty-slip marina with rentals galore—sailboats, paddleboats, Wave Runners, Jet Skis, and beach equipment.

Most important for your family is the outstanding year-round program called the Commodore Kids Club, offering supervised educational and entertaining options for ages four to twelve provided by fully licensed caregivers. Offered seven days a week, activities change daily and include nature walks, sand-castle building, face painting, arts and crafts, and G-rated video screenings. Full-day, half-day, and evening programs are available. Families with more than one child get to send the second child at half price. Call for current rates.

Kids also enjoy the game room with pinball, video, and Ping-Pong. This pro-gram is a real winner. We think your family will enjoy it enormously. Be sure to call for special holiday programs and value pack-ages that combine SeaWorld and other attractions' tickets, too. A very helpful staff is ready and waiting for your family. Like the slogan says, "Loews Loves Kids," and it shows! $$$$

For More Information

Coronado Visitors Bureau. 1047 B Avenue, 92118–3418; (619) 437–8788 or (800) 622–8300; www.coronado.ca.us.

La Jolla

Heading up the coast along Pacific Coast Highway 1 from Mission Bay and Pacific Beach will lead you directly into the tony suburb of La Jolla (say la-hoy-ya; it's Spanish for "the jewel"). This truly precious area is home of the University of California–San Diego (UCSD) and the distinguished Salk Institute for Biomedical Research. There is also some fabulous real estate along the beaches, coves, and caves; and trendy shopping and dining along downtown's Prospect Avenue, the Rodeo Drive of San Diego.

Birch Aquarium at Scripps Institution of Oceanography

2300 Expedition Way, off La Jolla Village Drive, on the campus of UCSD, overlooking La Jolla and the Pacific; (858) 534–3474; www.aquarium.ucsd.edu. Open daily 9:00 A.M. to 5:00 P.M. except Thanksgiving and Christmas. $$

These facilities are among the most prestigious world leaders in research and instruction. Opened in 1992, they replaced a smaller facility that had been operating since 1951. Inside the aquarium you can see more than 3,000 fish in thirty tanks, including a two-story, 70,000-gallon kelp forest with species from the waters of the West Coast, Mexico's Sea of Cortez, and the South Pacific. There is also a man-made interpretive tide pool. The innovative and interactive museum introduces the world's largest oceanographic exhibition, Exploring the Blue Planet. The bookshop has educational souvenirs and books for all ages on the science of the seas. This attraction strikes an educational counterpoint to the frenetic action of SeaWorld.

Museum of Contemporary Art, La Jolla

700 Prospect Street, La Jolla; (858) 454–3541; www.mcasd.org. Open 11:00 A.M. to 5:00 P.M. daily except Wednesday. Hours change seasonally.

Children can enjoy the outdoor sculpture garden and food court. Everyone will view outstanding examples of minimalist, conceptual, and California art in a beautiful setting.

La Jolla Walking Tours

910 Prospect Street; (719) 535–9636. Departs seasonally from the Colonial Inn. Call for current times and schedule.

Offers ninety-minute to two-hour walking tours of historic buildings and the La Jolla Cove area, teeming with sea and shore life.

For More Information

La Jolla Visitor Center. (Operated by the San Diego Convention and Visitors Bureau)

7966 Herschel Avenue, Suite A, 92037; (619) 236–1212.

North County–
Coastal Communities

Just north of La Jolla along the ocean, be sure to take the drive up Pacific Coast Highway 1/U.S. Highway 101 for a relaxing trip through some classic Southern California beach communities, inhabiting what the locals call North County. The charming seaside hamlets of **Solana Beach, Cardiff-by-the-Sea, Encinitas, Del Mar,** and **Leucadia** have miles of sandy beaches with rocky coves, cliffs above, and lots of friendly folks waiting to welcome you at the small shops, restaurants, and inns in these charming enclaves.

Torrey Pines State Beach and Reserve
North Torrey Pines Road, Del Mar; (858) 755–2063. Open daily 9:00 A.M. to dusk. $

This beach/reserve stretches between La Jolla and Del Mar. Enjoy one of just two places in the world where the Torrey pine tree grows (the other is Santa Rosa Island, near Santa Barbara). A visitor center has interpretive displays, and there are miles of great hiking and nature trails. The beach below is a favorite for swimmers; the cliffs above are a popular take-off spot for hang gliders.

Del Mar Fairgrounds & Race Track
2260 Jimmy Durante Boulevard, Del Mar; (858) 755–1141; www.sdfair.com.

This is where "the turf meets the surf" with two attractions. The San Diego County Fair runs here June 15 through July 4. Then thoroughbreds are off and running July through September. The combined facility is a gorgeous, 350-acre historic site overlooking the Pacific. More than a hundred events are held here each year. Call for this year's schedule. Del Mar Thoroughbred Club, (858) 755–1141 or (858) 793–5533 (info line); www.dmtc .com. Races held July through September, dark Tuesdays. Age 17 and younger **free** but must be accompanied by a parent. Camp Del Mar (www.campdelmar.com) is open every race day for children ages five through twelve. Supervised recreational activities while parents are at the club.

Quail Botanical Gardens
230 Quail Gardens Drive, just east of Interstate 5, Encinitas; (760) 436–3036; www.qb gardens.com. Open daily 9:00 A.M. to 5:00 P.M.; closed major holidays. First Tuesday of every month is free. $$

The gardens contain one of the world's most diverse plant collections, including California natives, exotic tropicals, palms, and bamboo. This site was formerly owned by avid plant collector and naturalist Ruth Baird Larabee, who donated her thirty-acre estate to the public in 1957. The gardens are open for self-guided tours as well as a super chance to see the namesake resident quails in a natural bird refuge.

Hot-Air **Ballooning**

North County is also famous for its hot-air balloon rides. Several companies offer sunrise and sunset flights that feature scenic views of the coastline, rolling hills, and reservoir-dotted valleys. Most companies fly year-round, weather permitting. Rides depart early in the morning or just before dusk and last about an hour. All pilots are FAA certified. Fares start around $135, but package and family plans are offered. Not advised for children age eight or younger. A Skysurfer Balloon Company (858) 481–6800; and California Dreamin' Balloon Adventures (760–438–9550 or 800–373–3359). Call for current prices and schedules.

For More Information

Del Mar Chamber of Commerce. 1104 Camino del Mar, 92014; (858) 755–4844; www.delmarchamber.org.

Encinitas Chamber of Commerce. 138 Encinitas Boulevard, 92024; (760) 753–6041 or (800) 953–6041; www.encinitaschamber.com.

Rancho Santa Fe

If you've had it with hype and just want to reeee-laaaax, the postcard perfect Spanish Colonial–style village of Rancho Santa Fe is known for its quiet, peaceful setting. Go 6 miles inland, amid magnificently fragrant eucalyptus trees. They were planted by the Santa Fe Railroad in hopes they would make great railroad ties—but the wood was too soft to even hold a spike! Today these trees provide a magnificent backdrop for the family-welcoming upscale village.

Where to Eat and Stay

Inn at Rancho Santa Fe, 5951 Linea Del Cielo; (858) 756–1131 or (800) THE–INN–1; www.theinnatranchosantafe.com. Third-generation hotelier Duncan Royce Hadden manages this family-owned and family-friendly inn. On the twenty-two manicured acres there are twenty-three cottages with eighty-nine individually styled accommodations, including many family suites—all set against a magnificent backdrop of eucalyptus. The entire clan can enjoy tennis, croquet on the front lawn, or a swim in the heated outdoor pool. The gym has your basic workout gear, and you can dine in the coffee shop, main dining room, or poolside. The inn even maintains a private guest cottage on the sand at Del Mar. You will feel like rich natives when you and your kids spend a day at the beach, then retreat to the inn. $$$$

Carlsbad

The picturesque beach community of Carlsbad (named for the famous Karlbad spa in Europe) is home to many coves and beautiful lagoons, as well as golf resorts, bistros, inns, and antiques emporiums. LEGOLAND California, a must-do family experience, opened in 1999.

LEGOLAND California (ages 2 to 12 recommended)

One Legoland Drive (just off Interstate 5, exit Cannon Road or Palomar Airport Road and follow signs); (760) 918–LEGO or (877) LEGOLAND; www.legoland.com. Open daily, hours vary seasonally, call for times. $$$$

Opened in March 1999 to well-deserved acclaim, this 128-acre park is the first LEGO-themed facility in the United States. It's worthy to note that Forbes.com named LEGOLAND one of the best theme parks in the world in 2003 and 2004. To celebrate the park's fifth birthday in 2004, five new attractions were added, including the Block of Fame (a gallery of famous busts made of LEGO), Coastersaurus (a Jurassic-themed roller coaster), Dig Those Dinos (an interactive archaeological site), Fun Town Fire Academy (families can test their teamwork), and Miniland USA—a tribute to the state of Florida out of, you guessed it, LEGO bricks! Thirty million plastic LEGO building blocks were used to create the 5,000 models that decorate the park. You and your kids won't believe what can be created out of those little blocks of plastic—and there's lots of opportunity for you to create, too! LEGOLAND is a hands-on, interactive experience for the entire family. No thrilling, chilling rides here—just forty attractions in nine themed "blocks" (The Beginning, Village Green, The Ridge, The Lake, Fun Town—our fave, The Garden, Castle Hill, Miniland, and Imagination Zone), plus restaurants and shops that mix education, a little bit of adventure, and a lot of fun! Be sure to schedule a day to really enjoy LEGOLAND at your kids' pace.

Biplane Rides and Aerial Dogfights/Barnstorming Adventures, Ltd.

6743 Montia Court; (760) 438–7680 or (800) SKY–LOOP; www.barnstorming.com. Open year-round during daylight hours. Call for prevailing winds, schedules, and fees.

Open-air flights in vintage cockpit biplanes and mock aerial combat in military-style aircraft could make for an unforgettable family adventure. All pilots are FAA-certified, and safety comes first, followed by fun! Since 1994, this family-owned business based at Palomar Airport has been committed to preserving and sharing aviation history. Tell "Tailspin Tom" and "Cash Register Kate" we sent you.

Flower Fields at Carlsbad Ranch

East of Interstate 5 at Palomar Airport Road and Paseo del Norte; (760) 431–0352; www.theflowerfields.com. Open March through April generally, during daylight hours. $$

Wear comfortable walking shoes as you and the kids traipse through more than fifty acres of gently sloping hillside covered with a rainbow of buttercups. An incredible sight!

Children's Discovery Museum of North Country (ages 2 to 12)
300 Carlsbad Village Drive #103, in the Village Faire shopping center, corner of Carlsbad Village Drive and U.S. Highway 101; (760) 720–0737. Open Tuesday through Sunday, generally noon to 5:00 P.M., with schedules varying seasonally. Be sure to call ahead. $

North County's first children's museum, this 3,000-square-foot facility opened in 1994 with a kids' supermarket, a medieval castle complete with costumes, and a variety of interactive displays. You'll also find a solar-powered toy train.

Where to Eat

Tip Top Meats & Deli, 6118 Paseo Del Norte, just off Interstate 5 at Palomar Airport Road; (760) 438–2620. Open daily 6:00 A.M. to 8:00 P.M. Don't be fooled by the name—this local favorite offers the best value for miles around. A full breakfast starts at $2.98 (one egg, home-fried potatoes, toast, and ham, bacon or sausage); burgers are $1.98; dinners start at $4.49 (prime rib roast, potatoes, cabbage, sauerkraut, soup or salad, and roll is only $6.98). Just enter through the market and proceed to the deli area, where you'll place your order. Pick a seat in the dining room and wait for your number to be called—and dig in to a tip-top meal! Say hi to owner "Big John" Haedrich for us! $

Where to Stay

Four Seasons Resort Aviara, 7100 Four Seasons Point, Carlsbad; (760) 603–6800; www.fourseasons.com/aviara. Located on a plateau overlooking the Batiquitos Lagoon, a wildlife sanctuary, and the Pacific Ocean, this opulent 331-unit property opened in August 1997 and is rated five-diamond by AAA. The adjacent Aviara Golf Club, designed by Arnold Palmer, opened in 1991 and is ranked in the top ten nationally by golf magazines. Your family can take part in three- or four-day golf

academies to see if you've got a Tiger Woods in the making!

Part of a 1,000-acre master planned community, the resort will remain more than 50 percent open space. In the Spanish Colonial–style main hotel, standard guest rooms are large (average 540 square feet) and feature five-star amenities.

The best feature for families is undoubtedly the Four Seasons' Kids for All Seasons program for ages five to twelve. Upon check-in, kids receive a personal invitation to visit the center and take part in kite flying, swimming and beach games, lagoon nature trail exploration, table games, and other supervised activities. The main pool area is very family-friendly with its adjacent kiddie pool now since the addition of a separate "quiet pool" and whirlpool. Your kids will receive a welcome cookie and milk turn-down treat on their first night as well as children's menus in all the restaurants. Cribs, strollers, high chairs, and playpens are all complimentary, along with a selection of toys to check out. The California Bistro serves three meals daily and should be your choice for the family. Or just indulge in twenty-four-hour room service. You deserve it! $$$$.

Grand Pacific Palisades Resort & Hotel, 5805 Armada Drive (exit Palomar Airport Road east from Interstate 5); (760) 827–3200; www.grandpacificpalisades

.com. Across the street from LEGOLAND, overlooking the Carlsbad Flower Fields and the Pacific Ocean, this should be your family's headquarters for fun in North County. You can leave your car in the hotel parking lot and walk across the street to the side entrance to LEGOLAND. Return during the day for naps and lunch breaks—an ideal way to plan your stay. The contemporary Mediterranean architecture of the hotel encloses ninety spacious hotel rooms and a seventy-one-unit time-share resort. A full-service restaurant, room service, two inviting outdoor heated pools and whirlpools, concierge services, a social activity director, a game room, and a fitness center—all staffed with friendly, helpful people—make this a grand place! $$$

For More Information

Carlsbad Convention and Visitors Bureau. P.O. Box 1246, 92018; (760) 434–6093 or (800) 227–5722; www .carlsbadCA.org.

Oceanside

Bustling Oceanside, at the mouth of the San Luis Rey Valley, is home base to the U.S. Marine Corps' Camp Pendleton (approximately 125,000 acres) and the ever-popular Municipal Pier—California's longest, which planks in at a whopping 1,942 feet. Check out the great fishing, seafood restaurants, and ice-cream shop located on this wooden wonder.

California Surf Museum

223 North Coast Highway, Oceanside; (760) 721–6876; www.surfmuseum.org. Open Thursday through Monday from noon to 4:00 P.M. (unless the surf is awesome!). Call for special events and seasonal operating hours. Free admission.

Everything you wanted to know about surfing—for the novice to learn and for the experienced to enjoy. A real kicked-back gem.

Helgren's Sportfishing

315 Harbor Drive South; (760) 722–2133. Open year-round; call for times and fees.

Take your choice of charter fishing vessels; half-day, full-day, and overnight trip options, as well as whale-watching cruises between December and February.

Mission San Luis Rey

4050 Mission Avenue, 4 miles east of town on State Route 76; (760) 757–3651. Open Monday through Saturday 10:00 A.M. to 4:30 P.M. and Sunday noon to 4:30 P.M. $

This "king of the missions" is number eighteen in the famous chain of twenty-one California churches begun by Father Serra. It's also the largest and has wooden double-dome construction. Picnicking facilities are available on the attractive grounds.

Where to Eat

101 Cafe, 631 South Coast Highway; (619) 722–5220; www.101cafe.net. Open daily from 6:30 A.M. to midnight. Established in 1928, this family diner serves up traditional American-style home-cooked meals. The hamburgers are the best and the milk shakes a dream. There are historic photos all over the walls. Old-fashioned cash only! (But an ATM is available on-site now.) $

Where to Stay

Oceanside Marina Suites, 2008 Harbor Drive North; (760) 722–1561 or (800)

252–2033; www.omihotel.com. Secluded at the tip of Oceanside's bustling harbor, the inn offers sixty-four one- and two-bedroom units with kitchens. Wonderful water views; many units have fireplaces and balconies. A pool, spa, and barbeque area are other highlights. This perfect family waterfront stopover is close to many North County attractions. $$

For More Information

Oceanside Visitor and Tourism Information Center. 928 North Coast Highway, Oceanside, 92054; (760) 721–1101 or (800) 350–7873; www.oceansidechamber.com.

Escondido and Vicinity

Inland from the Pacific, the north-south Interstates 5 and 15 run several miles apart, embracing gently rolling hillsides, forests, and streams that will make you pinch yourself and wonder, "Are we still in California?" In the center of it all is the city of Escondido. Other scenic communities scattered through inland North County include Fallbrook, San Marcos, Poway, Rancho Bernardo, La Costa, Vista, and Valley Center.

Heritage Walk and Escondido's Historical Society Museum

321 North Broadway in Grape Day Park, Escondido; (760) 743–8207; www.escondido historicalsociety.org. Open Thursday through Saturday 1:00 to 4:00 P.M. **Free.**

Includes a Victorian house, Indian metate (grinding stones), a circa 1888 Santa Fe Railroad depot, and the Bandy Blacksmith Shop.

California Center for the Arts

340 North Escondido Boulevard, Escondido; (760) 839–4138 or (800) 988–4253; www.artcenter.org. Call for current programs, schedules, and fees.

This center located on a twelve-acre campus has an art museum, a 1,500-seat concert hall, and art education programs for young people in a world-class facility. Also here is the Escondido Children's Museum, (760) 233–7755; www.escondidochildrensmuseum.org.

Iceoplex

555 North Tulip, Escondido; (760) 489–5550; www.iceoplex.com. Open daily at 8:30 A.M.; closing times vary. $$

This is a massive facility that boasts two Olympic-size ice-skating rinks, a fitness center, a spa, an Olympic lap pool, a Jacuzzi, a sauna, and a training room. You can chill out here after all your fun in the sun!

Westfield Shopping Town North County

272 East Via Rancho Parkway at Interstate 15, Escondido; (760) 489–2332; www.westfield.com. Open daily; call for seasonal hours.

With its 180 specialty shops, fifteen restaurants, and five major department stores, this is one of the largest indoor retail centers in the county. Your family will discover plenty to see, do, and eat here. (We think it makes a great stopover on the way to or from the Wild Animal Park.)

San Diego Wild Animal Park

15500 San Pasqual Valley Road, located 5 miles east of Interstate 15 on State Route 78, just outside Escondido; (760) 747–8702 or (760) 234–6541; www.wildanimalpark.com. Open every day beginning at 9:00 A.M. Closing times vary by season. $$$$

On 2,100 acres of prime sanctuary land, and without a doubt the showpiece of North County, the park was designed originally as a breeding facility for the San Diego Zoo (its sister facility). You and your family will want to spend a day here to see more than 3,000 wild animals roaming freely in settings that resemble their native habitats. Designed for the animals first and foremost, it is the only zoo where the guests are put in cages (specifically, into the comfortable Bush Line electric monorail, which glides above the habitats), while the animals roam unrestrained. You will see large herds of antelopes, gazelles, deer, rhinos, and exotic sheep and goats. Flocks of flamingos, pelicans, cranes, geese, ducks, herons, ostriches, vultures, and storks live in the big enclosures as well. Even the single-species exhibits—herds of African and Asian elephants, families of gorillas and chimpanzees—are large and natural. New in 2004 is a one-acre lion habitat; and returning is DINOS, a life-size robotic dinosaurs display.

The seventeen-acre Nairobi Village holds most of the visitor facilities, including restaurants, gift shops, and picnic areas. Plan to attend the bird show, wild animal show, and elephant demonstrations held here. And make some new friends in the petting kraal.

The Kilimanjaro Hiking Trail is a 1.75-mile walking safari where you can see rhinos, tigers, elephants, cheetahs, and giraffes up close and personal. Special photo caravan safaris will take you right into the middle of the habitats in a large, open-air truck for an additional fee. We cannot recommend this activity highly enough. The chance to pet a rhino or feed a giraffe as it bends over your head is a thrill of a lifetime. We really were impressed and amazed here.

Kit Carson Park/Queen Califia's Magical Circle

3333 Bear Valley Parkway, Escondido; (760) 839–4691; www.queencalifia.org or www.ci.escondido.ca.us/glance/parks/kitcarson/. Open from sunrise to sunset daily. **Free.**

The park was named after Christopher (Kit) Carson, the famous scout who guided Capt. John C. Fremont over the Sierra Nevada during an exploration expedition. This large regional day-use park features 100 developed acres and 185 undeveloped acres, beautiful walking/hiking trails, ball fields, lighted tennis courts, soccer fields, 3,000-seat outdoor amphitheater, three ponds, tot lot/playground, shaded picnic areas with tables/barbecues; Sports Center complex with pro shop, 20,000-square-foot skate park, two full-size roller hockey arenas, one full-size and one mini soccer arena.

Opened in October 2003, Queen Califia's Magical Circle in the Iris Sankey Arboretum is the only American sculpture garden created by the renowned French-American artist Niki de Saint Phalle. The garden's outside diameter measures 120 feet and is encircled by an undulating wall across which slither large, playful serpents decorated in colorfully patterned mosaics. The Snake Wall has one entrance into the garden—a mazelike passageway whose walls and floor are also decorated in bold patterns of black, white, and mirrored tiles. The garden takes its name from the legendary black Amazon queen, Califia, who was believed to rule a terrestrial island paradise of gold and riches. Be sure to include a visit to this amazing, unique structure to indulge your family's magical senses.

The Wave Waterpark

161 Recreation Drive off Broadway, Vista, 7 miles inland on State Route 78; (760) 940–WAVE; www.wave-waterpark.com. Open Memorial Day through Labor Day, 10:30 A.M. to 5:30 P.M. $$$

The state-of-the-art wave maker is called Flow Rider, one of only three in the United States. Your family's dudes (and dudettes) can body surf all day long and never have to wait for that perfect wave—because they're all perfect! Four wild waterslides, an underwater playground, an Olympic-size pool, and a picnic area make this inland water spot a great experience. It's a great value, too.

San Pasqual Battlefield State Historic Park and Museum

15808 San Pasqual Valley Road, Escondido; (760) 737–2201; www.parks.ca.gov. Open Friday through Sunday 10:00 A.M. to 5:00 P.M. **Free.**

The museum honors those who participated in the 1846 San Pasqual Battle during the Mexican-American War. See videos and exhibits regarding that historic time. A dramatic reenactment is held every December.

Antique Gas and Steam Engine Museum

2040 North Santa Fe Avenue, Vista; (760) 941–1791 or (800) 5–TRACTOR; www.agesem.com. Open daily from 10:00 A.M. to 4:00 P.M. $

Weekend threshing bees in June and October are really fun! Our kids were impressed with the blacksmith. Catch a bit of history at the museum. Forty acres of turn-of-the-last-century farming equipment, all maintained in working order. Kids can see actual corn, wheat, and oat crops harvested from the field and into the kitchen.

Where to Eat

Bates Nut Farm, 15954 Woods Valley Road, 3 miles east of Valley Center; (760) 749–3333; www.batesfarm.com. Open daily 9:00 A.M. to 5:00 P.M. This is a family favorite because of its **free** petting zoo, shady picnic grounds, fresh produce, and terribly tasty array of fruits, nuts, and candy. There are arts and crafts fairs each April and November; pumpkins predominate in October, and fir trees in December. $

Where to Stay

Welk Resort, Museum, and Dinner Theatre, 8860 Lawrence Welk Drive, 7 miles north of Escondido off Interstate 15; (760) 749–3000 or (800) 932–9355; www.welk resort.com. Museum open daily at 10:00 A.M.; closing times vary. **Free** admission to museum. Dinner theater performances offer musical variety for the whole family. Call for times, programs, and ticket prices. Not just for Grandma and Grandpa, with their memories of the legendary band leader, this 1,000-acre hideaway with only 132 spacious rooms has all the amenities for a super family vacation retreat. They include on-site golf, tennis, swimming pools, spa, and restaurants featuring kids' menus and all-you-can-eat buffets. Perfect for that multigenerational reunion! $$$$

For More Information

San Diego North County Convention and Visitors Bureau. 720 North Broadway, Escondido, 92025-1899; (760) 745–4741 or (800) 848–3336; www .sandiegonorthcounty.com.

Temecula Valley

The town of Temecula was founded in 1882 and served as an important stop on the Butterfield Stagecoach Route between San Bernardino and San Diego. Today it is a fast-growing community nestled between San Diego and Riverside Counties with some award-winning vineyards, fourteen wineries, horse ranches, seven golf courses, harvest festivals, and superb antiques shops.

Old Town Temecula (🏃) (🔒) (🍴)

Front Street between Moreno Road and Third Street. Open daily, hours vary.

Get a walking tour map and visit the Welty Building, jail, First National Bank, and G. Machado's store. Many of these historic buildings are antiques malls now, sure to delight shoppers. But there's no predicting how long they will grab your kids' attention (before they start acting like the proverbial bull in a china shop). Probably a half hour will do it.

Mission San Antonio de Pala

Pala Mission Road, north of State Route 76, Pala; (760) 742–1600. Open Tuesday through Sunday 10:00 A.M. to 3:00 P.M. $

A branch of the Mission San Luis Rey, it was built in 1816 as part of an inland chain of missions that never really developed. The chapel, gardens, and mineral room have all been restored. Very quaint.

Warner Springs Ranch

31652 Highway 79, Box 10, Warner Springs, 92086; (760) 782–4200; www.warnerhot springs.com or www.warnersprings.com.

With 25,000 acres nestled in the foothills of Palomar Mountain, Warner Springs Ranch offers your family plenty of room to roam. Stay in one of the 240 cozy bungalows (most with fireplaces); no phones or TVs. Miles of scenic walking, horseback riding, and hiking trails. Three pools (one is heated with hot spring water), eighteen-hole championship golf course, health spa, plus a private airport and glider school. High marks for the equestrian program, which is very kid friendly (kids age eight and older on trail rides, age six and older for riding lessons in the arena, and pony rides/animal-care sessions for really young children). Outstanding activities schedule means your kids will never say they're bored!

Where to Eat and Stay

Pala Mesa Resort, 2001 Old Highway 395, off Interstate 15, Fallbrook; (760) 728–5881 or (800) 722–4700; www.palamesa.com. This spacious golf resort is ideal for families, with its 133 connecting rooms, views of rolling hills, eighteen-hole golf course, and irresistible family-size swimming pool. You'll find plenty of outdoor recreation, including horseshoes, croquet, volleyball, tennis, badminton, a whirlpool, and a spa. Alexander's Restaurant is open 6:00 A.M. to 2:00 P.M. and 5:30 to 10:00 P.M. with a nice golf-course view. The early California decor will make you appreciate the reasonably priced children's menu even more. $$$$

Temecula Creek Inn, 44501 Rainbow Canyon Road, Temecula; (909) 694–1000 or (800) 962–7335; www.temeculacreek inn.com. Opened in 1969 and beautifully enhanced and enlarged in 2002, with 130 deluxe rooms and suites overlooking lush grounds that feature Native American art. Golf is king and queen here, with twenty-seven holes (rated 4-star by *Golf Digest*); plus tennis, swimming pools, fitness studio, Temet Grill. Excellent packages for families. $$$$

For More Information

Temecula Valley Chamber of Commerce. 27450 Ynez Road #104, Temecula, 92591; (909) 676–5090 or (888) TEMEC-ULA; www.temecula.org.

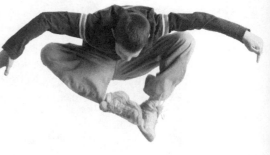

The Mountains (Back Country)

Don't miss the eastern portion of San Diego County, affectionately known by locals as the Back Country. Bisected by three main roads—State Routes 76, 78, and 79—the Back Country offers mountain peaks rising more than 6,000 feet, dazzling foliage in fall, snowfalls in winter (and sometimes even in April!), and desert flora year-round. This land of contrasts has fabulous hiking, biking, camping, and fishing options for your active times and plenty of bucolic beauty for your off-tour hours.

Palomar Mountain Observatory and State Park

From Oceanside, off State Route 76 (about 11 miles inland on County Road S6); (760) 742–2119. Open daily 9:00 A.M. to 4:00 P.M. Free.

For a grand perspective, ascend Mount Palomar (elevation 6,140 feet) to the observatory. Inside this striking white-domed structure, you'll find one of the world's largest scientific instruments—the 200-inch Hale Telescope. You and the kids can watch its inner workings and see a video at the museum nearby describing all the functions of this scientific wonder. Along with the observatory, enjoy the completely uncrowded State Park (760–742–3462 for general information) with thickly forested areas, wildlife, fishing, camping, and hiking trails.

For More Information

San Diego East Visitors Bureau. 5005 Willows Road, Suite 208, Alpine, 91901; (619) 445–0180 or (800) 463–0668; www.visitsandiegoeast.com.

Julian and Vicinity

For a piece of living history, continue toward the interior of North County along State Route 78, and you'll arrive at Julian. In the hills only 60 miles inland from Oceanside, Julian lies in the heart of the Cleveland National Forest. Some wooded areas were destroyed in the devastating fires of October 2003, but certainly not the pioneering, friendly spirit of this wonderful town. Beautiful downtown Julian looks much as it did a century ago. It was founded in 1870 by settlers Drew Bailey and his cousin Mike Julian, hence the name. A gold strike yielding nearly $5 million made the town of Julian famous back in the 1870s. When the gold rush ended, apples became the cash crop of choice. Now Julian is famous for hillside acres of apple orchards (Julian is known as Southern California's apple capital) and beautiful fields of spring wildflowers. The 2-block-long Main Street and surrounding area has everything you'll want within easy walking distance. Yes, you are still in Southern California (just an early 1900s version!).

Eagle Mining Company

North end of C Street, downtown; (760) 765–0036. Open daily 10:00 A.M. to 3:00 P.M., weather permitting. $$

Guided tours through this old gold mine will show you how those shiny, precious flakes were extracted from Mother Earth. A fascinating journey into the mountainside for the entire family.

Julian Pioneer Museum

2811 Washington Street; (760) 765–0227. Open Tuesday through Sunday 10:00 A.M. to 4:00 P.M. April through November, on weekends the rest of the year. $

Housed in a late 1800s structure, the museum shows you and the kids what life in early Julian was like.

Cuyamaca Rancho State Park

15027 Highway 79, south of Julian; (760) 765–0755. Open daily year-round. $$

Twenty-five thousand acres of beautiful terrain include pine, oak, and cedar trees; meadows; lakes; streams; and the Green Valley waterfall. Explore via 10 miles of trails for mountain biking, hiking, and horseback riding. You can see more than a hundred species of birds in the area, or perhaps even a mule deer or coyote. The park has a visitor center, gift shop, and a museum depicting the gold rush days at the Stonewall Mine during its 1886–1891 peak. We love just going for a simple picnic.

Mission Santa Ysabel

23013 Highway 79, Santa Ysabel; (760) 765–0810. Open daily 7:00 A.M. to dusk. Free.

You can take a self-guided tour of this charming satellite mission built in 1818. There is also an Indian burial ground and museum. It's a pleasant stopover on your way to Julian.

Seeing Julian in **Slow Motion**

Our favorite way to see Julian is by way of **Country Carriages** (760–765–1471), located right downtown on Main Street. To get your bearings on the area, begin with a ride on a horse-drawn carriage, all hitched up and ready to go. A thirty-minute clop-clop trip around town costs $25 per couple with two children—worth it for the history lesson alone. After your buggy ride, stay in the old-fashioned mood with an ice-cream treat at **Ye Olde Soda Fountain** at the **Julian Drug Store.** Kids of all ages love the chance to sit on the old-fashioned stools and see how such classics as an egg creme or black cow are made by hand.

Where to Eat

Dudley's Bakery and Snack Bar, On Highway 78 in downtown Santa Ysabel; (760) 765–0488; www.dudleysbakery.com. Open Wednesday through Sunday, hours vary seasonally. Here you will find an incredible selection of seventeen famous breads, plus cookies, pies, and yummy pastries. This is a great place to have breakfast or lunch with your family and pick up treats for later. Don't miss this place. It's usually jammed, so you won't be able to! $

The Julian Grille, 2224 Main Street; (760) 765–0173. Housed in a homey cottage, the restaurant serves lunch daily and dinner Tuesday through Saturday. The menu features steaks, pasta, and seafood your family will savor. $$

Where to Stay

Pine Hills Lodge and Dinner Theatre, 2960 La Posada Way, Julian; (760) 765–1100; www.pinehillslodge.com. Call for schedule and admission prices. A must-stop for vintage Back Country food and family entertainment. Every Friday and Saturday evening, a fantastic barbecue dinner of baked chicken and baby back ribs is accompanied by locally cast Pine Hills Players musical presentations. A variety of rustic and recently refurbished accommodations are offered in eighteen lodge and cabin units at reasonable rates. $$$

For More Information

Julian Chamber of Commerce. 2129 Main Street; (760) 765–1857; www.julianca.com.

Borrego Springs

This peaceful resort community is located inside the Anza-Borrego Desert State Park and has a wide variety of lodging, camping, dining, golf, and recreation options. The community hosts a Grapefruit Festival in April. The Borrego Days Festival in October includes a parade and an arts and crafts fair to welcome back snowbirds for the warm winter season. We think the best time to visit the area is during the spring, when desert wildflowers are in magnificent bloom.

Anza-Borrego Desert State Park

Approximately two hours east of downtown San Diego, just west of County Road S22 and surrounding the quaint town of Borrego Springs. The visitor center is located at 200 Palm Canyon Drive; (760) 767–4205 for general information or (760) 767–4684 for recorded wildflower information; www.anzaborrego.statepark.org. Open daily October through May 9:00 A.M. to 5:00 P.M.; rest of year open only on Saturday and Sunday. Camping fees vary and reservations are strongly suggested. $

This is the biggest state park in the United States, with 600,000 acres of wildly rugged mountains (highest elevation 6,000 feet) and desert (elevation 40 feet), along with flora, fauna, and fossils dating back 540 million years. You will see mesquite, yucca, and smoke trees, cacti, and thousands of native plants and flowers.

Finding **Hotel Values**

San Diego Hotel Reservations (800–SAVE–CASH; www.savecash.com) or Sights of San Diego Hotel Reservations (800–434–7894; www.booksandiego .com). Super helpful hotel reservation assistance at no charge. Firms represent 200-plus properties in the entire county and can book the price range, location, and style of hotel that's perfect for your family.

Start your visit at the magnificent 7,000-square-foot visitor center, built into the hillside, with exhibits, maps, natural history books, a twenty-minute video presentation, and volunteers who are eager to help your family plan your desert experience. There are nature walks, campfire programs, fossil programs, and guided hikes to choose from. The park is geared for off-road travel and exploration. The most dramatic and popular attraction is the spring wildflowers. Our favorite hikes include the Borrego Palm Canyon Nature Trail, a gentle 3-mile round-trip, as well as the Pygmy Trail, a 1-mile round-trip that leads to fifty short palm trees. Among the park's many other points of interest: the Box Canyon Historical Monument, Coyote Canyon, the Culp Valley Overlook, the Elephant Tree Discovery Trail, the Mason Valley Cactus Garden, and the Vallecita Stagecoach Station.

San Diego County, with its rich Spanish and Mexican heritage and American spirit, is a world-class destination with an ideal climate, fantastic natural wonders, and enough excitement to create a wonderfully satisfying family adventure. Adios!

Anza-Borrego **Junior Ranger Program**

This program will deepen your seven- to twelve-year-olds' appreciation of nature. It is the ultimate outdoor adventure for kids since parents are NOT allowed! On Saturday and Sunday during winter and spring, you can drop off your children at the visitor center for supervised activities in the park. Kids receive a log book to record their visit. Best of all, the Junior Ranger program is **Free!** Call the park for current times and a schedule at (760) 767–4205.

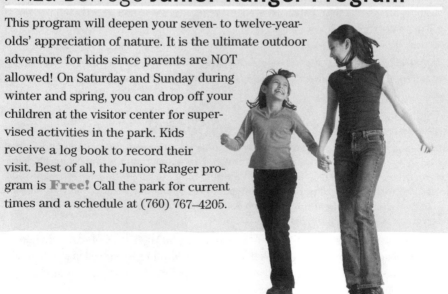

Where to Eat and Stay

La Casa Del Zorro Desert Resort, 3845 Yaqui Pass Road, Borrego Springs; (760) 767–5323 or (800) 824–1884; www.lacasa delzorro.com. Any of the two- or three-bedroom casitas (homes) will have you and your family feeling totally relaxed within hours at this forty-two-acre resort. Each bedroom has its own bath (such an advantage) and some casitas even have a private pool. This historic desert resort started in 1937 and is renowned as a haven of rest and tranquility. It is rated with four stars by Mobil and four diamonds by AAA. You can't go wrong choosing from any of the seventy-seven accommodations, in the value season starting as low as $60 per night. On the property, you'll find a putting green, three heated pools, whirlpools, and six lighted tennis courts. The restaurant serves all three meals daily, surrounded by beautiful views and early California decor. It's a great family destination getaway. $$$$

For More Information

Borrego Springs Chamber of Commerce. P.O. Box 420, Borrego Springs, 92004; (760) 767–5555 or (800) 559–5524; www.borregosprings.org.

Tijuana (Baja California, Mexico) Tourism and Convention Bureau. P.O. Box 434523, San Diego, 92143-4523, or call the office in Mexico direct by dialing 011 52 66/84–05–37, or access www.tijuana.com.

Crossing the Border into Mexico at Tijuana

Fifteen miles south of downtown San Diego is the border town of San Ysidro, California, the U.S. gateway to Tijuana, Baja California, and the rest of Mexico. San Ysidro, with its largely Hispanic population, provides services to American travelers bound for Baja as well as Mexican nationals leaving and entering California. This highly commercialized sector has signs in both English and Spanish. San Ysidro Boulevard leads directly to the border crossing. It's filled with Mexican-style stores, eateries, auto insurance dealers, pawn shops, and money-exchange houses. (Even though the U.S. dollar is widely accepted in Tijuana, you will need pesos farther into Mexico.) Keep in mind that Tijuana is the world's busiest port of entry with more than 60 million border crossings each year. The city itself is bursting with more than 1.2 million people in a semi-developed country with rapidly changing economics and politics.

You can cross the border on foot (we recommend you leave your car in one of the secured parking lots) or by car (not recommended for day trips, since you need to purchase Mexican auto insurance). The San Diego Trolley

(Blue Line) from downtown provides the easiest access since it terminates at the San Ysidro border crossing. The cost is only $2.50 each way (phone 619–234–1060 for schedules). Interstates 5 and 15 also terminate at the border, along with many of the amenities we take for granted.

Tijuana is a duty-free zone, which makes the city very popular for bargain shoppers seeking hand-crafted jewelry, pottery, and leather products. U.S. residents may return home with up to $400 worth of merchandise, including one liter of alcoholic beverages, 100 cigars, and 200 cigarettes (providing the person is twenty-one). Some merchandise, particularly fruits and vegetables, is not allowed into the United States. Tijuana's diverse shopping, dining, and entertainment options are not necessarily geared for everyone in your family, but the city does offer a sampling of cultural diversity and exposure to a bustling Mexican border town.

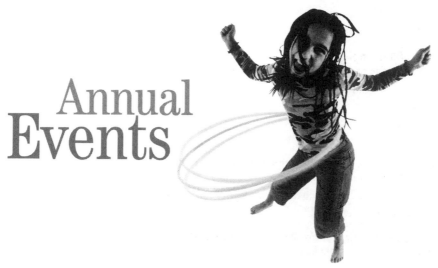

Annual Events

The Central Coast

The Central Coast covers a lot of wonderful territory, but your Southern California family fun has only just begun! These events are subject to change without notice. Please call ahead.

JANUARY

Winter Bird Festival—Morro Bay.
(805) 772–4467 or (800) 231–0592.
Guided tours of estuary and surrounding areas; plentiful bird-watching. **Free.**

FEBRUARY

Whale Celebration—Ventura.
(805) 644–0169.
Celebrate the annual gray whale migration with music and entertainment, environmental booths, and touch tanks in Ventura Harbor Village. **Free.**

International Film Festival—Santa Barbara.
(805) 963–0023.
Premieres and screenings of independent U.S. and international films; gala opening, workshops and seminars by film professionals. Admission fees vary.

Celebration of the Whales—Oxnard.
(805) 385–7545 or (800) 269–6273; fax (805) 385–7571.
Weekend celebration highlights gray whale migration; full-day trips, arts and crafts, and photo exhibit. **Free.**

MARCH

Taste of Solvang—Solvang.
(805) 688–6144 or (800) 458–6765; fax (805) 688–8620.

Food festival features dessert showcase, walking smorgasbords, world's largest Danish pastry, and entertainment. Fees vary.

APRIL

Ventura County Food and Wine Festival—Oxnard.
(805) 985–4852; fax (805) 994–4852.

Waterfront festival featuring fine foods from local restaurants accompanied by musical entertainment. Fees vary.

I Madonnari Italian Street Painting Festival—San Luis Obispo.
(805) 781–2777; fax (805) 543–1255.

Event features sidewalk and street pastel creations. **Free.**

Children's Day in the Plaza—San Luis Obispo.
(805) 781–2777; fax (805) 543–1255.

More than forty booths featuring spin art, water toys, face painting, and a petting zoo; singers, dancers, clowns, and jugglers. **Free.**

Presidio Day—Santa Barbara.
(805) 966–1279.

Celebration of early California arts, crafts, and music at historic 1782 Presidio Park. **Free.**

MAY

Garden Festival—San Luis Obispo.
(805) 781–2777; fax (805) 543–1255.

Floral displays and sale at a judges' show with speakers, exhibits, demonstrations, children's activities, music, and commercial and gardening booths. **Free.**

Annual California Strawberry Festival—Oxnard.
(805) 385–7578; fax (805) 486–2553.

Strawberry foods, contests, music, and arts and crafts.

I Madonnari Street Painting Festival—Santa Barbara.
(805) 569–3873.

More than 200 local artists and children create chalk paintings in front of the Old Mission; Italian market and entertainment. **Free.**

JUNE

Summer Solstice Celebration—Santa Barbara.
(805) 965–3396.

(See complete description on page 24.) **Free.**

Seafest—Ventura.
(805) 644–0169.

Celebrate the beginnings of summer with entertainment booths, environmental instruction, a chowder cook-off, and a children's harbor land and show.

Elks Rodeo and Parade—Santa Maria.
(805) 922–6006.

Calf roping, bull riding, bronco riding, steer wrestling, and barrel racing.

JULY

Fireworks by the Sea—Oxnard.
(805) 385–7545 or (800) 269–6273; fax (805) 385–7571.

Family-oriented daytime activities (arts and crafts, entertainment, and more), concluding
with a fireworks display over the water. **Free.**

Fourth of July Celebration—Ventura.
(800) 333–2989; fax (805) 698–2150.

Parade, street fair with 8 blocks of arts and crafts, food and entertainment; fireworks in
the evening. **Free.**

Santa Barbara County Fair—Santa Maria.
(805) 925–8824.

Country fair includes carnival, produce, livestock, and western music.

AUGUST

Olde Towne Fair—Lompoc.
(805) 736–4567 or (800) 240–0999.

Celebrate Lompoc's century-plus history with children's events, live music and entertainment, and an arts and crafts fair. **Free.**

California Mid-State Fair—Paso Robles.
(805) 239–0655 or (800) 909–FAIR; fax (805) 238–5308.

The Central Coast fair includes five stages of entertainment featuring top names daily,
PRCA rodeo, Destruction Derby, animal exhibits, arts and crafts, a working farm, wine tasting, pig races, and nightly dancing. Admission fees vary.

Annual Salsa Festival—Oxnard.
(805) 483–4542.

Salsa-making contest, 5k run, arts and crafts, dancing, music, and a carnival for children.
Free.

Old Spanish Days (Fiesta)—Santa Barbara.
(805) 962–8101.

(See complete description on page 25.) **Free.**

Ventura County Fair—Ventura.
(805) 648–3376 or (800) 333–2989; fax (805) 648–1012.
Traditional county fair features top-name entertainment, exhibits, livestock, motor sports, rodeo, food, and fireworks. Admission fees vary.

SEPTEMBER

Taste of the Town—Santa Barbara.
(805) 892–5556.
More than sixty local restaurants and wineries provide tastes of their best fare in the beautiful Riveria Research Park overlooking the city. Always held the first Sunday after Labor Day as a benefit for the local branch of the Arthritis Foundation. Ticket prices vary.

Simi Valley Days—Simi Valley.
(805) 581–4280.
Fair features a carnival, hoedown, barn dance, horse show, parade, 5k and 10k runs, food, and entertainment. Admission fees vary.

Danish Days—Solvang.
(805) 688–6636 or (800) 468–6765.
Celebration of Solvang's rich Danish heritage features Danish folk dancing, music, food, parade, and entertainment. **Free.**

California Beach Festival—Ventura.
(805) 654–7830 or (800) 333–2989; fax (805) 643–4555.
Three stages of entertainment, food, a surfing contest, and beach volleyball. **Free.**

OCTOBER

California Avocado Festival—Carpinteria.
(805) 684–0038.
Avocado celebration includes food, arts and crafts, music, and a flower show. **Free.**

Lemon Festival—Goleta.
(805) 967–4618; fax (805) 967–4615.
Family event featuring a lemon pie–eating contest, food, arts and crafts show, children's activities, farmers' market, and entertainment. **Free.**

NOVEMBER

Holiday Walk and Light the Downtown—Paso Robles.
(805) 238–4103; fax (805) 238–4103.
Lighted trees, candlelight caroling, farmers' market, and Santa and Mrs. Claus. **Free.**

DECEMBER

Winterfest—Solvang.
(805) 688–6144; fax (805) 688–8620.
Danish Village celebration features thousands of twinkling lights. **Free.**

Holiday Parade—San Luis Obispo.
(805) 541–0286; fax (805) 781–2647.

Holiday celebration includes floats, marching bands, youth organizations, and Santa Claus. **Free.**

Ventura Harbor Parade of Lights—Ventura.
(805) 644–0169 or (800) 333–2989.

Colorful parade of decorated lighted boats on Ventura Harbor. **Free.**

Christmas Lite Parade—Paso Robles.
(805) 238–4101; fax (805) 238–4029.

Christmas parade includes youth organization, merchant floats, bands, and Santa Claus. **Free.**

Holiday Boat Parade of Lights—Oxnard.
(805) 389–9495 or (800) 269–6273.

Lighted boat parade in the Channel Islands Harbor, holiday activities, and entertainment. **Free.**

Greater Los Angeles

The following list of Greater Los Angeles–area events is subject to change without notice. Please always call ahead to verify.

JANUARY

Tournament of Roses Parade—Pasadena.
(626) 449–4100; fax (626) 449–9066.

World-class parade of flowers features music and fantasy. The annual Rose Bowl game follows.

Dr. Martin Luther King Day Parade and Festival—Long Beach.
(562) 570–6816.

Parade, entertainment, and celebrations. **Free.**

Martin Luther King Jr. Celebration—Santa Monica.
(310) 434–4209; fax (310) 450–2387.

Interfaith celebrations with music, dramatic readings, and inspirational messages. **Free.**

Golden Dragon Parade—Los Angeles.
(213) 617–0396; fax (213) 617–2128.

Chinese New Year parade. Colorful floats, multicultural performances, arts and crafts. **Free.**

APRIL

Los Angeles Times Festival of Books.
(213) 237–5000; www.latimes.com.

More than 500 exhibitors and 400 authors, speakers, and celebrity presentations, plus a giant children's area, all take over the UCLA campus for the weekend. For the love of reading, don't miss this! **Free.**

Toyota Grand Prix—Long Beach.
(562) 436–3645 or (800) 4LB–STAY.

International field of world-class drivers and high-performance race cars negotiate the tight turns of the city in heated wheel-to-wheel competition.

Pasadena Spring Art Show—Pasadena.
(626) 795–9311; fax (626) 795–9656.

Fine arts and crafts, children's amusement area, international food court. **Free.**

Glory of Easter—Garden Grove.
12141 Lewis Street; (714) 971–4000; fax (714) 750–3836.

An annual Easter play with a cast of over 200 features special effects and live animals.

MAY

Cinco de Mayo—Los Angeles.
(213) 485–6855; fax (213) 485–5238.

Celebrate Mexico's 1862 victory over French forces in Pueblo, Mexico, with popular and traditional music, cultural presentations, dancing, and ethnic cuisine. **Free.**

Museums of the Arroyo Day—Los Angeles.
(626) 796–2898; fax (626) 304–9652.

Open houses for the Southwest Heritage, Lummis, Pasadena Historical, and Gamble House Museums, with each one offering activities, exhibits, and entertainment. **Free.**

Old Pasadena Summer Fest—Pasadena.
(626) 797–6803; fax (626) 797–3241.

Festival includes Taste of Pasadena, arts and crafts, children's activities, jazz festival, and entertainment. **Free.**

JUNE

San Fernando Valley Fair—Burbank.
(818) 557–1600; fax (818) 557–0600.

Live entertainment, rodeo, agricultural education, competitive exhibits, a carnival, arts and crafts, and an international food court.

Theater and Arts Festival—North Hollywood.
(818) 508–5115 or (818) 508–5156.

More than fifteen theaters host two days of live theater and entertainment, arts and crafts, food booths, and a children's court. **Free.**

JULY

Fireworks Extravaganza—Long Beach.
(562) 435–3511.
Features strolling entertainment and fireworks display. **Free.**

Celebration on the Colorado Street Bridge—Pasadena.
(626) 441–6333; fax (626) 441–2917.
Festival features bands, local restaurants, classic autos and motorcycles, art exhibits, and performance groups.

Art Festival—Malibu.
(310) 456–9025; fax (310) 456–0195.
Live music, food fair, orchid display and sale, pancake breakfast, and more than 200 artists on hand with exhibits. **Free.**

San Fernando Fiesta.
(818) 898–1200.
San Fernando's largest family event, including food, games, carnival rides, top-name Latin entertainment, and a consumer trade show. **Free.**

Fourth of July Celebration—Avalon.
(310) 510–1520.
Golf cart parade, dinner, and fireworks over Avalon Bay.

Lotus Festival—Los Angeles.
(213) 485–8745.
Experience a variety of Asian cultures, entertainment, art exhibits, ethnic cuisine, and children's activities.

Celebrate America—Santa Monica.
(310) 452–9209.
Celebrate July 4 Santa Monica style with music, booths, and spectacular fireworks. **Free.**

AUGUST

Catalina Ski Race—Long Beach.
(714) 994–4572.
World's largest water-ski race involving 110 boats pulling skiers from Long Beach's Belmont Pier to Catalina.

Taste of San Pedro—San Pedro.
(310) 832–7272; fax (310) 832–0685.
San Pedro restaurants present their signature entrees. Arts and crafts and a vintage car show are other highlights.

African Marketplace and Cultural Faire—Los Angeles.
(323) 734–1164; fax (323) 485–1610.

More than 2,000 performing artists, 300 vendors and exhibitors, 15 cultural and ethnic festivals, 7 stages of live performers, an international food court, and a children's village.

SEPTEMBER

Catalina Festival of the Arts—Avalon.
(310) 510–2700.

Exhibits include mixed media, photography, crafts, and sculpture. **Free.**

Los Angeles County Fair—Pomona.
(909) 623–3111; fax (900) 865–3602.

California's sensational county fair you can't miss! It takes at least a full day to visit the flower and garden exposition, midway, and various entertainments. Kids can participate in educational activities.

Greek Festival—Arcadia.
(626) 499–6943; fax (626) 449–6974.

Authentic Greek festival with food, pastries, folk dances, music, dance lessons, and children's games.

OCTOBER

Catalina Jazz Festival—Avalon.
(818) 347–5299; www.jazztrax.com.

Contemporary jazz musicians and instrumentalists perform in the renowned Catalina Casino ballroom.

Lobster Festival—Redondo Beach.
(310) 374–2171.

Lobster feed, dancing, entertainment, kids' games, Pirate Camp, crafts, and seafood specialty booths.

Scandinavian Festival—Santa Monica.
(626) 795–9311; fax (626) 795–9656.

Daylong smorgasbord celebrates the riches of Denmark, Finland, Iceland, Norway, and Sweden with food, music, imports, costumes, arts, crafts, and a raffle.

Industry Hills Pro Rodeo—City of Industry.
(626) 961–6892; fax (626) 961–0691.

PRCA rodeo event, petting zoo, clowns, food and beverages, and western-theme concessions.

Village Venture Street Fair—Claremont.
(909) 624–1681; fax (909) 624–6629.

Arts and crafts, food, costumes, pumpkins, children's parade, and Halloween-decorating contests. **Free.**

Oktoberfest—Huntington Beach.
(714) 895–8020; fax (714) 895—6011.
Old World village celebrates entire month with German food, drinks, and oompah bands.
Free.

Octoberfest—Pasadena.
(626) 795–9311.
Music, dancing, German food, games, and a pumpkin patch. **Free.**

Sabor De Mexico Lindo Festival—Huntington Park.
(323) 585–1155; www.hpchamber1.com.
Cultural celebration that pays tribute to the heritage of Mexico, through music, dancing, food, displays, and arts and crafts. The festival brings together more than 125 food, arts and crafts, and commercial exhibitors, plus concerts, live entertainment, two amusement and carnival areas, and a petting zoo. Three days and nights. **Free.**

NOVEMBER

Doo Dah Parade—Pasadena.
(626) 795–9311; fax (626) 795–9656.
Eccentric parade features unique performing groups and artist teams; includes wacky costumes and cars. **Free.**

The Fabulous Christmas Lane—Huntington Park.
(323) 585–1155; www.hpchamber1.com.
This parade features professionally built floats designed with the parade's annual theme. Giant character balloons, equestrians, marching bands, colorful dance ensembles, plus other specialty units.

DECEMBER

Main Street Merchants Holiday Festival—Santa Monica.
(310) 395–3648.
Sand sledding, face painting, and loads of holiday festivities kids will enjoy. **Free.**

Christmas Parade—Whittier.
(562) 696–2662; fax (562) 696–3763.
Bands, floats, horses, and Santa. **Free.**

Holiday Open House—Avalon.
(310) 510–2414.
Each year the Catalina Island Museum hosts open house at the Inn at Mount Ada, formerly the Wrigley Mansion. The mansion is exquisitely decorated for Christmas. The event culminates with a raffle of an all-expense paid stay at the inn to benefit the Catalina Island Museum. **Free.**

The Hollywood Christmas Parade.
(323) 469–2337.

This festive parade features celebrities, marching bands, classic cars, and, last but not least, Santa Claus!

The Glory of Christmas at the Crystal Cathedral—Garden Grove.
(714) 544–5697.

A blending of Christmas carols, live animals, flying angels, and special effects brings the nativity to life in this highly orchestrated stage show.

Orange County

The following list of Orange County events is subject to change without notice. Please call ahead to confirm.

FEBRUARY

Festival of Whales—Dana Point.
(800) 290–DANA.

Coastal whale-watching cruises and arts/crafts exhibition. **Free.**

MARCH

Swallows Day—San Juan Capistrano.
(949) 248–2048.

This fiesta celebrates the annual return of the swallows to Capistrano, featuring pageantry, entertainment, and food.

APRIL

Glory of Easter—Garden Grove.
(714) 971–4069.

This annual Easter play features special events, live animals, and a cast of more than 200 in the dramatic presentation of the last seven days of Christ on earth.

MAY

Strawberry Festival—Garden Grove.
(714) 638–0981.

Festival features strawberry dishes, including strawberry shortcake, pie, and tarts, entertainment, beauty contests, arts, crafts, and rides. **Free.**

JULY

Sawdust Art Festival—Laguna Beach.
(949) 494–3030; fax (949) 494–7390.

Laguna Beach becomes a magical village created by artists. The two-month (July and August) festival includes handcrafted treasures, entertainment, jugglers, storytellers, and jazz, country, rock, and contemporary musicians. Become an artist yourself by attending one of the many hands-on workshops.

Fourth of July Celebration—Huntington Beach.
(714) 536–5496; fax (714) 374–1551.

Red, white, and blue bash with a 5k run, parade, and fireworks. **Free.**

Festival of Arts and Pageant of the Masters—Laguna Beach.
(949) 494–1145 or (800) 487–3378; fax (949) 494–9387.

Colorful exhibit of fine, strictly original creations by 160 South Coast artists; includes the world-famous Pageant of the Masters "living pictures" performances.

Orange County Fair—Costa Mesa.
(949) 708–1543; fax (949) 641–1360.

This rural fair in an urban setting offers livestock, a carnival, a rodeo, commercial wares, themed attractions, and fiber arts.

AUGUST

U.S. Open of Surfing—Huntington Beach.
(714) 366–4584; fax (714) 366–9224.

Watch the best surfers in the world compete for a large sum. **Free.**

SEPTEMBER

Taste of Newport Beach—Newport Beach.
(949) 729–4400; fax (949) 729–4417.

Savor the cuisine of more than thirty Newport Beach restaurants; entertainment.

OCTOBER

Oktoberfest—Huntington Beach.
(714) 895–8020.

Old World Village features German food, drink, and oompah bands. **Free.**

NOVEMBER

Sawdust Art Festival Winter Fantasy—Laguna Beach.
(949) 494–3030; fax (949) 494–7390.

Unique holiday arts and crafts festival features 150 artists and craftspeople from around the country, with artist demonstrations, hands-on workshops, children's art activities, continuous entertainment, Santa Claus, and a snow playground. Continues through December.

DECEMBER

Glory of Christmas—Garden Grove.
(949) 544–5679.

Live Nativity scene includes animals, flying angels, holiday music, and pageantry.

Christmas Boat Parade—Newport Beach.
(949) 729–4400 or (949) 729–4417 or (800) 94–COAST.

More than 200 illuminated and decorated boats cruise the harbor. **Free.**

Christmas at the Mission—San Juan Capistrano.
(949) 248–2048.

Holiday celebration includes music, entertainment, and refreshments. **Free.**

The Inland Empire and Beyond

The following list of events in the Inland Empire is subject to change. Please always call ahead.

FEBRUARY

Civil War Reenactment—Calico.
(760) 254–2122 or (800) TO–CALICO.

Features living-history displays, drills, and music.

Whiskey Flats Days—Kernville.
(760) 376–2629 or (800) 350–7393; fax (760) 376–4371.

Parade, carnival, rodeo, gunfighters, various contests, frog jumping, arts and crafts, a petting zoo, and much to eat. **Free.**

MARCH

Calico Hullabaloo—Calico.
(760) 254–2122 or (800) TO–CALICO.

Relive the rough-and-ready days of old Calico with greased-pole climbing, arm wrestling, and lots more.

Redlands Bicycle Classic—Redlands.
(909) 798–0865.

Thousands of cyclists from around the world compete. **Free.**

Winterfest—Mammoth Lakes.
(760) 934–6643 or (800) 367–6572.

Winter celebration with cross-country ski races, snowmobile competition, and fun rides for the kids.

APRIL–MAY

Ramona Pageant—Hemet.
(909) 658–3111 or (800) 645–4465; fax (909) 658–BOWL.

Unique outdoor pageant portrays the lives of the Southern California mission-period Indians and Hispanics. Play adapted from Helen Hunt Jackson's 1884 novel *Ramona*.

Indian Pow Wow—Kernville.
(760) 376–2696 or (800) 350–7393.

A celebration of American heritage, dancers, drumming, Native American foods, arts and crafts. **Free.**

Orange Blossom Festival—Riverside.
(800) 382-8202.

This citrus celebration takes place in downtown Riverside. Besides three entertainment stages, citrus cooking demonstrations, and arts and crafts booths, the festival has a children's grove and a living-history village.

MAY

May Trout Classic—Big Bear Lake.
(909) 585–6260 or (800) 4–BIG–BEAR.

Fishing competition.

Spring Aire Arts and Crafts Faire—Big Bear Lake.
(909) 585–3000; fax (909) 584–2886.

Show features hundreds of handcrafted items. Vendors, raffles, and loads of antiques.

JUNE

Huck Finn's Jubilee—Victorville.
(760) 245–2226.

River celebration and campout relives the life and times of Huckleberry Finn. Raft building, parade, big-top circus, hot-air balloon rides, music, crafts, and more. **Free.**

JULY

All Nations Pow Wow—Big Bear.
(909) 584–9394 or (800) BIG–BEAR.

American Indians from across the United States participate in traditional dancing and crafts.

Fourth of July Festivities—Mammoth Lakes.
(760) 924–2360 or (800) 367–6572.

Fireworks (of course!), a parade, a pancake breakfast, an arts and crafts show, a chili cook-off, a quilt show, and a horseshoe tournament. What, no barbecue?

July 4 Fireworks Over the Lake—Big Bear.
(909) 866–2112 or (800) BIGBEAR.
Barbecue, entertainment, and spectacular fireworks.

Jazz Jubilee—Mammoth Lakes.
(760) 934–2478; fax (760) 934–2478.
World-class jazz bands perform outdoors.

Sierra Summer Festival—Mammoth Lakes.
(760) 934–3342 or (800) 367–6572.
Music festival spotlights master's classes, plus chamber, pop, and folk music.

AUGUST

Labor Day Arts and Crafts Festival—Mammoth Lakes.
(760) 873–7242.
More than seventy arts and crafts booths in an outdoor setting, along with entertainment, kids' activities, and lots of food.

SEPTEMBER

Apple Harvest—Oak Glen.
(909) 797–6833.
Southern California's top apple-growing region is the site for this event, with apple picking, a candy factory, hay rides, crafts on display, an art show, and (yum!) barbecues. **Free.**

Eastern Sierra Tri-County Fair and Wild West Rodeo—Bishop.
(760) 873–3588.
Old-fashioned country-fair fun, with exhibits, a carnival, pig races, pony rides, a petting zoo, horse shows, and a PRCA rodeo.

Fall Festival Arts and Crafts—Big Bear Lake.
(909) 585–3000; fax (909) 584–2886.
Hundreds of handcrafted items on display.

Fiesta Days—Morongo Valley.
(760) 363–7242.
A small-town fair that offers music, food, and arts and crafts. **Free.**

Kern County Fair—Bakersfield.
(805) 833–4900; fax (805) 836–2743.
Family entertainment par excellence, a livestock show, a carnival, agricultural and floricultural exhibits, plus an auction.

Rodeo Stampede—Barstow.
(760) 252–3093; fax (760) 252–3093.
PRCA rodeo.

OCTOBER

Calico Days Festival—Calico.
(760) 254–2122 or (800) TO–CALICO.

Go back in time to Calico's glory years with a Wild West parade, a gunfight, stunts, burro races, rock pulling, and games circa the 1880s.

Desert Empire Fair—Ridgecrest.
(760) 375–8000.

Five-day event with 4-H competition, arts and crafts, entertainment, a rodeo, a demolition derby, and a livestock auction.

Mardi Gras Parade—Barstow.
(760) 256–8657.

Halloween parade includes floats, bands, horses, clowns, costumed children, plus contingents from the military, fire, and sheriff's departments.

Oktoberfest—Big Bear Lake.
(909) 866–4607.

Music, singing, dancing, contests, arts and crafts, food, and games in a mountain setting. *Wunderbar!*

Wild West Daze Rodeo—Kernville.
(760) 378–3157.

Wild horse races, bull riding, saddle bronco-ing, bareback riding, steer decorating, barrel racing, and mutton busting.

NOVEMBER

Gem and Mineral Society Show—Ridgecrest.
(760) 377–5192.

Dozens of gem and mineral exhibits, plus field trips. Educational.

Harvest Fair—San Bernardino.
(909) 384–5426; fax (909) 384–5160.

Re-creation of an 1881 Old West town, with a country/bluegrass show, crafts, and a unique car show.

DECEMBER

Children's Christmas Parade—Victorville.
(760) 245–6506; fax (760) 245–6505.

More than 150 holiday-theme floats, bands, novelty vehicles, and marching by equestrian units. **Free.**

Christmas Parade—Lone Pine.
(760) 876–4444; fax (760) 876–4533.

Old-fashioned Christmas parade with (you guessed it) Santa Claus.

Festival of Lights—Riverside.
(909) 683–7100 or (909) 683-2670.

Holiday lighting of the historic Mission Inn and surrounding downtown locations. Entertainment and specialty booths. **Free.**

The Deserts

The following list of events planned in the deserts is subject to change without notice. Please always call ahead to verify.

JANUARY

Palm Springs International Film Festival—Palm Springs.
(760) 322–2930; fax (760) 322–4087.

More than 150 international films with a special awards gala honoring industry greats.

FEBRUARY

South West Arts Festival—Indio.
(760) 347–0676 or (800) 44–INDIO; fax (760) 347–6069.

Marketplace for contemporary and traditional southwestern art; 150 acclaimed artists showcase fine and craft art.

McCormicks Exotic Antique Car Show and Auction—Palm Springs.
(760) 320–3290; fax (760) 323–7031.

Display and auction of 300 classic, antique, and special-interest cars.

Riverside County Fair and National Date Festival—Indio.
(760) 863–8247 or (800) 811–FAIR; fax (760) 863–8973.

The festival features exhibits of dates and produce; fine arts; floriculture; gems and minerals; a livestock show; and pig, camel, and ostrich races.

MARCH

La Quinta Arts Festival.
(760) 564–1244; fax (760) 564–6884; www.LQAF.com.

Takes place at Center for the Arts (south of Highway 111). This art extravaganza is now in its twenty-first year. Stunning art creations from more than 270 juried artists. Families will enjoy the Children's Art Garden, with activities for ages seven through twelve (must be accompanied by an adult). It all takes place thirty minutes from downtown Palm Springs in a dramatic desert setting at the base of the Santa Rosa Mountains. Live entertainment and tastes of Coachella Valley's great restaurants.

State Farm Cup and Newsweek Champions Cup—Indian Wells.
(760) 340–3166; fax (760) 341–9379; www.champions-cup.com.

Prestigious tennis event featuring top male and female professionals.

MAY

Grubstake Days—Yucca Valley.
(760) 365–6323; fax (760) 365–0763.

Parade, carnival events, dancing, demolition derby, games, food, hometown crafts booths, children's activities, PRCA rodeo; takes place Memorial Day weekend. **Free.**

DECEMBER

Festival of Lights Parade—Palm Springs.
(760) 778–8415 or (800) 927–7256.

Illuminated bands, floats, and automobiles make this one of the desert's top holiday events.

Tamale Festival—Indio.
(760) 342–6532 or (800) 44–INDIO; www.tamalefestival.org.

This very popular food festival is held the first weekend in December. Tamale Land has children's activities. A carnival is open throughout the event.

Golf Cart Parade—Palm Desert.
(760) 346–3263 or (800) 873–2428.

More than one hundred golf-cart floats with dazzling decorations.

Joshua Tree National Park Festival—
Twentynine Palms.
(760) 367–5522.

Exhibits and sales by more than twenty artists.

San Diego County

The following list of events is subject to change without notice. Please call in advance to confirm dates and times.

MARCH

Shamrock Festival—San Diego.
(619) 233–4692; fax (619) 233–4148.

St. Patrick's Day block party in San Diego's Gaslamp district with live music, Irish entertainment, food, and face painting. **Free.**

APRIL

Santa Fe Market—San Diego.
(619) 299–6055; fax (619) 296–1570.

Festival of southwest American Indian arts and crafts including guest artists and cultural demonstrations. **Free.**

Encinitas Street Fair—Encinitas.
(760) 943–1950.

More than 300 vendors, children's rides, face painting, clowns, arts and crafts. **Free.**

MAY

Fiesta Cinco De Mayo—San Diego.
(619) 299–6055; fax (619) 296–1570.

Mexican celebration in Old Town includes nonstop entertainment and food booths. **Free.**

Carlsbad Village Faire—Carlsbad.
(760) 434–8887.

One-day street fair features 800 booths; arts, crafts, antiques, international foods, and live entertainment.

JULY

San Diego County Fair—Del Mar.
(858) 792–4262; fax (858) 792–4453.

Annual county fair featuring world-class entertainment, rides, exhibits, livestock, and food.

Fourth of July Parade and Celebration—Coronado.
(800) 622–8300.

Includes fireworks and demonstrations by the U.S. Navy. **Free.**

An Old-Fashioned Fourth of July—San Diego.
(619) 220–5423.

Activities include hayrides, music, entertainers, dancing, sack races, and pie-eating contests. **Free.**

Fourth of July Freedom Days—Oceanside.
(760) 722–1534; fax (760) 722–8336.

Parade, street fair, festivities, fireworks, and music at the outdoor beach amphitheater. **Free.**

AUGUST

Latin American Festival—San Diego.
(619) 299–6055; fax (619) 296–1570.

Latin American crafts, artists, demonstrations, entertainment, and food booths. **Free.**

SEPTEMBER

Fall Fiesta—Old Town San Diego.
(619) 220–5422.

Celebrating the Hispanic heritage of Alta California with foods, crafts, music, and dance. **Free.**

Harbor Days—Oceanside.
(760) 721–1101; fax (760) 722–8336.

Celebrate a festival of crafts and events at the beautiful Oceanside Marina and Harbor. **Free.**

OCTOBER

Oktoberfest—Carlsbad.
(760) 434–6093 or (800) 227–5722.

Patriotic, traditional German music; children's games and lots of German food.

NOVEMBER

Community Tree Lighting—Julian.
(760) 765–1857; fax (760) 765–2544.

Old-fashioned Christmas tree lighting, costumed carolers, living Nativity pageant, and horse-drawn carriage rides. **Free.**

Festival of Lights—San Diego.
(619) 299–6055.

Celebration includes dances from around the world and dramatic Nativity scene lighting. **Free.**

DECEMBER

Holiday of Lights—Del Mar.
(858) 755–7161; fax (858) 792–4453.

Holiday light display featuring more than 200 themed entries including Santa's elves, Twelve Days of Christmas, and a magical forest. **Free.**

Holiday in the Park—San Diego.
(619) 220–5422; fax (619) 220–5421.

Candlelight tours of museums and historic homes featuring period decorations and entertainment.

Mission Christmas Faire—Oceanside.
(760) 721–1101; fax (760) 722–8336.

More than 200 booths, amusement rides for children, and entertainment. **Free.**

Harbor Parade of Lights—Oceanside.
(760) 721–1101; fax (760) 722–8336.

Lighted boat parade through the oceanside harbor. **Free.**

Index

About the Authors

Coauthors Laura Kath and Pamela Price have more than fifty years combined travel and life experience in sunny Southern California. Pamela resides in Palm Springs when she is not traveling and writing/broadcasting about her experiences. She is the author of *100 Best Spas of the World* (The Globe Pequot Press) and consults with her niece and nephew, Mari and David Price, for the hottest trends in family travel.

Laura is the author of twelve nonfiction books and president of Mariah Marketing, her Santa Barbara County–based consulting business. She is a member of the International Food, Wine & Travel Writers Association and the Society of Incentive Travel Executives.

This dynamic duo blends the best of real-life family travel experience with the most up-to-the-minute visitor information—making this book a must-read.